Edward K. Chung, M.D., Director of the Heart Station at Thomas Jefferson University Hospital in Philadelphia, is a world-renowned cardiologist and medical professor. He has published many books and hundreds of medical articles about the heart, and he has delivered numerous lectures at many universities, colleges, and various health organizations world-wide.

A Healthy Heart Handbook

ONE HEART, ONE LIFE

EDWARD K. CHUNG, M.D.

A SPECTRUM BOOK

Prentice-Hall, Inc., Englewood Cliffs, New Jersey 07632

Library of Congress Cataloging in Publication Data

Chung, Edward K.
    One heart, one life.

    "A Spectrum Book."
    Bibliography: p.
    Includes index.
    1. Heart—Diseases.   2. Heart—Diseases—
Prevention.   I. Title.
RC672.C45   616.1'2   81-19953
                                  AACR2

ISBN 0-13-634642-1

ISBN 0-13-634634-0 {PBK.}

To my wife, Lisa, and my children, Linda and Christopher.

1   2   3   4   5   6   7   8   9   10

This Spectrum Book can be made available to businesses
and organizations at a special discount when ordered in
large quantities. For more information, contact: Prentice-
Hall, Inc.; General Publishing Division, Special Sales;
Englewood Cliffs, New Jersey 07632.

Editorial/production supervision by Eric Newman
Cover design by Jeannette Jacobs
Manufacturing buyer: Cathie Lenard

Prentice-Hall International, Inc., *London*
Prentice-Hall of Australia Pty. Limited, *Sydney*
Prentice-Hall of Canada, Ltd., *Toronto*
Prentice-Hall of India Private Limited, *New Delhi*
Prentice-Hall of Japan, Inc., *Tokyo*
Prentice-Hall of Southeast Asia Pte. Ltd., *Singapore*
Whitehall Books Limited, *Wellington, New Zealand*

CONTENTS

27

PREFACE

After publication of my forty-two medical textbooks (including audiovisual materials) and more than 400 papers in the field of heart disease, I believe there is a true need for a complete book on the heart for the general public. This thought was further supported by the fact that I see so many cardiac (heart) patients who die needlessly. Heart attack (myocardial infarction) means definite damage to the heart, but not necessarily death to the patient.

In addition, numerous patients and members of their families suggested the need for a concise and readable book on the heart for lay people, and this suggestion was further endorsed by my wife, who is also a physician (Medical Director, U.S. Public Health Service, Philadelphia) who treats many cardiac patients.

It is important to realize that each of us has only one heart; if it goes, there is no spare. That is the reason my book is entitled *One Heart, One Life*—in order to emphasize this essential fact. We are all aware of the fact that should we break an arm or leg, the other limb, when forced, can do most of the work of the broken one. With the heart, however, there is no "other one." Some organs, such as our lungs and kidneys, come in pairs, so the loss of one is not always crippling or fatal—not so for the heart.

In the United States alone, more than 1 million people die annually from various heart diseases; among them, a heart attack is the cause of death in 600,000 people. Without a doubt, heart disease is the most common cause of death—accounting for more deaths than all other diseases combined. Unfortunately, more than half the 600,000 deaths from heart attack occur before the patient reaches the hospital, where the chances for survival and recovery would have been much greater. Immediate medical attention without delay is a key issue. In many cases, a few minutes means the difference between life and death.

Many people believe that extensive damage to the heart accounts for the deaths. However, in many cases of heart attack, the heart is only minimally damaged. In other words, the damage to the heart is often not enough to cause death when proper and immediate medical attention is given. Heart attacks don't have to be fatal—many patients die from a heart attack needlessly, primarily because of delayed medical attention.

Sudden death often occurs even if the damage is minimal because of electrical failure (heart rhythm disturbance)—either too fast, too slow, or no heartbeat. When immediate medical attention is provided, electrical failure is often prevented, and even if it should happen, the heart rhythm disturbance can easily be corrected. Sudden death from electrical failure is somewhat comparable to the way a clock or watch sometimes stops ticking even though it is otherwise in good condition. After the heart stops (cardiac arrest), it may be restarted by simple cardiopulmonary resuscitation, which can be learned without much difficulty.

More than 80 percent of the deaths from heart attack occur within the first twenty-four hours after onset of symptoms; and many die within the first hour. Therefore, the first twenty-four hours, particularly the first few hours after a heart attack, are truly the critical time that will determine the difference between life and death in many cases.

There are various reasons why medical attention is frequently delayed. First of all, many patients and their families misinterpret heart attack symptoms or warning signs. Chest pain is commonly taken very lightly and often misjudged as "gas pain," "indigestion," "common cold or flu," or even "nervousness." Without seeking medical attention, some people may take an antacid or aspirin. Others foolishly fail to seek medical attention without any reason, even when the symptoms are unmistakably typical of a heart attack. Some individuals may even deny to themselves that they are having chest pain. Some patients often hold off medical attention because they believe that a heart attack means "the end" of their lives, and many expect to lead the life of a semiinvalid even when they are lucky enough to recover from a heart attack. Obviously, their judgments are incorrect.

When the general public is adequately informed and stimulated, unnecessary delays in seeking medical attention can be minimized or even avoided. When proper and immediate medical attention is given, many patients with heart disease may be able not only to prolong their lives but also to improve their quality. Lack of adequate guidelines often causes serious consequences for the marriage, work, sports, and quality of life in addition to the life expectancy of cardiac patients. When adequate education is provided for the general public, much confusion and needless anxiety for patients and families can be reduced or even eliminated.

Needless to say, the prevention of a heart attack is far more desirable if possible. A heart attack can be prevented, particularly at an early age in many cases, when various known risk factors are eliminated or controlled. The common risk factors include hypertension (high blood pressure), obesity (overweight), elevated fat (cholesterol or triglyceride) content in the blood, smoking, diabetes mellitus (sugar in the blood), stress, taking birth control pills, and a family history of heart attack. Prevention is the best way to reduce or prevent death and sickness from heart disease, and prevention requires an *informed* and *motivated* public. A reliable source (*New England Journal of Medicine*, July 13, 1978) clearly indicates that less-educated patients (eight years of schooling or less) had more than three times the risk of sudden death, compared with those with a higher education among 1,739 men after recovery from a heart attack over a three-year period. Inadequate understanding of their heart disease with a lack of motivation was considered the main reason for a higher death rate among the less-educated group.

Millions of Americans have started exercise programs in all age groups, but the exercise should be performed intelligently. Sudden vigorous physical exercise, even in apparently healthy individuals, may be harmful if it is beyond the capacity of a person's heart function. This is particularly true for patients with known heart disease and for individuals with known risk factors. An exercise (stress) ECG test using a motor-driven treadmill under medical supervision is highly recommended before any vigorous or competitive exercise in order to determine the individual's capacity. The most dangerous exercise is shoveling snow on a very cold day, especially if you are rushing (e.g., to clear out a parked car).

In addition to heart attack, there are many other forms of heart disease. In this book, all common heart diseases (such as congenital malformations, rheumatic heart disease, heart diseases from infection, toxic substances, or trauma) are discussed fully. Many commonly asked questions (such as "How can I prevent a heart attack?" "Is exercise good for the heart?" "What should we do when a heart attack is suspected?" "How effective is coronary bypass surgery?" "How much sexual activity is allowed after a heart attack?" "How important is it to treat high blood pressure?" "Who will need an artificial cardiac pacemaker?" "What is a heart murmur?") are clearly answered in simple language. In fact, everything the general public always wanted to know about the heart is fully discussed. Over 80 percent of various congenital heart defects are cured by open heart surgery today, and the patients return to normal lives. Coronary bypass surgery, likewise, can not only prolong life but also provide a productive and enjoyable life. Similarly, artificial heart valves or heart pacemakers are often life-saving measures when they are placed at the proper time. The proven fact is that more than 250,000 Americans with artificial cardiac pacemakers live productive lives.

Needless to say, the purpose of this book is by no means to replace the personal doctor's advice. Rather, it is to supplement his or her medical advice. It should provide a better understanding of the heart condition and the personal doctor's recommendations and stimulate patients to ask more meaningful and useful questions of their physicians. The healthy individual should make every effort to stay in good health. *One Heart, One Life* is written for healthy people, as well as cardiac patients, in the hope that common questions that affect all of us may be answered. This book is an attempt to educate the general public about one organ none of us can ignore. What the heart is and does, many different heart conditions (prevention, diagnosis, and treatment), and various contributing factors to heart disease are discussed in simple language.

My sincere appreciation is expressed to Ms. Lynne Lumsden, editor-in-chief, and Mr. Eric Newman, senior production editor, of Spectrum Books, Prentice-Hall, Inc., for the publication of this book.

I am truly grateful to my wife, Lisa, and our children, Linda and Christopher, for their patience and understanding during the preparation of this book.

Lastly, I will always owe deep gratitude and appreciation to my father, Dr. Il-Chun Chung, who has always provided guidance and inspiration for me.

ABBREVIATIONS

A_2. Aortic second heart sound
AF. Atrial fibrillation
BP. Blood pressure
CABS. Coronary artery bypass surgery
CAD. Coronary artery disease
CCU. Coronary care unit
CHF. Congestive heart failure
CPR. Cardiopulmonary resuscitation
DC shock. Direct-current shock
ECG. Electrocardiogram
ER. Emergency room
ICCU. Intermediate coronary care unit
IHSS. Idiopathic hypertrophic subaortic stenosis

LBBB. Left bundle branch block
MI. Myocardial infarction
NG. Nitroglycerin
P_2. Pulmonic second heart sound
RBBB. Right bundle branch block
RHD. Rheumatic heart disease
SBE. Subacute bacterial endocarditis
SSS. Sick sinus syndrome
VF. Ventricular fibrillation
VPC. Ventricular premature contraction
WPW syndrome. Wolff-Parkinson-White syndrome

1

INTRODUCTION

The heart is located in the chest anteriorly (toward the front) between the two lungs, supported by the diaphragm (Figure 1.1); its average weight is approximately 11 ounces (oz) (350 grams [g]). The heart is composed of muscle (the medical term *myocardium* is commonly used to designate heart muscle; *myo* means "muscle"; *cardium* means "heart"), and it consists of four chambers. The four chambers include two pumping chambers (left and right ventricles) and two receiving chambers (left atrium and right atrium). The left atrium receives blood from the lungs, whereas the right atrium receives blood from the rest of the body. The two atria (the term *atria* is plural for *atrium*) fill the ventricles completely by squeezing blood into the ventricles before their pumping cycle begins. The right ventricle pumps blood to the lungs, while the left ventricle pumps blood to the rest of the body. This circulatory system is illustrated in Figure 1.2. The pumping cycle (the mechanical event of the heart) of the ventricles is synchronous to the electrical event of the heart. The heart produces heartbeats (about 60 to 100 beats/min. in adults) spontaneously through the natural pacemaker, called the "sinus node," situated in the right atrium (Figure 1.3). The sinus node in the heart is comparable to a generator in an automobile. Each heartbeat initiated by the built-in generator—the sinus node—can be felt as a "pulse" by placing the fingers on the wrist; each is also audible through a stethoscope on the chest wall.

In addition, the heart has four valves that open and close rhythmically, synchronous to each heartbeat, to maintain constant blood circulation in the entire

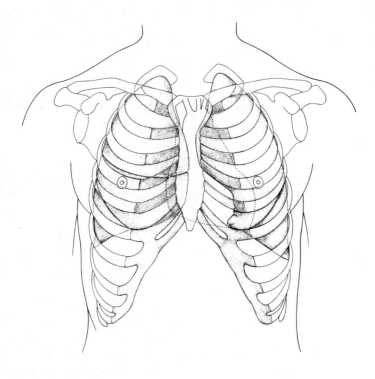

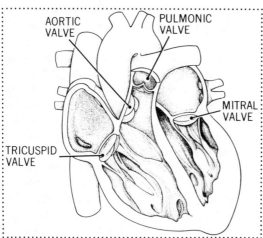

FIGURE 1.1. Anatomy of the heart. (Medical illustration by Larry Stein.)

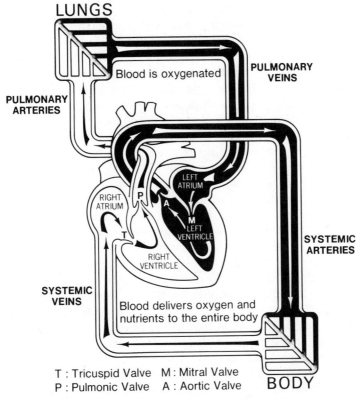

LUNGS

Blood is oxygenated

PULMONARY
VEINS

PULMONARY
ARTERIES

LEFT
ATRIUM

RIGHT
ATRIUM

P A

M
LEFT
VENTRICLE

T

RIGHT
VENTRICLE

SYSTEMIC
ARTERIES

SYSTEMIC
VEINS

Blood delivers oxygen and
nutrients to the entire body

BODY

T : Tricuspid Valve   M : Mitral Valve
P : Pulmonic Valve   A : Aortic Valve

FIGURE 1.2. Blood circulation through the heart. (Medical illustration by Larry Stein.)

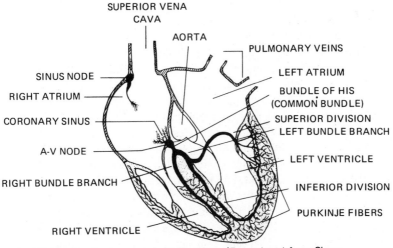

SUPERIOR VENA
CAVA

AORTA

PULMONARY VEINS

SINUS NODE

LEFT ATRIUM

RIGHT ATRIUM

BUNDLE OF HIS
(COMMON BUNDLE)

CORONARY SINUS

SUPERIOR DIVISION
LEFT BUNDLE BRANCH

A-V NODE

LEFT VENTRICLE

RIGHT BUNDLE BRANCH

INFERIOR DIVISION

PURKINJE FIBERS

RIGHT VENTRICLE

FIGURE 1.3. Conduction system of the heart. (Reproduced from Chung,
E.K.: *Principles of Cardiac Arrhythmias,* Second Edition, Baltimore,
Williams & Wilkins Co., 1977.)

3

body. When any of these four valves is damaged in any way (commonly as a result of rheumatic fever), the heart is unable to function adequately. Damage of the heart valves may be due to a variety of causes, including infections, inflammation, trauma, heart attack, congenital malformation, and so forth. When the heart valve malfunction is significant, the heart eventually fails to pump properly, leading to congestive heart failure (CHF). The term *CHF* is used when congestion occurs because the heart muscle pumps less efficiently than normal, so that the decreased strength of the muscle results in a backdrop of blood behind the heart. The two most common findings in CHF include shortness of breath (dyspnea) and fluid retention, or edema (e.g., swelling of ankles or congestion in the lungs). Although digitalis (commonly known as the "heart pill") and many other medications are effective against CHF, in increasing the pumping action, the damaged heart valve eventually should be replaced with an artificial heart valve for complete recovery. It should be remembered that replacement of the damaged valve may not be effective when heart function is markedly deteriorated because of delayed medical attention. Thus, it is essential to seek medical care early.

Likewise, various congenital heart defects ("congenital cardiac malformations," meaning heart diseases at birth) can be repaired by means of heart surgery. When heart surgery is performed early in life for most common congenital heart defects, the success rate is nearly 100 percent, with negligible mortality (death rate), and normal life is expected in most cases. If surgery for congenital heart disease is delayed, however, various complications may occur, and premature death cannot be avoided in many cases.

There are two major coronary arteries, the right coronary artery and the left main coronary artery, with numerous branches (Figure 1.4) that supply blood to the heart muscle itself. When these coronary arteries are normal in healthy individuals, increased pumping action (e.g., during various muscular activities—walking, running, love making, eating) causes the coronary arteries to enlarge so that a larger amount of blood is delivered to the heart muscle in order to meet increased demands. When significant narrowing occurs in the coronary arteries, usually as a result of atherosclerosis (hardening of the arteries), however, the increased demands of the blood supply on the heart muscle cannot be accomplished. Under these circumstances, the patient begins to experience chest pain—called "angina pectoris."

Typical anginal pain is usually triggered by physical exercise and/or emotional stress, but some cases (a special type of angina) may produce chest pain even at rest or during sleep, particularly during a bad dream. Anginal pain may be experienced as a viselike, constricting sensation (tightness) or a pressurelike feeling in the entire chest, or only in the left side or midsection of the chest. Anginal pain is often transmitted to the neck, throat, jaw, cheeks, teeth, shoulders, arms, or hands (commonly left-sided) and even to the midsection of the abdomen or to the back between the shoulders. When anginal pain is felt primarily in unusual locations, the patient may often misinterpret it as another disease, such as stomach upset, indigestion, gallbladder disease, toothache, and even appendicitis. Anginal pain is often associated with a pale face, cold sweat, shortness of breath, palpitations, and ab-

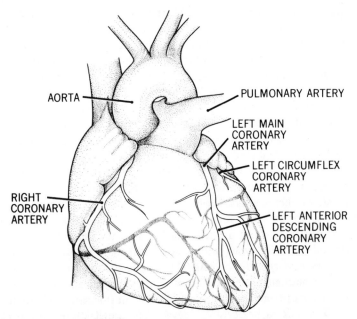

FIGURE 1.4. Normal coronary arteries. (Medical illustration by Larry Stein.)

normal heart rhythm. Typical anginal pain usually lasts from a few minutes to ten or twenty minutes, but it may last longer than that. It is important to remember that a heart attack should be suspected immediately when the pain lasts longer than this and when it persists even after resting. A hallmark of anginal pain in most cases is its prompt relief upon resting. In addition, typical anginal pain is usually relieved promptly by taking nitroglycerin (NG—a small, white tablet) sublingually (placed under the tongue).

When one or more coronary arteries are completely blocked and no more blood flow is possible, a portion of the heart muscle will become dead—called a "myocardial infarction" (*myo* means "muscle"; *cardial* means "heart"; and *infarction* means "dead tissue"). Many physicians use the term *MI*, a common abbreviation for myocardial infarction (heart attack). The nature of chest pain due to a heart attack is often similar to that of angina pectoris, but the intensity and the duration of the pain are much greater in the former. A characteristic feature of chest pain in heart attack is that it is *not* relieved by resting and/or by taking NG. In addition, in a heart attack the chest pain often occurs even during rest. In most cases of heart attack, the patient requires a narcotic, such as morphine injection, for severe and persisting chest pain. Such chest pain is often described as a "crushing sensation in the chest" or a "knife-stabbing sensation of the chest." On rare occasions, however, proven heart attack victims may experience only minimal symptoms (e.g., a mild pressure sensation or slight discomfort in the chest), or the patient may even be totally symptom free (called a "silent MI"—about 10 percent

5

of all heart attack cases). Chest pain in a heart attack is often associated with a cold sweat, pale or gray-colored face, severe shortness of breath, great anxiety, a feeling of impending death, nausea, belching, vomiting, palpitations, abnormal heart rhythm, and shock. Of course, some patients may lose consciousness as a result of severe anxiety, intense chest pain, electric failure (very fast or slow heart rhythm, or cardiac arrest), shock, CHF, or any combination of these. Sudden death may occur unless immediate and proper medical attention is provided under these circumstances. As a rule, heart attack is suspected strongly when the chest pain is *not* relieved by more than two or three NG pills in any patient with known angina pectoris. Medical attention should be sought without delay when the aforementioned symptoms (either singly or in combination) are experienced in any individual, even by someone with no history of heart disease.

Even though the heart attack means that a portion of the heart muscle is dead from lack of blood supply through the blocked coronary artery (or arteries), many patients can recover from a heart attack completely and may be able to return to their full activities when proper and immediate medical treatment is provided. The term *coronary artery disease* (CAD) or *coronary heart disease* is commonly used to designate angina pectoris as well as MI. It can be said that angina pectoris is a precursor of heart attack in many cases, but it is impossible to predict when a patient with angina pectoris will develop an actual MI. Although many patients can be treated medically, the result of coronary artery bypass surgery (CABS) is extremely favorable today for victims of severe angina pectoris as well as of MI, especially in young people, when proper medical attention is provided early and a good surgical team at an up-to-date facility is available.

Healthy individuals have normal blood prossure (BP), which rises briefly during physical exercise or emotional stress. The BP has two readings—systolic and diastolic pressure. The first component is a pressure measured during the pumping phase—referred to as "systolic pressure" (pressure during contraction of the ventricles), whereas the second component is a pressure measured during the filling (expansion) phase—referred to as "diastolic pressure" (pressure during dilation or expansion of the ventricles). For instance, a BP of 130/90 mmHg means systolic pressure of 130 mmHg with a diastolic pressure of 90 mmHg.

When the BP is abnormally elevated, it is called "hypertension" (*hyper* means "increased"; *tension* means "pressure"). Elevated diastolic pressure is more serious than systolic pressure. When hypertension persists, the heart has to work harder than usual, and eventually many patients develop enlargement of the heart as a compensatory mechanism. In advanced cases of hypertension, when proper treatment is not given, the heart is unable to pump sufficiently, and subsequently CHF occurs. In addition, hypertension may be associated with many other serious complications, such as heart attack, stroke, and kidney (renal) failure, even in young people. Therefore, good control of hypertension under constant medical supervision is essential. Unfortunately, the exact cause of hypertension is not fully understood in many cases.

In some individuals, the heart muscle itself may be damaged by various causes, including toxic substances such as alcohol. The term *cardiomyopathy* is used to designate heart muscle disease (*cardio* means "heart"; *myo* means "muscle"; and *pathy* means "disease"). Again, the exact cause of cardiomyopathy, in some cases, is not clearly known. Sooner or later, many patients with advanced cardio-myopathy will develop CHF, which may lead to death.

Healthy people maintain a regular and stable heart rhythm initiated by the natural (intrinsic) pacemaker—called the "sinus node" (Figure 1.3). Normal heart rhythm initiated by the sinus node is called "normal sinus rhythm." However, the heart rhythm may become extremely rapid or slow, and at times the heart may stop beating (cardiac arrest) altogether. There are many excellent drugs available for various types of abnormal heart rhythms (arrhythmias or dysrhythmias). In some cases with extremely rapid heart rhythm, electric shock may be required (direct-current shock or cardioversion) in order to restore normal heart rhythm. When heart rhythm is very slow or the heart stops beating, an artificial cardiac pacemaker with a battery power source must be used in order to maintain an ideal heart rate. It should be remembered that there will not be enough pumping action when the heart rhythm is extremely fast or slow. As a result, the patient may faint or develop CHF; even sudden death may occur unless immediate and proper medical attention is provided. Approximately 250,000 people live with artificial pacemakers in America alone, and 25,000 to 40,000 new patients annually will require an artificial pacemaker implantion.

There are many types of heart diseases, including various congenital heart defects, heart disease from infections or inflammations, heart disease from a variety of injuries, heart disease from toxic substances, CAD, hypertensive heart disease (from high blood pressure), and cardiomyopathies (heart muscle diseases). In America alone, about 30 million people suffer from some type of heart disease, and among them 3 million are victims of heart attack annually. Every year more than 1 million people die from heart diseases in the United States alone; among them, heart attack is the most common (600,000 people) cause of death. Thus, death from heart disease accounts for more deaths than all other diseases combined.

Although heart attack is estimated to be much more common in men than in women, CAD has been accounting for more than 200,000 deaths a year among American women, a death toll 60 percent greater than that from cancer. It has been estimated that men have thirteen times as many heart attacks as do women up to age forty-five. Men still have approximately twice as many heart attacks as women do between ages forty-five and sixty-two. However, after age sixty-two, women are just as susceptible as men to heart attack. Recent experiences clearly indicate that some young women (below forty-five or even younger than thirty), especially those who smoke and/or use oral contraceptives (birth control pills), may have a higher chance of suffering a heart attack.

It is unfortunate that more than half the 600,000 deaths from heart attack occur before the patient reaches the hospital, where chances for survival with good recovery would have been much greater. Immediate medical attention without delay is the key issue. In many instances, a few minutes mean the difference between life and death. It is a general misbelief that deaths result from extensive damage to the heart. Indeed, in many instances, the heart is only minimally damaged. In many cases damage to the heart is not enough to cause death when proper and immediate medical treatment is provided. Numerous patients die from heart attack needlessly because of delayed medical attention. It is truly regrettable that many heart attack victims die much too young with hearts still capable of functioning. Sudden death commonly occurs even if heart damage is only minimal as a result of electrical failure (heart rhythm disturbances). When immediate medical attention is provided, electrical failure is easily prevented; even if it should occur, heart rhythm disturbances can readily be managed. Permanent damage to the brain often occurs when that organ receives inadequate or no blood supply as a result of electrical failure of the heart. Consequently, permanent brain damage may lead to a semiinvalid, vegetative life even if the patient recovers from the heart attack.

It is reasonably certain that delay in seeking medical attention can be minimized or even avoided when the public is adequately informed and stimulated. Many heart attack victims may be able not only to prolong, but also to improve the quality of, their lives when proper and immediate medical attention is provided. In fact, many patients recover from heart attack fully and return to previous activities (e.g., work, sports, sexual activities). A heart attack can be prevented in many cases, especially in young people, when various risk factors are eliminated or properly controlled. The common risk factors are hypertension, obesity, (overweight), high fat (cholesterol or triglyceride) content in the blood, emotional stress, use of oral contraceptives (birth control pills), and a family history of heart attack (the heredity factor). Except for the heredity factor, all risk factors can be eliminated or treated properly.

Although there is a controversy among cardiologists (heart specialists) regarding the exact value of physical exercise in relation to heart function, exercise is considered definitely beneficial for many people when it is performed intelligently with proper medical guidance. It should be emphasized, however, that sudden, vigorous physical exercise, even in apparently healthy people, may be harmful when it is performed beyond the capacity of their heart function. This is especially true after age forty-five, in patients with known heart disease, or in individuals with known risk factors. Under these circumstances it is advisable, therefore, that an exercise (stress) ECG test using a motor-driven treadmill under direct medical supervision be performed before any vigorous or competitive exercise is undertaken in order to assess the individual's heart capacity.

Although alcohol is not exactly considered a risk factor for CAD, it is definitely harmful for patients with known heart disease. It has been shown that as little as 2 oz of alcohol a day may increase damage to an already damaged heart and that it may significantly reduce the pumping action of the heart. In addition, alcohol may cause abnormal heart rhythms that further damage the heart, and even sudden death may occur. Alcohol may also increase the level of fat (triglycerides) content in the blood and may cause hypertension, which predisposes to heart attack. The fact that alcohol causes cardiomyopathy has been stressed previously. Needless to say, alcohol may cause permanent damage to other organs, including the liver and the brain. Furthermore, alcohol may produce beriberi heart diseases (heart disease from a vitamin B deficiency), which is a form of cardiomyopathy.

It is well documented that cigarette smoking is one of the major risk factors for heart attack. The public is well aware of the message on every pack of cigarettes: "Warning: The Surgeon General has determined that cigarette smoking is dangerous to your health." For any individual who has had a heart attack or suffers from angina pectoris, smoking is not merely hazardous but actually suicidal. Likewise, cigarette smoking is more harmful when other risk factors are present. Therefore, without a doubt, it is absolutely essential to stop smoking under these circumstances. Nonetheless, it seems that abandoning the bad habit of smoking is very difficult unless the individual is highly motivated. Thus, in-depth education of the public through providing necessary information is extremely important in order to stimulate and guide them.

It should be emphasized that expert medical opinions may differ slightly in some areas, and it is helpful for the patient and family members to understand this fact. However, fundamental therapeutic goals are essentially the same among all physicians. When there is full cooperation with mutual understanding between physicians, other medical and paramedical personnel, and a highly motivated general public, the highest therapeutic goals can be achieved. The aim will be toward a productive life with full recovery from heart attack and other major heart diseases by minimizing or preventing unnecessary complications, including death. By all means, the healthy individual should make every effort to stay in good health. High motivation with sufficient stimulation and knowledge regarding heart diseases is especially important to prevent heart attack and other serious heart diseases. By maintaining motivation and achieving knowledge, needless deaths may be avoided, particularly in young people.

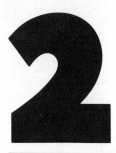

THE NORMAL HEART
AND ITS FUNCTION

The shape of the human heart closely resembles that of a thick cone rather than the common drawing of a Valentine heart. The heart, situated in the chest between the right and left lungs, is well protected by the chest wall and rib cage (Figure 1.1). The normal heart is about the size of a fist but may grow to weigh as much as a pound in a highly trained athlete.

The heart is surrounded by a tough, protective membrane known as the *pericardium* (*peri* means "around"; *cardium* means "heart"). When an infection or inflammatory process (from virus or bacteria) involves the periocardium, the disease is called "pericarditis." Similar, the term *myocarditis* is used to designate infectious process or inflammation involving the myocardium. When there is fluid accumulation in the pericardial sac as a result of severe infection, heart failure, or some other disease (e.g., myxedema or hypothyroidism—poor function of the thyroid gland), the term *pericardial effusion* is used to designate this disease process. Of course, heart function will be diminished when the patient develops myocarditis or pericarditis.

The heart, consisting of four chambers, has two large chambers (lower chambers) that are called "ventricles"; their main function is pumping blood. The right ventricle pumps blood to the lungs to be loaded with oxygen, whereas the left ventricle pumps the oxygen-rich blood to supply oxygen and important nutrients throughout the body. Thus, the heart is not really one pump but two. The right ventricle is situated almost in front of the left ventricle rather than exactly on the right and left side in the chest if one looks at the heart head on. The left ventricular muscle mass is approximately two and a half to three times thicker than the right ventricular muscle mass. And the electrical energy of the left ventricle is about ten times greater than that of the right ventricle. Two smaller chambers (the left atrium and the right atrium) are located above the two ventricles. The terms *atrium* and *auricle* are used interchangeably. The main function of the two atria is to receive blood from the entire body and the lungs. The atria push the received blood down to the ventricles. Therefore, the term *pumping chambers* is appropriate for the ventricles, whereas the term *receiving chambers* may be used for the atria.

There is a muscular wall between the right and left atria—called the "atrial septum." Similarly, another muscular wall is situated between the right and left ventricles—called the "ventricular septum." Some infants are born without these muscular walls—called "atrial septal defect" and "ventricular septal defect," respectively. Atrial septal defect and ventricular septal defect are the most common forms of congenital heart defect.

There are four valves in the heart. The *mitral valve* is situated between the left atrium and the left ventricle. The *aortic valve* is located at the outlet of the left ventricle. These two valves close and open harmoniously and rhythmically for the circulation of the left half of the heart. The circulation of the other half is carried out by the *tricuspid valve* and the *pulmonic* (pulmonary) *valve.* The tricuspid valve is located between the right atrium and the right ventricle; the pulmonic valve is situated at the outlet of the right ventricle. Blood is pumped by the right ventricle to the lungs via the pulmonary arteries following closure of the tricuspid valve and opening of the pulmonic valve in order to pick up oxygen (oxygenated blood); this process is essential for life (refer back to Figures 1.1 and 1.2). The oxygenated blood returns to the left atrium via the pulmonary veins, and again the blood is pushed down to the left ventricle through the mitral valve (Figures 1.1 and 1.2). The blood, now fully loaded with oxygen and important nutrients, is pumped by the left ventricle, following closure of the mitral valve and opening of the aortic valve, and is carried to all parts of the body via the aorta and its branches (elastic muscular tubes). The aorta is the largest trunklike artery, with a diameter about equal to that of a large garden hose. From the aorta, many arteries, including the coronary arteries, branch off to take fresh blood (blood loaded with oxygen and nutrients) to all parts of the body. After delivering the oxygen and nutrients throughout the body, the used blood returns to the right atrium through two large vessels, the *inferior vena cava* and the *superior vena cava.* The inferior vena cava collects blood from the area of the body below the heart, whereas the superior vena cava receives blood from above the heart (Figure 1.2). Thus, the left ventricle is responsible for pumping oxygenated blood with nutrients throughout the entire body and for bringing the used blood back to the right atrium. Complete circulation of the cardiovascular (heart and blood vessels) system takes about ten to fifteen seconds.

The rhythmic and continuous cardiovascular circulation (the mechanical event of the heart) is controlled by the electrical events initiated by the natural (intrinsic), built-in pacemaker of the heart—called the "sinus node" or the "sino-atrial node" (Figure 1.3). The sinus node is a small bundle of muscle fibers that contain numerous pacemaker cells; it is located in the right atrium at the junction of the superior vena cava (Figure 1.3). The sinus node constantly receives signals from nerve centers in the brain and spinal cord that respond to the body's demands under various circumstances. In addition, the sinus node is closely controlled by hormones released by the adrenal and thyroid glands. In simple terms, the heart's sinus node is comparable to an automobile's generator. The sinus node fires the electrical impulses regularly, at about 60 to 100 beats/min. in adults, for as long as one maintains normal heart function.

When the electrical impulse is fired by the sinus node, it spreads the right atrium in a wavelike fashion from top to bottom. This electrical event is called "right atrial depolarization"; it is followed by "left atrial depolarization" in a similar manner. Both right and left atrial depolarizations produce a P wave on the electrocardiogram (*electro* means "electrical"; *cardio* means "heart"; *gram* means "recording"; an *electrocardiogram* (ECG) is a recording of the eletrical activity of the heart). The electrical events of the heart are illustrated in Figure 2.1. After both atria are fully activated (depolarized), the heart impulses reach the atrio-ventricular (A-V) node, another bundle of muscles, which is located in the upper portion of the wall or septum between the two ventricles (Figure 1.3). The electrical impulse, then, soon passes down the bundle of His (A-V bundle or common bundle) and down the right and left bundle branches with numerous His-Purkinje fibers to activate the ventricles (Figure 1.3). During ventricular activation (depolarization), a large wave forms on the electrocardiogram—termed the "QRS complex" (Figure 2.1). Following ventricular depolarization, the ventricles become relaxed. This stage, called "ventricular repolarization," produces the T wave on the ECG (Figure 2.1). The entire electrical event, initiated from the sinus node to the end of the ventricular repolarization process, produces the P wave, the QRS complex, and the T wave on the ECG (Figure 2.1). This entire electrical process is one cardiac (heart) cycle.

When the electrical event of the heart is disturbed in any way, abnormal cardiac (heart) rhythm is produced. There are many types of abnormal heart rhythm—too fast, too slow, or irregular rhythm or no heartbeat at all. The term *cardiac arrhythmia* or *cardiac dysrhythmia* is commonly used to designate a variety of abnormal heart rhythms. CAD (angina pectoris and heart attack) is the most common cause of abnormal heart rhythms, but many other heart diseases may be associated with rhythm abnormalities. Abnormal heart rhythms may also be caused by other diseases (e.g., hyperthyroidism—abnormally increased function of the thyroid gland) and by excessive ingestion of coffee, tea, cola drinks, and alcohol and by cigarette smoking. Abnormal heart rhythms (depending upon the type and the underlying disease process) may cause a variety of symptoms, such as palpitations, a feeling of skipped heartbeats, shortness of breath, chest pain, fainting, and shock. Sudden death may also occur in some cases when the heart rhythm is extremely fast or slow, or when the heart stops beating altogether, unless immediate

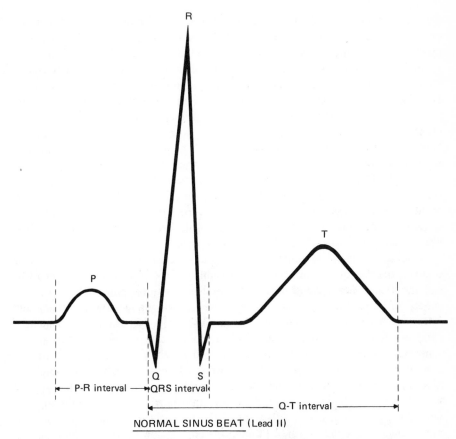

R

P

T

Q

S

— P-R interval —→ QRS interval

Q-T interval

NORMAL SINUS BEAT (Lead II)

FIGURE 2.1. Various electrocardiographic complexes. (Reproduced from Chung, E.K.: *Principles of Cardiac Arrhythmias,* Second Edition, Baltimore, Williams & Wilkins Co., 1977.)

medical attention is provided. There are many effective medications available for abnormal heart rhythms, but some cases require electric-shock treatment or an artificial cardiac pacemaker.

As described previously, the electrical events of the heart occur harmoniously and rhythmically, synchronous to the mechanical events. That is, the atrial contraction is caused by the atrial activation (depolarization), and it occurs immediately before the opening of the mitral and tricuspid valves. The ventricular contraction is caused by the ventricular depolarization (activation)—the QRS complex on the ECG (Figure 2.1).

During these mechanical events, two distinct heart sounds are created, primarily by the closure of various heart valves. The sounds are readily audible through a stethoscope. When the two ventricles begin to contract, the tricuspid and mitral valves close abruptly. Then the pulmonic (pulmonary) and aortic valves

(Figure 1.2) open, and the leaves of these two valves vibrate from the sudden rise of pressure as the blood forces them to expand. The heart sound created primarily by the closure of the tricuspid and mitral valves is called the "first heart sound"; it is often expressed as "lub" when the entire heart sounds are depicted as "lub-dub." Soon after the first sound fades away, the pressure within the ventricles falls low enough for the aortic and pulmonic valves to close, and the tricuspid and mitral valves open. The heart sounds caused primarily by the closure of the pulmonic and aortic valves is called the "second heart sound," often expressed as a "dub." Since the diastole (the expansion period of the ventricles) lasts longer than the systole (the contraction period of the ventricles), there is a silence after each heart cycle. Consequently, normal heart sounds can be expressed as "lub-dub"–silence–"lub-dub"–silence–etc. Occasionally, vibrations of the ventricular wall can be heard as that chamber fills with blood pouring from the atria during the expansion period (diastole) of the ventricles. This heart sound, called the "third heart sound," is relatively common in young people.

As far as the precise timing of heart sounds is concerned, the first heart sound occurs a fraction of a second after the beginning of the QRS complex on the ECG, and the second heart sound practically corresponds to the end of the T wave. A variety of heart diseases produce abnormal heart sounds in terms of timing and intensity. When any heart valve fails to close properly, when the opening of the valve is narrower than usual, or when blood backs up into the atria or the ventricles, an abnormal noise will be produced by the damaged valve(s). The abnormal noise created by a damaged or diseased heart valve is termed the "heart murmur." There are many types of heart murmurs depending upon which valve is damaged and the nature of the damage. In general, the heart murmur heard during the expansion period (diastole) of the ventricle is termed "diastolic murmur," whereas the murmur heard during the contraction period (systole) is called "systolic murmur." Heart murmurs are also common in various congenital heart malformations (e.g., ventricular septal defect, atrial septal defect). Physicians may be able to diagnose various heart valve diseases or congenital defects by analyzing the nature of heart murmurs. Slight or faint heart murmur is not uncommon in healthly people, but a loud murmur nearly always indicates heart disease. A very loud heart murmur may even be heard without a stethoscope.

The normal heart with a rate of 70 beats/min. pumps a little more than 2.5 fluid oz of blood per stroke, which adds up to 6 quarts of output per minute. As a result, the heart pumps about 5,500 quarts of blood daily, weighing six tons. However, the heart is capable of pumping as much as 35 quarts/min. when necessary, such as during vigorous physical exercise (e.g., running, competitive sports). Heart rate increases markedly during various physical activities. Maximum heart rate may become as fast as 180 to 200 beats/min. during intense physical exertion by a healthy individual with a resting heart rate of 60 or 70 beats/min. Each heartbeat is transmitted all the way to the periphery of the blood circulation as it is felt as a pulse on the wrist, neck, or ankle artery.

The cardiovascular system is well coordinated so that the blood supply to any particular portion of the body is regulated according to that portion's needs. For instance, the stomach and the rest of the digestive system require an additional blood supply during and after meals. When digestion is completed, extra blood flow to the digestive system shuts off, and the extra blood supply becomes available to other parts of the body. During physical work, larger amounts of blood are supplied to the arms and legs. During physical exertion, there is an increase in the amount of oxygen used by the tissues. For a larger oxygen supply, the heart's output of blood has to be increased, primarily through a faster heart rate, a more rapid rate of breathing, and an increase in the oxygen extracted from the bloodstream by organs and tissues. The heart's output is also increased through a decrease in the resistance to blood flow near the extremities of the cardiovascular system. The resistance of the blood flow to the extremities is reduced because the blood vessles that supply the working muscle tissue are enlarged. If an individual is in good physical condition, his or her oxygen can be supplied at a slower rate than in an individual in poor physical health.

As far as nervous control of the heart is concerned, there are two separate nervous systems that link the heart and brain—the *sympathetic* (accelerator) *nerve* releases *noradrenaline,* whereas the *vagus* (inhibitory) *system* tends to slow the heart. The major effect of the vagus system is to depress the frequency of heart impulses fired by the sinus node. To continue the automobile analogy, the sympathetic nerve functions like an accelerator and the vagus nerve acts like the brake. Thus, the nervous system controls the heart function according to the needs of the human body. The maintenance of normal contractile (pumping) force in the heart primarily depends upon the influence of the sympathetic nerve. This sympathetic nerve increases the pumping action of the heart muscle and increases the heart rate. When the pumping action of the heart is diminished and the blood supply becomes inadequate to the demands (for oxygen and other nutrients) of the tissues, the condition is called "congestive heart failure" (CHF)—meaning a weakened heart. In other words, the reduced output of blood by a weakened heart in CHF is not enough for the demands of tissues. CHF may be caused by any type of heart disease, including hypertensive, coronary, valvular, and congenital heart diseases and cardiomyopathy (heart muscle disease). CHF is usually manifested by fluid accumulation in various parts of the body, including leg edema, congestion of the liver causing enlargement, and congestion in the lungs. Congestion in the lungs (pulmonary congestion) due to CHF may lead , in advanced cases, to the life-threatening condition called "pulmonary edema." In the old medical textbooks, the term *dropsy* was often used to describe CHF. In patients with CHF, the usual complaint is shortness of breath (dyspnea) on exertion, and it is often associated with fatigue, weakness, and leg edema. For CHF, digitalis (often called the "heart pill") and many other drugs are used to increase the heart's pumping action. However, the direct cause of CHF should be corrected by surgery if possible. For instance, the only solution to congenital heart disease is surgical repair of the defect. Similarly, significant valve damage must be replaced with an artificial heart valve.

The heart contains two major coronary (heart) arteries—the right coronary artery and the left main coronary artery, with numerous small branches (see again Figure 1.4). These coronary arteries, like arteries that supply blood to other parts of the body, branch off from the aorta. The heart must receive necessary nutrients constantly from these coronary arteries, rather than from blood passing through the heart chambers. The coronary artery is relatively small, with a diameter of about 2mm to 3mm (2/25 in. to 3/25 in.) in normal hearts. In normal hearts, the diameter (caliber) of the coronary arteries enlarge to supply larger amounts of blood to the heart muscle when more pumping action is needed. However, when the caliber of the coronary arteries is narrowed (usually as a result of atherosclerosis), only an inadequate blood supply to the heart muscle is possible. The narrowing of the coronary artery is called "coronary artery stenosis," which may be symptom free in early stages of the disease or in mild cases. When the narrowing of the coronary artery progresses further (Figure 2.2), the patient begins to experience chest pain, especially during physical exertion. This entity, as mentioned earlier, is called "angina pectoris."

When atherosclerosis becomes far advanced, one or more coronary arteries may be completely blocked (Figure 2.2) so that a portion of the heart muscle receives no blood at all. This stage of CAD is called "myocardial infarction" (MI). Dead heart muscle becomes scar tissue when an MI is healed. In lay terms, a heart attack means an MI. Many heart attack victims recover completely when proper medical treatment is provided immediately. Whenever necessary, coronary artery bypass surgery (CABS) may be carried out for patients with severe angina pectoris or MI, especially young people. Surgical results are extremely favorable, and more people undergo CABS every year.

FIGURE 2.2. Coronary artery stenosis—various stages. A: Normal coronary artery. B: Early stage. C: Advanced stage. D: Far-advanced stage. E: Complete occlusion. (Medical illustration by Larry Stein.)

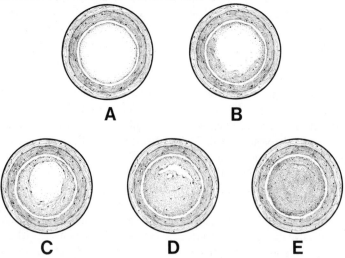

The healthy heart maintains normal blood pressure (BP), which is comparable to maintaining water pressure in a household plumbing system or air pressure in automobile tires. The kidneys receive about 25 percent of the blood supply pumped by the heart each minute, and they play an important role in controlling BP and fluid balance in the body. The BP usually rises briefly during physical exercise or emotional excitement, but it does not depend on the heart rate itself. By and large, BP tends to increase when one gets older. The term *hypertension* (*hyper* means "increased"; *tension* means "pressure") is used when BP is abnormally elevated. The fact that hypertension is one of the most important predisposing factors for heart attack is well known. Therefore, good control of hypertension is essential in preventing serious complications.

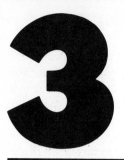

HEART ATTACK

Approximately 3 million Americans suffer from heart attack (myocardial infarction, or MI) annually. Without a doubt, heart attack is the number one killer; it is the cause of death for over 600,000 people annually in the United States. Unfortunately, more than half the 600,000 deaths from heart attack occur before the patient reaches the hospital, where chances for survival would have been much greater. Immediate and proper medical attention is extremely important; a few minutes make the difference between life and death in many cases. As mentioned earlier, many heart attack victims die needlessly with only minimal heart damage, primarily because of delayed medical attention. Sudden death often occurs even if the damage is minimal because of electric failure of the heart—heart rhythm disturbances called "cardiac arrhythmias." Serious heart rhythm disturbances can be prevented or corrected with immediate and proper medical attention.

Medical attention is often delayed because patients and their families simply misinterpret the symptoms of a heart attack. Chest pain is commonly misjudged as indigestion or gas pain, and some people take an antacid without seeking medical attention. Other individuals foolishly fail to seek medical attention even when the symptoms are unquestionably typical of a heart attack. Unnecessary delays can be minimized or even avoided through education and motivation. Many patients with heart attack can prolong and improve the quality of their lives with immediate and proper medical treatment. Because of improved medical and surgical treatment, many individuals may return to their full activities (e.g., work, sports, sexual activity) after recovery from a heart attack.

It is important to remember that a heart attack can be prevented, especially in young people, when various risk factors are eliminated or controlled. Common risk factors include high blood pressure (hypertension), obesity (overweight), elevated fat (cholesterol or triglycerides) content in the blood (hyperlipidemia), cigarette smoking, diabetes mellitus, stress, birth control pills (oral contraceptives) and family history (hereditary or genetic factor) of a heart attack (see Table 3.1). Only a highly motivated and properly informed individual can use willpower to control or eliminate these factors. For example, it seems extremely difficult to quit smoking (one of the worst risk factors) unless one is highly motivated. It should be stressed that these factors are closely interrelated; a combination of them disproportionately speeds up the incidence of heart attack. For example, many obese people have hypertension, hyperlipidemia, *and* diabetes. When obesity is well controlled by sensible eating habits, other risk factors may disappear spontaneously or become minimized. And although taking birth control pills is considered only a minimal risk factor by itself, when it is combined with cigarette smoking, the chance of suffering a heart attack even at an early age is extremely high. Other than heredity, gender, and age, all these risk factors can be controlled or eliminated.

The term *coronary artery disease* (CAD) or *coronary heart disease* includes *angina pectoris* and *myocardial infarction* (MI–heart attack). "Angina" means constricting pain, and "pectoris" refers to the chest. Angina pectoris (often called "angina") occurs when significant narrowing of the coronary arteries (Figure 2.2) is produced by atherosclerosis (hardening of the arteries) so that blood supply to the heart muscle (the myocardium) is diminished. Typical angina is usually triggered by physical exertion and/or emotional stress. When one or more coronary arteries are completely blocked and no more blood flow is possible, a portion of the heart muscle dies—called an MI (heart attack). In many patients a heart attack is preceded by angina pectoris, although a heart attack may occur suddenly without any warning sign or symptom in apparently healthy individuals.

TABLE 3.1. Risk Factors for Coronary Artery Disease.

MAJOR FACTORS	MINOR FACTORS OR FACTORS CLOSELY LINKED TO HEART DISEASE
Heredity	Oral contraceptives (birth control pills)
Advanced (old) age	Type A personality
Male sex	Inactive (sedentary) living
Hypertension (high blood pressure)	Coffee, tea, and alcohol
Hyperlipidemia (elevated blood contents of cholesterol or triglycerides)	Gout (elevated blood contents of uric acid)
Obesity (overweight)	
Cigarette smoking	
Stress	
Diabetes mellitus	

In this chapter, every aspect of heart attack is described in detail. They include causes, common risk factors, symptoms, diagnosis, complications, medical treatment, surgical treatment, home care after discharge from the hospital, and prevention.

CAUSES OF HEART ATTACK

The major cause of heart attack is atherosclerosis (hardening of the arteries) that involves one or more coronary arteries. Atherosclerosis means that fatty deposits like cholesterol build up in the lining of an artery. The terms *arteriosclerosis* and *atherosclerosis* have been used interchangeably for the same disease process, but the latter has been more popular in recent years.

Atherosclerosis is a long-standing disease process that starts very early in life, but it does not become apparent as a disease entity until it is far-advanced. In the very early stage of atherosclerosis, there may be a thin, yellowish, fatty streak in the artery, usually no more than half an inch long and an eighth of an inch wide. When the disease progresses further, the fatty deposit increases in size and becomes harder, as calcium may be deposited in it. As the fatty deposits enlarge, the diameter of the coronary artery becomes progressively narrowed so that blood flow is reduced. In some cases of advanced atherosclerosis, a blood clot is produced in an area of marked narrowing, frequently leading to complete blockage of the coronary artery. The end result, needless to say, is MI (heart attack). Under this circumstance, the term *thrombosis* is used to designate the blood clot that blocks the coronary artery. This disease process, atherosclerosis, is comparable to the corrosion and mineral deposits that take place in an old plumbing pipe. Although atherosclerosis may involve diffusely many arteries, the disease process often involves certain portions of the artery system more than others. Thus, some coronary arteries may be completely normal whereas others may show marked narrowing from advanced atherosclerosis.

As described previously, there are two major coronary arteries—the right coronary artery and the left coronary artery, with its many branches (Figure 1.4). Like other arteries, the coronary arteries branch off from the aorta (Figure 1.2). Sufficient blood supply with necessary nourishment is constantly carried to the heart muscle through the coronary arteries. When more blood is needed, such as during physical exercise, the heart has to work harder—beating faster and pumping more strongly to meet the increased demand.

In spite of a continuous and progressive disease process from atherosclerosis, many individuals experience no symptoms at all until the narrowing of the coronary artery becomes profound. When the narrowed artery is unable to supply sufficient blood with necessary nourishment to the heart muscle, the first symptom of CAD occurs: The patient experiences chest pain—angina pectoris. Significant narrowing means that the original diameter of the coronary artery is reduced by more than 70 percent. It is rather unusual to experience angina when the narrowing is less than 50 percent of the total original diameter of the artery.

The first angina attack is usually triggered by vigorous or sudden physical activity (such as climbing a flight of stairs, shoveling snow, playing a competitive sport) and/or emotional excitement. Under these circumstances, the blood supply is not sufficient for the increased demand because of the narrowed coronary artery. When the narrowing of the artery is so marked that little or no blood circulation is possible, the patient will develop MI (heart attack). Of course, a heart attack is the end result when there is a complete blockage of the coronary artery. Progressive changes in the coronary artery due to atherosclerosis are illustrated in Figure 2.2. As emphasized earlier, MI means that a portion of the heart muscle is dead because of a lack of blood supply through a blocked coronary artery (Figure 3.1). Once an MI takes place, the death of muscle tissue is irreversible; when it heals, it becomes scar tissue. The complete healing process after heart attack takes approximately four to six weeks.

Many patients with angina pectoris experience no symptoms as long as they are in a resting state, because the narrowed coronary artery is capable of supplying sufficient blood to maintain minimal activity. However, angina will be observed during extraordinary physical activities because the narrowed coronary artery cannot supply blood for increased demand. Therefore, the typical angina attack is characterized by exertional chest pain. For the same reason, the electrocardiogram, or ECG (the graphic recording of the electrical activity generated by the

FIGURE 3.1. Heart muscle showing infarcted area (damaged heart muscle from heart attack). (Medical illustration by Larry Stein.)

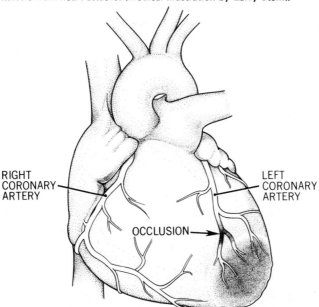

heart—see Chapter 24), is often (up to 75 percent with proven angina pectoris) normal in the resting state in spite of marked narrowing of the coronary artery. When physical exercise is performed (such as the treadmill exercise ECG test—see Chapter 24) by the patient with angina pectoris, the ECG is often abnormal, and the patient often experiences typical angina pain simply because the demand exceeds the available blood supply. Exercise-induced ECG change and angina pain are somewhat comparable as a phenomenon to an old automobile that can run at a low speed without any difficulty but that runs very poorly when the driver tries to accelerate beyond certain speed, because the fuel line is clogged.

In some patients with slowly progressing CAD, reserve (collateral) coronary arteries may develop to compensate for the inadequate blood supply to the heart by the diseased coronary artery. When adequate collateral circulation is produced to bypass the narrowed coronary artery, some individuals may be completely symptom-free for a long time despite marked narrowing of the coronary arteries. However, most patients eventually develop symptoms of angina when the disease process is far advanced. Although some individuals develop heart attack suddenly as the very first indication of CAD, without experiencing angina pain in the past, there have been warning signs that were misinterpreted as symptoms of other problems—indigestion, gas, gallbladder disease, or the like—when one looks back for possible signs of CAD.

Atherosclerosis may involve arteries of other organs, including the brain, kidneys, intestines, and legs. When the blood supply to the brain is impaired by a narrowed or blocked artery, brain function becomes abnormal. There may be impairment of speech, vision, coordination, or balance in mild cases. When the blood supply is cut off entirely to a portion of the brain, the patient develops a *cerebrovascular accident* (stroke). Weakness or paralysis of one side of the body is often observed in patients with stroke, and in severe cases, the patient may become unconscious. Fortunately, various signs and symptoms of stroke are often transient.

When the kidney (renal) arteries are involved in atherosclerosis, the patient often develops high blood pressure and slowly progressing impairment of kidney function until full-blown kidney failure occurs. The term *abdominal angina* is used when atherosclerosis affects the arteries supplying blood and nourishment to the intestinal tract. Abdominal pain due to abdominal angina typically occurs after meals because the blood supply to the intestinal tract necessary for digestion is impaired. The arteries that supply the blood to the legs are often involved in the atherosclerotic process, and this causes pain in the calf muscle or hip while walking. This disease process is termed "claudication," and the pain typically disappears upon resting. It is not uncommon for atherosclerosis to involve diffusely many arteries in the body. This type of diffuse atherosclerotic process is called "generalized atherosclerosis," which simply means that many arteries involving many organs show hardening from atherosclerosis.

Although atherosclerosis is a slowly progressing process—considered an "aging process" in some situations—it can progress much faster than usual, even in young people, under certain conditions. Factors that speed up the development of CAD are the risk factors, and they are summarized in Table 3.1.

As mentioned previously, atherosclerosis is the major cause of CAD, but less commonly CAD may be produced by other disease processes or trauma. Some individuals may be born with an abnormal coronary artery (congenital anomaly of the coronary artery). In this case, CAD may manifest itself even in children or young adults. Various chest traumas may cause heart attack when the coronary artery is damaged. The trauma that causes a heart attack is commonly open trauma (trauma with wound), but it may be blunt trauma (trauma without a visible wound). The best example of trauma-induced CAD is a steering-wheel chest injury in automobile accidents. Of course, surgical injury to the coronary artery may cause a heart attack in some cases. Many types of infections or malignancies (e.g., cancer) may involve the coronary artery in rare cases.

Coronary artery spasm has become a known clinical entity, and angina pain may be produced solely by spasm without fixed narrowing of the coronary artery. However, in many such cases, an underlying, fixed, coronary narrowing often coexists. Coronary artery spasm is discussed in detail in Chapter 4.

RISK FACTORS

Although any individual may suffer a heart attack at any time regardless of age, sex, nationality, race, or social background, some factors are known definitely to influence the development of atherosclerosis, which frequently causes CAD at an early age. These risk factors appear in Table 3.1. Various risk factors are cumulative. In other words, the more risk factors present, the more likely it is that the individual will suffer CAD (angina or heart attack) at an early age. And many risk factors are closely interrelated; for example, when one factor is eliminated or well controlled, at the same time, other risk factors often improve or even disappear altogether. Of course, it requires high motivation with sufficient knowledge to control or eliminate various risk factors.

Although the chance of suffering a heart attack is greater for those with a previous heart attack than for those who have never had one, it is by no means true that everyone with a history of heart attack will inevitably have another attack. In fact, not uncommonly, many people, after recovery from a first heart attack, reduce significantly their chances of having another attack, possibly even below the chances of those who never had any evidence of CAD. This can be accomplished by reducing or even eliminating various risk factors under careful medical supervision, because individuals with previous heart attack, with unforgettable, life-threatening, and painful experiences, will often have deeper concerns and interests about their health than healthy people. Of course, high motivation with proper medical guidelines is indispensable for the prevention of a second heart attack.

Heredity (Genetic) Factor
(Family History of Heart Attacks
at an Early Age)

It has been shown that certain families have higher chances than others of suffering a heart attack at an early age. For example, if one or both parents, brothers or sisters, or one or both grandparents have had heart attacks early in life, there is a greater probability that other family members will have a heart attack at a young age unless great effort has been exercised to reduce the risk. Although the heredity factor is considered uncontrollable, in many types of diseases, it is not a simple matter of inheritance. In a precise sense, the higher incidence of early heart attacks in some families is by no means clearly hereditary in all aspects. In many cases, it is rather environmental, habitual, or traditional; therefore, these aspects can be modified as needed. For instance, family members are often equally obese because certain families may have inherited a tendency to be overweight or because they have a tendency to overeat. Family eating habits that are transmitted from parents to children are traditional rather than hereditary.

Another good example is smoking habits. When one or both parents smoke, their children are more likely to smoke than are the children of parents who do not smoke.

As far as nationality or racial inheritance is concerned, white American men have been considered the subgroup with the greatest chance of suffering from heart attacks, even at an early age. However, nationality or race per se does not seem to be a key factor for predisposition to a heart attack. For example, the incidence of heart attacks in Asian countries (e.g., Japan, Korea) is lower than in any other country in the world, but the heart attack incidence among the first and second generations of Asian descendants born in America is almost equal to that of other Americans. In other words, American-Asians have a much higher incidence of heart attack than Asians born in their native countries. Similarly, the incidence of a heart attack among American blacks and whites is almost the same. These observations strongly suggest that cultural and environmental factors influence greatly the incidence of heart attack, rather than the nationality or racial inheritance factor.

Advanced (Old) Age

As described earlier, aging is one of the most important factors in the development of atherosclerosis—hardening of the arteries—because atherosclerosis is considered a part of the aging process. The degree of atherosclerosis is usually minimal up to the age of forty-five or fifty, but its development speeds up progressively and rapidly thereafter, especially after age sixty.

Male Sex

By and large, the incidence of heart attack is much higher in men than in women, but by no means are women immune to atherosclerosis. It has been shown that men have about thirteen times as many heart attacks as do women up to the age of forty-five. Between the ages of forty-five and sixty-two, men still have approximately twice as many heart attacks as women. However, the chance of suffering a heart attack after the age of sixty-two, is almost equal among men and women.

The statistics show that CAD has been accounting for more than 200,000 deaths per year among American women, a death toll 60 percent greater than that of cancer. It should be remembered that the chance of suffering a heart attack increases markedly when any woman smokes and/or takes oral contraceptives, even at an early age.

Hypertension (High Blood Pressure)

It is a well-known fact that hypertension (high blood pressure) is one of the major and most common risk factors for CAD. A detailed discussion of hypertension appears in Chapter 5.

Hyperlipidemia (Elevated Blood Contents of Cholesterol and/or Triglycerides)

Hyperlipidemia (elevated blood contents of cholesterol and/or triglycerides) is known to be one of the major and most common risk factors for the development of CAD. Cholesterol and triglycerides, which are fatty materials, must be present in the bloodstream of all healthy individuals, because these substances are essential fuel sources that are used by many cells of the body. When the body requires energy, the fats can be mustered and carried in the bloodstream as triglycerides to the areas where the energy is required. Cholesterol is contained in practically every cell of the human body, and it plays the role of regulating the nourishment that is carried into and out of the cells through the cell membranes. The brain contains a large quantity of cholesterol that is essential for various brain functions. Cholesterol is also an important material in the production of corticosteroids (hormones of the adrenal gland) as well as sex hormones. In addition, cholesterol has an important role in the digestion of fats.

When cholesterol and triglyceride levels in the blood are elevated beyond normal values, however, this is definitely abnormal, and it speeds up the process of atherosclerosis in various arteries, including the coronary arteries. On the other hand, many individuals with malnutrition, particularly in underdeveloped countries, have lower than normal values of these fatty materials. In some people, an abnormally high blood content of cholesterol and triglycerides is a result of a hereditary predisposition, whereas the majority of such cases are simply the end results of overeating foods containing large quantities of these fatty materials. Cholesterol contents of common foods are listed in Table 3.2, and low-cholesterol and low-fat diets are shown in Table 3.3.

The values of these blood lipids can be measured with simple tests and expressed in numbers. The test should be performed after fasting for at least fourteen hours. Customarily, the test is done in the morning before breakfast, after overnight fasting. Only a small sample of blood drawn from a vein is required.

TABLE 3.2. Cholesterol Content of Common Foods
(Cholesterol Content in Milligrams of 100-Gram Portions
of Common Foods).

FOODS	CHOLESTEROL CONTENT
Egg white	0
Margarine, vegetable fat	0
Milk (skimmed)	3
Milk (whole)	11
Creamed cottage cheese	15
Ice cream	45
Chicken (raw)	60
Mutton	65
Margarine (2/3 animal fat)	65
Cheese spread	65
Fish fillet	70
Pork (raw)	70
Lamb (raw)	70
Beef (raw)	70
Veal (raw)	90
Lard and animal fat	95
Cheddar chesse	100
Cream cheese	120
Shrimp	125
Crab	125
Heart (raw)	150
Lobster meat	200
Oysters	200 or more
Butter	250
Sweetbreads	250
Liver (raw)	300
Caviar or fish roe	300 or more
Kidney (raw)	375
Egg (whole)	550
Egg yolk (frozen)	1,280
Egg yolk (fresh)	1,500
Brain (raw)	2,000 or more
Egg yolk (dried)	2,950

TABLE 3.3. Low-Cholesterol/Low-Fat Diet.

ALLOWED	EXCLUDED
Beverages (Non-dairy) Coffee, tea, carbonated beverages, fruit juice, vegetable juice, decaffeinated coffee.	Sugar-sweetened beverages.
Dairy Products 1 pint fat-free skim milk, fat-free buttermilk, dried nonfat milk, evaporated skim milk, dry (non-fat) cottage cheese, yogurt made from skim milk, skim milk cheese (Saprago).	Whole milk, whole milk products, canned whole milk, all creams (sour and sweet), evaporated milk (whole), ice cream, ice milk, sherbert, commercial whipped toppings, cream substitutes, cream cheese, all hard cheese (except skim milk Saprago).
Breads French, Italian, white, rye, whole wheat, pumpernickel, matzo, saltines, graham crackers, baked goods containing no whole milk or egg yolk and made with allowed fat.	Quick breads, coffee cake, pancakes, sweet rolls, waffles, muffins, donuts, egg bread, cheese bread, commercial mixes containing dried eggs and whole milk, biscuits, cornbread, French toast, hot rolls, corn chips, potato chips, cheese crackers, other flavored crackers.
Cereals Whole grain ½ cup serving, refined grain cereal ½ cup serving, ¾ cup serving of cold cereal, rice, macaroni, noodles, flour, spaghetti.	Sugar-coated cereals.
Desserts Custard made from skim milk and egg allowance, fruit allowed, gelatin desserts, skim milk yogurt, water ice, fruit whips, puddings made with skim milk, frostings made with allowed fat, skim milk, and no egg yolks, junkets made with skim milk, angel food cake mixes.	Commercial cakes, commercial pies, commercial cookies, commercial mixes (cake and cookies), frozen cream pies, coconut, coconut products.
Fats Corn oil margarine, corn oil, cottonseed oil, safflower oil, soybean oil, sesame seed oil, sunflower seed oil, peanut oil, 1½ tsps. of mayonnaise may be substituted for 1 tsp. oil, soft safflower margarine (liquid safflower oil—not hardened, partially hardened or hydrogenated—should be the first listed ingredient; the first listed item on the label indicates the predominant ingredient).	Butter, lard, chicken fat, coconut oil, olive oil, hydrogenated margarine, hydrogenated shortening, all other fats not listed, salt, pork, suet, bacon, and meat drippings, gravies unless made with polyunsaturated fat, sauces, such as cream sauce, etc., unless made with allowed fat and skim milk.

TABLE 3.3 (continued).

ALLOWED	EXCLUDED
Fruit	
Fresh, frozen, or canned (at least 1 serving citrus fruit or juice).	Heavily sweetened fruits or juices.
Meat, Poultry, Fish	
Limit as recommended; usually 5 oz. daily. Lean beef, leg of lamb (baked, broiled, roasted or stewed without fat), lean veal, chicken (without skin), turkey (without skin), fish (except those excluded), egg white, peanut butter, cornish hen (without skin), squab (without skin), tuna or salmon (water packed), cottage cheese made with skim milk.	Egg yolk, luncheon meat, cold cuts, hot dogs, sausages, bacon, goose, duck, poultry skin, shellfish (crab, oyster, lobster, scallops, shrimp, clams), fish roe (caviar), all organ meats (heart, liver, brains, kidneys), all fatty meats, regular fried meats and fried fish unless fried with allowed oils, ham, corned beef, regular ground beef, or hamburger, spare ribs, pork and beans, meats (canned or frozen in sauces or gravies), frozen or packaged dinners, frozen or packaged prepared products (convenience foods).
Potato or Substitute	
White potato, sweet potato, 1 cup hominy, macaroni, noodles, rice, spaghetti.	Fried potatoes, potato chips, creamed potatoes.
Salad Dressings	
Vinegar, lemon juice, corn oil, zero dressing.	Any others.
Soups	
Fat-free clear boullion, fat-free clear consomme, fat-free broth, fat-free vegetable soup, cream soup made with skim milk, packaged dehydrated soups.	Any others.
Sweets	
Hard candies, jam, jelly, marmalade, honey, sugar, syrup (containing no fat), gum drops, mint patties (no chocolate, butter, sugar, syrup).	Candies made with milk, chocolate, butter, or cream. Fudge made with whole milk and butter or other animal fat.
Vegetables	
Any fresh, frozen, or canned, cooked without saturated fat.	Buttered, creamed, or fried vegetable unless prepared with allowed fat.
3 or more servings daily (include 1 yellow or leafy green vegetable), 1 raw.	Omit strongly flavored vegetables if they cause distress.
Miscellaneous	
Herbs, mustard, sugar, spices, pickles, salt, cocoa.	Olives, white sauce, gravy, commercial popcorn, chocolate fudge, nuts,

For best results, it is advised that one eat one's usual diet (regardless of its nature) for several weeks before the test. Although the exact normal values of blood lipids vary slightly among different medical institutions and laboratories, the normal ranges of cholesterol and triglycerides in America are from 150 to 300 mg percent and from 10 to 170 mg percent, respectively. Medical investigators have reported that the incidence of CAD is seven times higher in individuals with cholesterol values above 259 mg percent than in those with values below 200 mg percent.

Cholesterol and triglyceride values are often both elevated in the blood; but the cholesterol level may be high when the triglyceride value is normal, and vice versa. Of course, the risk of suffering a heart attack is greater when both cholesterol and triglyceride values are high than when only one of them is elevated. It has been pointed out that the elevation of triglyceride levels is more closely linked to the development of atherosclerosis than the elevation of cholesterol.

The practical way to distinguish between saturated and unsaturated fats is as follows. The saturated fats, which tend to increase cholesterol contents in the blood, are fats that harden at room temperature. Gravy fat is such an example. Saturated fats are contained in various meats, especially pork, beef, and lamb, and in butter, cream, whole milk, and cheese made from cream and whole milk. On the other hand, saturated vegetable fats are contained in various solid and hydrogenated shortenings and in coconut oil, cocoa butter, and palm oil, which commonly is used to make cookies, pie fillings, and nondairy milk and cream substitutes. Polyunsaturated fats, which tend to lower cholesterol contents, remain in liquid form at room temperatures. Common examples of polyunsaturated fats include corn oil, sesame seed oil, and soybean oil. Another type is monounsaturated fats (e.g., olive oil), which have little or no effect on cholesterol levels in the blood.

Elevation of blood triglyceride levels may be hereditary, but it is often associated with overweight. Ingestion of large amounts of sugar and alcohol causes increased blood levels of triglycerides. In addition, excessive stress is an important factor in producing high triglyceride contents in the blood. For example, business executives, politicians, lawyers, and physicians have a tendency to have high triglyceride levels because of excessive stress in their roles that cannot be avoided in many cases.

For the prevention and actual reduction of hyperlipidemia, the intake of various foods containing large amounts of cholesterol or triglycerides (e.g., egg yolk, lobster, shrimp, pork, beef, butter, cheese) should be minimized. In order to eliminate saturated fats, soups can be cooled off by placing them in the refrigerator after cooking, then skimming off the solid fat floating on top before reheating. In addition, consumption of sugar and alcohol should be minimized, and unnecessary stress must also be avoided if possible. Reduction of weight alone is often sufficient to reduce mild elevation of blood lipids in obese individuals. Detailed descriptions of various diets are found in Chapter 19. An in-depth discussion about alcohol in relation to heart disease is found in Chapter 23.

Various drugs to reduce blood lipid contents are available, but none of them seem fully satisfactory. Among them, clofibrate (Atromid-S) is most commonly used (see Chapter 17). In general, low-fat, low-cholesterol (see Table 3.3), and low-sugar diets, with low intake or avoidance of alcohol, are advisable for those who have hyperlipidemia or have recovered from a heart attack.

Obesity (Overweight)

As described previously, obesity (overweight) is one of the major and most common risk factors in the development of CAD. Mild obesity (less than 20 to 30 percent above the ideal body weight; see Table 3.4) is probably not sufficient to produce atherosclerosis process early in life, however. Medical study has demonstrated that the chance of suffering from CAD was 2.8 times greater for individuals who were 30 percent overweight within a ten-year period than among those who were 10 percent or more underweight.

Obese individuals have many other risk factors, such as hyperlipidemia, inactivity, hypertension, and diabetes mellitus, and all these factors accelerate the process of atherosclerosis. Remember that all risk factors have cumulative effects. When there is significant overweight, it simply means that the heart has to work harder to provide adequate circulation for the extra fatty tissues. This is comparable to an individual carrying a large sandbag every day unnecessarily. When the heart has to work harder for the extra fatty tissues for some time, it may progressively enlarge to compensate for the extra work loads. Then, eventually, the heart is unable to keep up the constant work, and this leads to CHF. CHF simply means that the heart is too weak to maintain adequate blood circulation. CHF is, of course, a serious problem that further aggravates heart diseases, including CAD (see Chapter 6).

In addition, overweight has adverse effects on many other diseases. According to life insurance data, the mortality (death) rate increases progressively and rapidly with the degree of overweight. In other words, the heavier the individual, the higher that person's chance of getting many diseases, including heart attack, at an early age. Consequently, the probability of death at an early age becomes greater.

When the individual with obesity reduces weight, all other risk factors will improve or may even disappear spontaneously, and he or she becomes healthier. However, overweight is not easily controlled unless the individual is highly motivated and properly informed about the serious nature of the problem. Many Americans enjoy eating rich foods containing large amounts of cholesterol, triglycerides, and sugar without realizing the serious nature of obesity.

The most important step in losing weight is to cut down food intake for life. In addition, everyone has to eat a proper diet (such as low-cholesterol and low-fat meals—see Table 3.3) in order to prevent obesity. Lowering calorie intake is essential for obese people. The caloric contents of foods and beverages are shown in Table 3.5, and caloric requirements for various activities are listed in Table 3.6. In addition to a reduced intake and a properly chosen diet, a well-designed exercise

TABLE 3.4. Desirable Weights for Men and Women (Ages 25 and Over).

MEN

Height (with shoes, 1-in. heels)		Weight in pounds (as ordinarily dressed)		
Feet	Inches	Small frame	Medium frame	Large frame
5	2	112-120	118-129	126-141
5	3	115-123	121-133	129-144
5	4	118-126	124-136	132-148
5	5	121-129	127-139	135-152
5	6	124-133	130-143	138-156
5	7	128-137	134-147	142-161
5	8	132-141	138-152	147-166
5	9	136-145	142-156	151-170
5	10	140-150	146-160	155-174
5	11	144-154	150-165	159-179
6	0	148-158	154-170	164-184
6	1	152-162	158-175	168-189
6	2	156-167	162-180	173-194
6	3	160-171	167-185	178-199
6	4	164-175	172-190	182-204

WOMEN

Height (with shoes, 2-in. heels)		Weight in pounds (as ordinarily dressed)		
Feet	Inches	Small frame	Medium frame	Large frame
4	10	92-98	96-107	104-119
4	11	94-101	98-110	106-122
5	0	96-104	101-113	109-125
5	1	99-107	104-116	112-128
5	2	102-110	107-119	115-131
5	3	105-113	110-122	118-134
5	4	108-116	113-126	121-138
5	5	111-119	116-130	125-142
5	6	114-123	120-135	129-146
5	7	118-127	124-139	133-150
5	8	122-131	128-143	137-154
5	9	126-135	132-147	141-158
5	10	130-140	136-151	145-163
5	11	134-144	140-155	149-168
6	0	138-148	144-159	153-173

Reproduced with permission from Metropolitan Life Insurance Company, *Statistical Bulletin* 40: November-December 1959.

TABLE 3.5. Caloric Content of Common Foods and Beverages.

FOODS	AMOUNTS	CALORIES
Soups		
Bouillon or consomme	1 cup	30
Chicken noodle	1 cup	65
Vegetable beef or chicken	1 cup	70
Clam chowder	1 cup	85
Tomato	1 cup	90
Cream soups	1 cup	150
Split pea	1 cup	200
Vegetables		
Lettuce	3 small leaves	3
Radishes	2 small	4
Cucumber	1/2 medium	5
Celery	1 large stalk	5
Cabbage (raw)	1/2 cup	12
Cauliflower	1/2 cup	15
Squash (summer)	1/2 cup	15
Beans (green)	1/2 cup	15
Green pepper	1	20
Cabbage (cooked)	1/2 cup	20
Asparagus	6-7 stalks	20
Carrots	1/2 cup or 1 medium	25
Eggplant	1/2 cup or 2 slices	25
Spinach	1/2 cup	25
Tomato (canned or cooked)	1/2 cup	25
Tomato (raw)	1 medium	30
Beets	1/2 cup	30
Broccoli	1 large stalk	30
Squash (winter)	1/4 cup	45
Peas	1/2 cup	55
Corn	1/2 cup	70
Beans (lima)	1/2 cup	80
Potato chips	10	100
Potato (white)	1 medium	100
Potato (sweet)	1 medium	200
Beans (kidney)	1/2 cup	335
Meat, Fish, and Poultry		
Shrimp (canned)	4 to 6	65
Bacon	2 strips	100
Frankfurter	5 1/2 × 3/4 inches	125
Beef liver (fried)	2 ounces	130
Rib lamp chop	1 medium	130
Bluefish (baked)	3 ounces	135
Salmon (drained)	2/3 cup	140
Whole lobster	1 pound	145
Tongue or kidney	average portion	150
Tuna fish (canned, drained)	2/5 cup	170
Veal cutlet (unbreaded)	3 ounces	185
Fish (cod, haddock, mackeral boiled or baked)	average portion	190
Chicken	6 ounces	190

TABLE 3.5 (continued).

FOODS	AMOUNTS	CALORIES
Breaded fish sticks (fried)	4 ounces	200
Turkey	3 1/2 ounces	200
Loin pork chop	1 medium	235
Ham (smoked or boiled)	2 slices	240
Hamburger patty	3 ounces	245
Ground beef	3 ounces	245
Trout	average portion	250
Roast leg of lamb	3 ounces	250
Sardines (drained)	4 ounces	260
Salami	2 ounces	260
Bologna	4 ounces	260
Beefsteak	3 ounces	300
Roast beef	3 ounces	300
Cereals, Breads, Crackers		
Saltine	1 (2 inches square)	15
Ritz cracker	1	15
Ry-Krisp	1 double square	20
Puffed wheat	1 cup	45
Bread, (rye, white, whole wheat)	1 slice	70
Hard roll	1 average	95
Other dry cereal	average portion	100
Farina (cooked)	3/4 cup	100
Egg noodles (cooked)	1 cup	100
Biscuit	1 (2-inch diameter)	110
Pancakes	2 medium	130
Muffin	1 medium	130
Oatmeal (cooked)	1 cup	135
Danish pastry	1 small	140
Bun, cinnamon with raisins	1 average	185
Rice (cooked)	1 cup	200
Macaroni or spaghetti, cooked	1 cup	200
Waffles	1 medium	230
Flour	1 cup	400
Desserts		
Jell-O	1 serving	65
Cookie—plain	3 inch diameter	75
Sponge cake	2 X 2 3/4 X 1/2 inches	100
Angel food cake	1/12 cake	115
Doughnut (plain)	1	130
Brownie	2 inches square	140
Fruit ice	1/2 cup	145
Cream pie	1/6 pie	200
Chocolate pudding	1/2 cup	220
Lemon meringue pie	1/6 pie	280
Chocolate layer cake	1/12 cake	350
Fruit pie	1/6 pie	375
Dairy Products		
Light cream (sweet or sour)	1 tablespoon	30
Heavy cream	1 tablespoon	50

TABLE 3.5 (continued).

FOODS	AMOUNTS	CALORIES
Whipped cream	1 tablespoon	50
Butter	1 pat	60
Egg (plain)	average	80
Skim milk	1 cup	90
Buttermilk (from skim milk)	1 cup	90
Cottage cheese	1/2 cup	100
Cheese	1 ounce or slice	100
Butter	1 tablespoon	100
Egg (fried or scrambled)	average	110
Yogurt	1 cup	120
Whole milk	1 cup	160
Evaporated milk	1/2 cup	170
Ice cream	1/6 quart	200

Fruits

Olive	1 large	8
Cantaloupe	1/3 medium	35
Peach (fresh)	1 medium	45
Pear (fresh)	1 medium	45
Tangerine	1 large	45
Plums (fresh)	2 medium	50
Apricots (raw)	2 to 3	50
Applesauce (unsweetened)	1/2 cup	50
Grapefruit	1/2 medium	55
Cherries (fresh)	15 large	60
Orange	1 medium	70
Peach (canned in syrup)	2 halves, 1 tbsp. juice	70
Pear (canned in syrup)	2 halves, 1 tbsp. juice	70
Apple	medium	75
Plums (canned in syrup)	2 medium	75
Apricots (canned or dried)	halves, 4 to 6	85
Banana	medium	85
Fruit cocktail (canned)	1/2 cup	90
Pineapple (canned in syrup)	1 slice	90
Applesauce (sweetened)	1/2 cup	95
Cherries (canned in syrup)	1/2 cup	100
Prunes (cooked with sugar)	5 large	135
Raisins (dried)	1/2 cup	200
Avocado	1/2 small	250
Cranberry sauce	1/2 cup	250

Snacks

Peanut or pistachio nut	1	5
Pickles	1 large sour	10
Pickles	1 average sweet	15
Butternut	1	25
Walnuts, pecans, filberts, cashews	4 whole	40
Chocolate creams	1 average size	50
Brazil nut	1	50
Popcorn	1 cup popped	55
Potato chips	10 or 1/2 cup	100
Chocolate bar	1 small	155
Chocolate nut sundae	average size	270

TABLE 3.5 (continued).

FOODS	AMOUNTS	CALORIES
Miscellaneous		
Spices and herbs		0
Boiled dressing (cooked)	1 tablespoon	30
Catsup or chili sauce	2 tablespoons	35
Sugar, white	1 tablespoon (3 teaspoons)	50
French dressing	1 tablespoon	60
Jam or jelly	1 tablespoon	60
Cheese sauce	2 tablespoons	65
Brown gravy	1/2 cup	80
Chocolate sauce	2 tablespoons	90
Peanut butter	1 tablespoon	100
White sauce (medium)	1/4 cup	100
Mayonnaise	1 tablespoon	100
Margarine	1 tablespoon	100
Salad oil, olive oil, etc.	1 tablespoon	125
Butterscotch sauce	2 tablespoons	200
Beverages		
Coffee or tea (plain)		0
Tomato juice	1/2 cup	25
Grapefruit juice (unsweetened)	1/2 cup	40
Pineapple juice	1/2 cup	55
Apple juice or cider	1/2 cup	65
Ginger ale	8 ounces	70
Prune juice	1/2 cup	85
Grape juice	1/2 cup	90
Cola drink	8 ounces	95
Cocoa made with milk	1 cup	175
Chocolate milk	8 ounce glass	185
Eggnog (without liquor)	1 glass	235
Ice cream soda	average size	255
Chocolate malted milk	1 glass	450
Alcoholic Beverages		
Wine	1 wine glass	75
Brandy	1 brandy glass	80
Gin	1 jigger	115
Beer	8 ounces	120
Whiskey	1 jigger	120
Rum	1 jigger	125
Cocktail	1 cocktail glass	150

program is also very important in maintaining an ideal body weight. Diet and the heart, and exercise and the heart are discussed later, in Chapters 19 and 21. There are various medications available for reducing weight (primarily by cutting down appetite), but none of them is satisfactory, and many of these drugs have significant side effects (see Chapter 17).

Cigarette Smoking

Cigarette smoking is the most common risk factor for CAD. A detailed discussion of cigarette smoking is found in Chapter 22.

TABLE 3.6. Caloric Requirement (Calories Per Hour) for Various Activities (For Average Adults—150 Pounds).

CALORIES	ACTIVITIES
80	Resting (supine) or sleeping
100	Resting (sitting)
140	Standing
120-140	Driving automobile
180	Housework (average)
210	Walking (2.5 mph), bicycling (5.5 mph)
220-230	Gardening, canoeing (2.5 mph)
250-270	Golf (power cart), bowling, billards, lawn mowing (250 calories for power mowing and 270 calories for hand mowing)
300-350	Walking (3-3.5 mph), calisthenics, swimming (¼ mph), fencing (social), rowboating (2.5 mph), volleyball, square dancing, badminton (social), horseback riding (trot), roller skating, dancing (fox-trot), tennis (doubles), golf (carrying clubs)
350-400	Table tennis (vigorous), ice skating (10 mph), sawing or chopping wood, digging ditch
400-500	Walking or jogging (5 mph), badminton (competitive), tennis (singles), water skiing, touch ball, climbing mountain (100 feet/hr.)
600-700	Running (5.5 mph), squash and handball (social), bicycling (13 mph), skiing (10 or more mph), basketball (vigorous), fencing (competitive)
800-900	Running (10 mph), many competitive sports

Stress

It has been suggested by various medical studies that excessive psychological stress predisposes individuals to CAD. Human life is full of stress, but not every stress is harmful. Joyful emotional stress is not likely to aggravate CAD. Unpleasant stress such as experiencing unusual fear, insecurity, frustration, or dissatisfaction related to one's occupation is considered a risk factor. Excessive stress is often encountered in the Western world, particularly in the United States, and that stress is considered an important risk factor responsible for the high incidence of heart attack in America, compared with many underdeveloped countries. The higher incidence of heart attack among Asian-Americans than among native Asians supports the importance of stress as a risk factor.

It has been demonstrated that psychosocial stress may cause elevation of triglyceride levels in the blood. Of course, increased triglycerides in the blood predispose one to the development of atherosclerosis at an early age. From available information, unnecessary stress is harmful, and it should be avoided to help prevent CAD.

Diabetes Mellitus

Diabetes mellitus (often simply called "diabetes") is a disease, often inherited, in which the body is unable to handle ingested carbohydrates (sugars and starches) properly because of lack of insulin production by the pancreas or ineffective use of the hormone. In some cases, diabetes mellitus develops as a result of trauma to the pancreas or surgical removal of the pancreas for various medical reasons. Although diabetes may affect children (called "juvenile diabetes"), more commonly it appears later in life (called "adult-onset diabetes"). Most people with adult-onset diabetes are obese.

Cholesterol contents in the blood tend to be more elevated in diabetic individuals than in nondiabetic people, and the incidence of hypertension is about two times higher in diabetics. According to one study, the chance of suffering from CAD was 1.4 times greater in diabetic men between ages thirty and fifty-nine than in nondiabetics. The incidence of getting CAD was even greater (2.5 times) in diabetic women than in nondiabetics. Furthermore, the risk of death from coronary artery disease in diabetic men and women was 2.3 times and 5.7 times greater, respectively, than in nondiabetics.

It is extremely important to detect diabetes early and to treat it properly because not only is diabetes itself a serious disease; it is also one of the major risk factors for CAD. Furthermore, many diabetic individuals have other risk factors, such as obesity, hypertension, and hyperlipidemia. Diabetic diets are discussed in Chapter 19.

Oral Contraceptives (Birth Control Pills)

Although medical investigators have reported that the incidence of blood clots in the blood vessels of various organs is higher in women taking oral contraceptives (birth control pills), many millions of women use them without serious side effects. Therefore, taking oral contraceptives alone seems to be only a minor risk factor for CAD. However, the risk becomes considerably higher when there is one or more other risk factors present, such as smoking, hypertension, a family history of heart attack at an early age, hyperlipidemia, obesity, or a history of blood clots in the legs, lungs, or the heart itself. The risk seems particularly higher for women who take birth control pills and smoke or who have suffered blood clots anywhere in the body in the past. Thus, birth control bills should definitely be avoided under these circumstances. It is rather foolish to use birth control pills when the risk of CAD or blood clots elsewhere in the body is high for women with other risk factors. The risk of CAD from oral contraceptives further increases in women over the age of thirty or thirty-five.

If any woman taking birth control pills experiences chest discomfort, difficulty in breathing, spitting up blood, pain in the legs, or the like, she must consult a physician immediately or go to a hospital emergency room (ER) without delay.

Type A Personality

Personality is shown to influence somewhat one's chances of getting a heart attack. In America, personality is classified arbitrarily into two types—Type A and Type B—but many individuals do not belong exactly to either Type A or B. It has been suggested that people with Type A personality are coronary prone.

Individuals with Type A personality are always time conscious, and they are compulsive about work and their success. They often get frustrated and extraordinarily angry when their colleagues or friends do not meet their time schedule. These individuals constantly remind themselves not to waste time. Many executives, professional people (e.g., college professors, physicians, lawyers), and politicians are Type A personalities in that they are usually ambitious, aggressive, and competitive, with an intense drive. Individuals with Type A personality have little or no time for friendships, and they much prefer to have their associates' respect than friendship. They have a tendency to tackle excessive work loads beyond their capacity in order to make sure that no time will be wasted. They try to complete all their work as soon as possible, and want to accomplish everything themselves. They set up so many deadlines for various tasks according to their own guidelines because of their productivity-conscious character. Individuals with Type A personality are often frustrated and disappointed about their accomplishments because of their very high goals and excessive work loads. Most of them are perfectionists with extremely large egos.

People with Type A personality do not enjoy watching television programs showing sports, soap operas, dramas, and the like; instead, they prefer to watch talk shows or news shows, in hopes that they can improve their productivity and success.

Although it is difficult, everyone has to try hard to modify Type A personality in order to reduce the risk of suffering a heart attack. One should not set goals that are beyond one's capacity. One should avoid as many deadlines as possible, and must learn that it is neither necessary nor possible to do everything by oneself. People should prepare their minds to yield a victory to others by assessing their own capacity. There is no reason to be a winner at all times.

People should avoid continuous and consecutive appointments with little time in between. They should take more time out to enjoy friends and family. It is wise not to feel that one must do something important all the time for the sake of productivity. People have to learn how to enjoy life rather than punish themselves. It is a common observation that many people who enjoy their work and lives seem to live longer and more peacefully. The best example of this is that many artists and musicians who enjoy every moment of their lives live long (up to eighty or ninety years), often without any disease. It is important to remember that no one can enjoy life as much as before when the body is no longer able to function properly because of any disease, particularly heart problems. When one regrets one's behavior, it may be too late.

Inactivity (Sedentary Living)

Inactivity (sedentary living) is considered a risk factor because lack of exercise seems to accelerate the development of atherosclerosis leading to CAD at an early age. Physical activity, exercise, and the heart are discussed in Chapter 21.

Coffee, Tea, and Alcohol

Coffee, tea, and alcohol are *not* exactly risk factors for CAD, but they are closely related to heart function, particularly when the heart is already diseased. Coffee and tea are agents (containing caffeine) that can stimulate the heart to beat much faster than usual or to beat irregularly in some individuals. Various abnormal heart rhythms are often harmful and potentially dangerous when the heart is considerably damaged (e.g., after recovery from a heart attack). Therefore, consumption of a large quantity of coffee or tea is not advisable for those with known heart disease, particularly CAD, or for individuals with known heart rhythm abnormality. Similarly, ingestion of large amounts of cola drinks may cause heart rhythm abnormalities. Alcohol and the heart are discussed in Chapter 23.

Gout (Elevated Blood Contents of Uric Acid)

Although it is not uniformly agreed upon by physicians, elevated uric acid levels in the blood seem to increase the risk of CAD. According to one medical study, the risk of CAD is reported to be 1.6 times greater among individuals with elevated uric acid levels than in those with normal uric acid levels.

SYMPTOMS

In general, there are three patterns in developing a heart attack. Most commonly, the heart attack is preceded by a history of angina pectoris for weeks, months, or even years. The second most common pattern is the sudden development of heart attack in apparently healthy individuals with no history of angina pectoris. The least common pattern is the so-called silent MI which means a painless heart attack. The nature and location of chest pain in both angina pectoris and heart attack are very similar or even identical, but the pain is much more intense and lasts much longer in a heart attack. Chest pain in a heart attack is not relieved by rest and/or NG (a small, white tablet of nitroglycerin that should be placed under the tongue).

The term *angina pectoris* means a constricting pain in the chest as a result of insufficient blood supply to the heart muscle by virtue of narrowed coronary artery(ies). The narrowing of the coronary artery, as repeatedly stressed, is almost always (in more than 95 percent of cases) due to atherosclerosis. Insufficient blood supply to the heart muscle is called "myocardial ischemia"; it occurs when the demand for circulation to the heart muscle exceeds the blood supply through the narrowed coronary artery. In the resting state, the heart muscle receives enough blood and nourishment, even though the coronary artery is narrowed, because only minimal blood supply is needed for minimal activity. Therefore, there is no symptom (e.g., chest pain) at rest in patients with angina pectoris.

On the other hand, blood supply is no longer adequate during extraordinary activities. At this time, the patient with angina pectoris experiences chest pain. Typical angina, therefore, is expressed as exertional chest pain. Commonly, angina is triggered by walking up a hill or upstairs, walking on a very cold day, carrying or pushing a heavy object, engaging in sexual intercourse, shoveling snow, raking leaves, eating heavy meals, and so forth.

In addition, angina may be triggered by emotional stress, anxiety, or excitement, such as watching exciting television programs or movies. In some cases, the patient with angina pectoris may wake up at night because of chest pain triggered by bad dreams.

The angina may be expressed in many ways, in location as well as in quality and nature. It is often expressed as chest discomfort or a pressure sensation in the chest, rather than as actual chest pain. Angina may be expressed as a viselike, constricting sensation, heaviness, or a burning or pressurelike feeling in the entire chest, midportion, or left side of the chest; it is commonly felt in the area behind the breastbone. The angina is frequently transmitted to various locations including the neck, jaw, gums, teeth, cheeks, shoulders, arms, elbows, and hands. At times, angina may radiate to the upper or midsection of the abdomen, back between the shoulders, and even behind the ears. Not uncommonly, it may be felt primarily at the already mentioned locations with no actual pain in the chest. Thus, some patients with angina visit dentists, otolaryngologists (physicians specializing in diseases of the ears, nose, and throat), and opthalmologists (eye doctors) because of unusual locations of angina. Therefore, pain or any type of discomfort above the umbilicus (navel) may be an expression of angina pectoris, especially in individuals with known heart disease or known risk factors.

Some patients may experience numbness or tingling sensations in the shoulders, arms, wrists, elbows, or fingers, with or without the aforementioned chest discomfort. In some cases, various forms of abnormal heart rhythms, a choking sensation in the throat, shortness of breath, and weakness may be associated with angina.

Typically, angina lasts from less than a minute to a few minutes, but it may last up to ten or twenty minutes. It is rather unusual for angina to last more than twenty minutes. Therefore, heart attack should be suspected when angina lasts more than twenty minutes. In addition, typical angina subsides immediately upon resting and/or when NG is taken sublingually. When the angina is not relieved by rest, and/or when the pain is not relieved by two tablets of NG, the possibility of a heart attack should be strongly considered. As a rule, chest pain from angina pectoris or heart attack does not get worse from taking a deep breath.

Heart Attack Preceded by Angina

Over one-third of patients with heart attacks give a history of alteration in the pattern of angina, sudden onset of atypical angina, or an unusual feeling described as "bad indigestion" in the chest. A heart attack should be considered a strong possibility when chest discomfort or pain does not go away upon resting, and when it is not relieved by two or more tablets of NG. By and large, the pain is much more intense and lasts longer in a heart attack than in angina. Impending heart attack should be considered when angina occurs more frequently than before, and when chest discomfort or pain is provoked by physical activity that did not cause angina before. The most serious kind of angina is atypical angina (variant angina, unstable angina, crescendo angina, or Prinzmetal's angina) that occurs at any time (even at rest or during sleep), unrelated to physical exertion. Because of its unusual nature, it is termed "atypical or variant angina." Atypical angina is considered a precursor of impending heart attack in many cases (see Chapter 4).

When NG is required, one must be sure that the drug has been kept in a cool (though not necessarily in the refrigerator) and dark place (such as a brown bottle) and that is not more than six months old. The reason for this is that NG will lose its potency considerably when the drug is too old, or has been exposed to sunlight for a long time. Also, one must be certain that NG is placed under the tongue and allowed to dissolve. It should not be swallowed or chewed but left to dissolve in the mouth. If the NG tablet is fresh, its effect is almost immediate, and the usual angina subsides within a few minutes (not more than five minutes). The second tablet of NG should be placed under the tongue if there is no obvious effect on the angina from the first tablet within five minutes. If the second tablet is still ineffective, a heart attack should be suspected, and immediate medical attention must be sought.

In addition to agonizing chest pain, many patients with a heart attack frequently develop cold sweats; nausea; vomiting; cough; wheezing; shortness of breath; light headedness; fainting; very rapid, slow, or irregular heart rhythm; and a feeling of impending death. Some patients develop profound shortness of breath from CHF or pulmonary edema (see Chapter 6). Some others may collapse suddenly from shock (see Chapter 7) or abnormal heart rhythms, particularly ventricular fibrillation. Ventricular fibrillation is commonly preceded by ventricular tachycardia (very rapid beating of the ventricles), and ventricular fibrillation frequently leads to cardiac arrest and death unless immediate and proper treatment is given. Therefore, it is essential to seek medical attention immediately when a heart attack is suspected.

Heart Attack without a History of Angina Pectoris

Some individuals develop a heart attack suddenly without any history of angina or any warning signs. This is, of course, a most frightening experience. The heart attack victim will experience intense chest pain as described previously, and the pain is often associated with profuse cold sweats, marked weakness, severe short-ness of breath, nausea, vomiting, dizziness, heart rhythm abnormalities, and faint-ing. Many heart attack victims feel a fear of impending death. Some patients lose consciousness instantly because of severe chest pain, intolerable anxiety, shock, or CHF, but most commonly they collapse as a result of electric failure (extremely rapid or slow rhythm or no heartbeat at all). At this point, simple cardiopulmonary resuscitation (CPR; see Chapter 15) can be applied immediately, with a little experience. Of course, rapid transportation to a hospital ER is imperative for immediate medical attention.

A heart attack is often triggered by extraordinary physical activities (e.g., shoveling snow), as seen in angina pectoris and/or intense emotional stress or excite-ment. In addition, many heart attack victims (particularly younger people) have one or more risk factors (see Table 3.1) that may not previously be known to the patient.

Silent Myocardial Infarction (MI)

In 5 percent to 15 percent of heart attack cases, the usual chest pain may be absent or minimal. This is called a "silent MI," a painless heart attack. In other patients with heart attack, the typical chest pain may be masked by immediate complications, including pulmonary edema, severe CHF, shock, syncope (fainting), and so on.

Although a silent MI is a known entity, in many cases the heart attack is *not* truly silent. In other words, many patients may be able to recall various symptoms of a heart attack when they look back on their history more carefully. It is also interesting that so-called silent heart attack seems much more common among individuals with minimal education (less than a high school education) than among highly educated people. This strongly suggests that the various symptoms of heart attack have frequently been misinterpreted as other problems, such as indigestion, stomach or gallbladder trouble, or that various symptoms have simply been ignored. Of course, every individual has different responses to the intensity of chest pain.

Silent MI often causes sudden death. Even when the victim survives the heart attack, various complications (discussed later in this chapter) often follow because physical as well as emotional rest for at least two to three weeks is essential for the healing process of damaged heart muscle after a heart attack. Remember that it usually takes four to six weeks for complete healing of heart muscle after a heart attack.

Among the complications, ventricular aneurysm is most commonly observed in patients with silent MI, as a result of a lack of the necessary resting period. Ventricular aneurysm means that that the ventricular wall (the muscle layer of the pumping chamber of the heart) stretches, then bulges (blows up like a balloon); and finally, it often ruptures (blows up). When the ventricular aneurysm occurs, the probability of ventricular rupture is great, and most of the victims die in this circumstance. Ventricular rupture following the development of ventricular aneurysm is comparable to a worn-out automobile tire's blowing up. Of course, many people with silent MI die from various heart rhythm abnormalities from the lack of the necessary resting period after heart attack. When there is no clinical history suggesting a past heart attack, the evidence of previous heart attack can be documented by the ECG (see Chapter 24) or on postmortem (autopsy) findings.

WHAT THE PATIENT AND FAMILY SHOULD DO WHEN A HEART ATTACK IS SUSPECTED

When an individual experiences chest pain during physical exercise, he or she must stop all activities and sit down to rest. Patients with known CAD should place one tablet of NG under the tongue. In most cases, mild angina is relieved by rest and/or a tablet of NG within a few minutes. If the chest discomfort is not relieved by NG within five minutes, the second NG should be taken immediately. If the chest discomfort still persists after the second NG tablet, a heart attack or an impending heart attack should be suspected.

The patient or whoever is at hand should arrange immediate transportation to a nearby hospital ER. When the chest pain is very intense in apparently healthy individuals, again, a heart attack should be suspected, and immediate medical attention is essential. The patient or companion should dial the local emergency telephone number (911 is the common number in many large cities in the United States). If there is no such number available in the area, the patient or friend must call the fire department, police department, rescue squad, or an ambulance. When there is an immediate response, the patient must be transported to the nearest hospital ER. If no immediate response is obtained from the phone calls for any reason, the patient may be moved quickly to the ER either by personal car or taxi, whichever is convenient, rather than wasting a moment. It is also a good idea to inform the family physician simultaneously. It is not advisable for the patient to drive a car when a heart attack is suspected; someone else has to drive. It is preferable to transport the patient in a vehicle equipped with necessary medical facilities and trained medical or paramedical personnel so that proper treatment can be provided enroute to the ER.

The first 911 emergency system went into service in 1968 in New York City. Since then, the system has spread to all parts of the country. There are now about 800 such systems serving nearly 50 million people in America, including such large cities as New York, Philadelphia, Detroit, Boston, Seattle, Los Angeles, and Chicago. Recently, laws have been passed in seven states requiring all their communities to have 911 installed by the late 1980s, and legislation is pending in several other states. In large cities, a 911 call is automatically routed to a central public-service answering point that typically serves the entire city. There, after determining the nature of the emergency, a dispatcher transfers the call to the fire department, the police, or an emergency medical service (Figure 3.2). However,

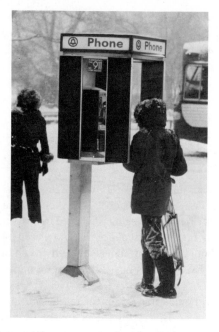

FIGURE 3.2. Public telephone booth showing 911 emergency calling system. (Reproduced with permission through the courtesy of AT&T Company, New York, New York.)

the emergency service was not originally adopted on any large-scale basis in the suburbs, and the reason for this is fairly easy to understand. In a large, sprawling, suburban county, a single telephone office can serve a number of towns, and the problems associated with forwarding calls from a central answering point to the appropriate municipal emergency service had been too great to permit the wide use of the 911 system.

The Western Electric manufacturing arm of the American Telegraph and Telephone Company has unveiled an expanded version of its 911 service that makes it possible for even the most widespread county to offer residents a central emergency number. The new, expanded 911 system (E911) designed by Bell Laboratories and made by the Western Electric Company, automatically displays the caller's phone number on a console in front of a dispatcher (Figure 3.3). Working from the phone number, the dispatcher can cross-check the address and send the necessary help. The E911 system uses software and associated computer hardware to route an emergency call automatically to the locality from which it originated. In the near future, the E911 service will be able to display immediately not only the phone number but also the address from which the call originated.

Many people make emergency calls and then, because of panic, a language problem, or simple unfamiliarity with the area, are unable to tell the dispatcher where they are. With the new system, the dispatcher immediately knows the caller's phone number and can go to work from there. An example of the problem that this system avoids occurred for an 82-year-old woman in Alameda County, California. Seconds away from a heart attack, she dialed 911. Before she could give her name or address, she fell to the floor. Thanks to the improved version of the 911

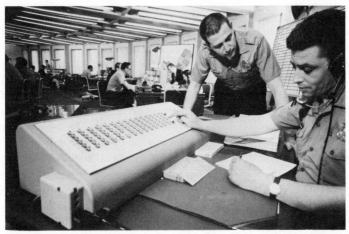

FIGURE 3.3. Communications center in the New York City Police Department showing Extended 911 emergency calling system (E911). (Reproduced with permission through the courtesy of AT&T Company, New York, New York.)

emergency communication system, however, the 911 dispatcher was able to determine the woman's address quickly, and a rescue team and ambulance arrived on the scene shortly. E911 is also technically capable of storing other information, such as the fact that a particular person is a potential heart attack victim. This information can then be displayed when an emergency call is received from that person's number. In an emergency, every second counts. With the 911 system, people can contact the necessary dispatcher faster, and help can arrive more quickly.

The patient may take a third and even a fourth NG tablet at five- to ten-minute intervals while waiting for an ambulance to arrive. It should be noted that NG is *not* habit-forming. While the patient is being transported to the ER, his or her ECG and other important signs (e.g., blood pressure) may be monitored when the vehicle is equipped with medical facilities. Emergency CPR and necessary injections can be provided if needed during transportation. The ideal ambulance for the cardiac patient is a mobile coronary care unit (mobile CCU) that is fully equipped with all necessary medical facilities with full trained personnel (a physician and/or cardiac nurse). A mobile CCU is an extension of the ordinary hospital CCU (discussed later in this chapter). Mobile CCUs are available in many European countries and the U.S.S.R. In America, mobile CCUs are not as popular as in other countries for various reasons and are available only in selected areas (such as Los Angeles, Seattle, New York City).

When the patient with suspected heart attack develops cardiac arrest before the ambulance arrives, proper CPR (such as mouth-to-mouth resuscitation and external cardiac massage) should be given. Even someone who has not learned how to give CPR may be able to restore normal heart rhythm by applying any stimulus, such as a mild blow by the fist, to the patient's chest. It may be too late to wait for medical or paramedical personnel to arrive for the treatment of cardiac arrest.

Therefore, it is strongly recommended that every individual, regardless of occupation, learn the proper technique for applying CPR. Simple CPR is relatively easy to learn, even for lay people, and it is often a life-saving measure.

As soon as the patient arrives at the hospital, an ER physician should be notified. The patient or a companion should clearly indicate the problem to the physician—suspected heart attack. Unless the ER physician is promptly and clearly informed about the urgent nature of the disease (suspected heart attack), unnecessary delay in treatment may occur even in the hospital ER. The ER physician will evaluate the patient quickly by taking a history of the symptoms, performing a physical examination (such as measuring blood pressure and listening to heart sounds), and assessing the ECG findings as well as necessary blood test results (see Chapter 24). When the diagnosis of heart attack is established or suspected, the patient will be admitted to the CCU for further evaluation and treatment.

Immediate medical attention is essential because a few minutes may determine the difference between life and death in many patients with heart attack. More than 80 percent of deaths in heart attack victims occur during the first twenty-four hours, many within the first hour. In many cases, death occurs even when the heart is only minimally damaged. That is, the heart need not have died because the damage to this muscle was not enough to cause death. It has been shown that the incidence of sudden death is *not* closely related to the area of damaged heart muscle from heart attack. In most cases, sudden death from heart attack occurs as a result of electric failure. The electric failure causing death is usually ventricular fibrillation (VF), which frequently leads to cardiac arrest (no heartbeat at all). VF is commonly preceded by a very rapid beating of the ventricles (ventricular tachycardia).

Even when these life-threatening heart rhythm abnormalities occur, they can be successfully treated in many cases if medical attention is sought immediately. Heart rhythm abnormalities can be treated at the scene of the attack by specially trained ambulance attendants or other paramedicals. Of course, they can be treated by physicians or nurses in the hospital ER, in the mobile CCU or hospital CCU, or in the patient's room at the hospital. The brain will suffer permanently when its blood supply is cut off for four minutes or more from cardiac arrest. Therefore, when treatment of cardiac arrest is delayed for any reason, permanent brain damage is often unavoidable, even if heart function is restored and the patient is able to recover fully from the heart attack itself. If the brain damage is permanent, the victim will have to live as a semiinvalid.

DIAGNOSIS

As soon as the patient is seen in the hospital ER and a heart attack is suspected through clinical background alone, medication (usually morphine or Demerol injection) is given to ease chest discomfort, and oxygen will be administered either by mask or through a nasal tube. In addition, a small needle connected to a plastic tube and a bottle containing glucose (sugar) solution (most commonly 500 cc of 5 percent dextrose in water) will be inserted into the vein. Through this, medication (such as that for rapid or irregular heart rhythm) can simply be injected into the plastic tube connected to the needle in the vein whenever needed. When medication is administered directly into the bloodstream via the vein, its effect is prompt. In other words, it takes the medication only a few seconds to go from the vein to the heart.

In addition, electrodes will be placed on the chest wall and connected to the cardiac monitor that displays the ECG. Through the display of the heart's electrical activity on the cardiac monitor, it is possible to appreciate various types of abnormal heart rhythm; thus, any necessary treatment (medications, direct-current shock, or artificial pacemaker) can be applied as needed. The electrodes for the cardiac monitor may be affixed to the patient in the ER before the patient is transferred to the CCU or after the patient is admitted to the CCU, depending upon clinical circumstances. Various types of treatment may also be given in the ER or in the CCU, as judged by the physician. In some cases, the ER physician may request a consultation with a cardiologist (a heart specialist) for further evaluation.

It is *not* essential to establish the diagnosis of heart attack in every case in the ER. When a heart attack is strongly suspected or angina seems to be getting worse, the patient will be hospitalized even without definite diagnosis of a heart attack.

Symptoms

With acute MI, in typical cases, the diagnosis can be established without much difficulty on the basis of characteristic symptoms, as described previously in this chapter (see "Symptoms").

Physical Findings

A physician can detect various abnormal findings by examining the patient with a heart attack, but none of them are diagnostic:—rather, they are supportive. Depending upon the severity of the heart attack and the presence or absence of various complications (e.g., heart failure, abnormal heart rhythm, shock—discussed later in this chapter), various physical findings may be present. They may include rapid and/or irregular (at times, too slow) pulse, fever, rapid breathing (tachypnea), pulmonary rales (wet, bubbling sounds in the lungs from fluid accumulation), gallop rhythm (triple heart sounds) and various abnormal heart rhythms, hypotension (lower than normal blood pressure—a sign of shock), heart murmurs, clammy skin, grayish skin color, appearance of marked air hunger (shortness of breath or dyspnea), anxiety, and fear.

Fever is usually *not* present at the beginning of a heart attack and during prolonged shock. However, the temperature may rise to 37.8 to 39.4° C (100 to 103° F). Temperature above 103° F is rather unusual. Fever may last for twenty-four hours, or it may persist for three to seven days. Many patients with a heart attack may not have an appreciable fever.

Pulmonary rales (bubbing sounds) are heard in the chest through a stethoscope when there is fluid accumulation in the lungs and air passage during breathing through the airway filled with fluid is impaired. Pulmonary rales are one of the common signs of CHF (see Chapter 6). Gallop rhythm (triple heart sounds—resembles the sound of a horse running) is also a common sign of CHF. Heart murmur (abnormal noise generated by blood flow through the damaged heart valve or by abnormal communication in the muscular wall between the heart chambers) is usually *not* heard in patients with heart attack unless there is a serious complication. That is, heart murmur occurs in patients with heart attack when there is considerable damage in the heart valves (commonly, damage in the tissue structures surrounding and supporting the mitral valve—papillary muscle dysfunction or rupture of the chordae tendineae) or perforation of the ventricular septum (a hole in the muscular wall between the right and left pumping chambers).

Laboratory Findings

Without a doubt, the most important tool, and an indispensable one, in establishing the diagnosis of a heart attack is the ECG. When there is significant damage to the heart in patients with acute heart attack, the ECG reveals characteristic findings (Figure 3.4).

FIGURE 3.4. Myocardial ischemia, injury, and infarction (scheme). (Reproduced from Chung, E.K.: *Electrocardiography: Practical Applications With Vectorial Principles,* Second Edition, Hagerstown, Md., Harper & Row Publishers, 1980.)

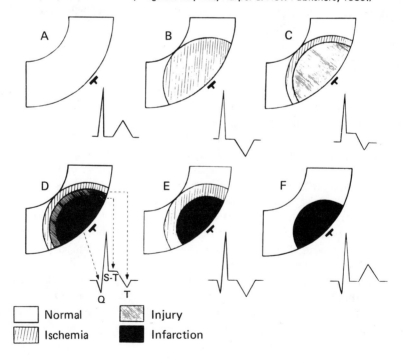

The next important laboratory test for the diagnosis of acute MI is a determination of serum (blood) enzymes. The most reliable and specific serum enzyme is creatine phosphokinase (CPK) isoenzyme, MB fraction which appears earliest in the serum; when determined every two hours, its elevated value gives an estimate of the magnitude of the heart damage. Normal values of CPK for male and female are 5 to 55 mU/ml, and 5 to 35 mU/ml, respectively. MB fraction per total CPK is 0 to 5 percent.

Other serum enzymes valuable for the diagnosis of heart attack include serum glutamic oxaloacetic transaminase (SGOT) and serum lactic acid dehydrogenase (LDH). SGOT activity increases in 6 to 12 hours, reaches a peak in 24 to 48 hours, and returns to normal in 3 to 7 days. LDH begins to rise within 24 to 48 hours, and it may remain elevated for 5 to 10 days. Normal values of SGOT and LDH are 10 to 40 units/ml and 60 to 120 units/ml, respectively.

In addition to the determination of the serum enzymes, some other blood tests may be valuable, although not necessarily diagnostic of a heart attack. For instance, leukocytosis (increased white blood cell counts) up to 20,000 cells/cu mm often occurs on the second day and returns to a normal count within one week (normal white blood cell counts: 4,800 to 10,800/mm^3). Another example is the sedimentation rate, which is normal at the beginning of the heart attack, but which rises on the second or third day and remains elevated for one to three weeks. Normal values for the sedimentation rate of male and female are 1 to 13 mm/hr. and 1 to 20 mm/hr., respectively.

Other laboratory tests, including Holter monitor ECG, exercise ECG, echocardiogram, myocardial imaging, cardiac catheterization, coronary arteriography, and chest X-ray, are discussed in Chapter 24.

DIFFERENTIAL DIAGNOSIS (HOW TO DISTINGUISH HEART ATTACK FROM OTHER DISEASES)

As emphasized repeatedly, various symptoms of a heart attack may, superficially or at times, closely simulate those of many other diseases involving the heart or other organs. A common mistake that many members of the general public make is to interpret the chest discomfort of a heart attack very lightly—as indigestion, some sort of stomach trouble, gallbladder trouble, or even a chest cold. Whenever any suspicion or possibility of a heart attack is raised, medical attention should be sought without delay. Remember that a few minutes can mean the difference between life and death in many heart attack victims. When pain or discomfort occurs in some unusual location, such as the jaw, gum, teeth, behind the ears or eyes, and so forth, the patient may erroneously go to the dentist or to doctors specializing in eye or ear diseases. Recall that pain from heart attack may be located anywhere above the umbilicus (navel).

From the physician's viewpoint, likewise, a heart attack may resemble many other diseases. For example, a heart attack sometimes closely simulates acute pericarditis (inflammation involving the pericardium—a sac surrounding the heart). In pericarditis, fever often precedes the onset of chest pain, which is predominantly pleuritic in nature (more superficial in nature). The chest pain in pericarditis is relieved considerably by holding one's breath and leaning forward, and it becomes worse upon swallowing. The friction rub (scratch-quality noise in the chest) appears early, and it is loud diffusely over the chest through careful auscultation (listening to the chest with a stethoscope). Differential diagnosis is clearly made with the various laboratory findings (see Chapter 24).

Another disease that often simulates a heart attack is pulmonary embolism (blood clots in the lungs). Acute pulmonary embolism also causes chest pain, often indistinguishable from that of a heart attack, as well as hypotension (lower than normal blood pressure), dyspnea, distended neck veins, and so on. But pulmonary embolism often produces hemoptysis (spitting up blood), and thrombophlebitis (painful and swollen tissues over inflamed veins with thrombosis—blood clots) is frequently found in the legs, the groin, and the lower abdomen. Physicians can distinguish between pulmonary embolism and heart attack from various laboratory studies, particularly ECG changes (see Chapter 24) and the lung scan. In the lung scan test, a radioactive material is injected into the circulation of the lungs, and those areas of the lungs having blood clots are then revealed.

Dissecting aneurysm (a tear involving the inner layer of the aorta; see Figures 1.1 and 1.2) may cause chest pain very similar to that of a heart attack. In this disease, the violent chest pain is often of maximum intensity at the onset. The pain characteristically spreads up or down the chest and back over a period of hours. Very important clinical manifestations of dissecting aneurysm include changes in pulses, changing aortic murmurs, and left pleural effusion or cardiac tamponade (see Chapter 13). Differential diagnosis from a heart attack is usually made from ECG and chest X-ray findings.

Since emotionally disturbed people without any heart disease may experience chest pain (called "functional" chest pain) very similar to coronary (cardiac) pain, various differential points between functional and coronary chest pain are summarized in Tables 3.7 and 3.8.

COMPLICATIONS OF HEART ATTACK

Although many heart attack victims recover without any unusual problems, some patients, particularly with massive MI, may develop various complications. There are three major complications, including cardiac arrhythmias, CHF, and shock. These complications are closely interrelated, and one often leads to or aggravates others. These complications directly influence morbidity and mortality. In other words, unless these complications are immediately and properly treated, death is often unavoidable.

TABLE 3.7. Differential Diagnosis Between Coronary and Functional Chest Pain.

	CORONARY	FUNCTIONAL
Age	Older persons (age above 45)	Young (age: 20-40)
Sex	Common in male	Common in female
Etiology	Coronary artery disease (atherosclerosis)	Psychologic insecurity and maladjustment
Precipitating factors	Exercise (eating, working), excitement, stress	Spontaneous or emotional
Hereditary	Family history of coronary heart disease and/or hypertension	Family history of psychoneuroic disorder
Initial symptom	Chest pain, pressure sensation, tightness in the chest	Anxiety, dyspnea, hyperventilation
Feeling of palpitation	Often present, and may be associated with tachyarrhythmias	May be present without true cardiac arrhythmias
Objective signs of heart disease	Present	Absent
Fever	May be present (up to 102°F.)	May be present but rarely exceeds 100.5° F.
Fainting	Often present	May be present but transient
Shock	Often present in acute myocardial infraction	Absent
Heart failure	Often present	Absent
Chest x-ray	Often shows cardiomegaly or signs of congestive heart failure	Normal
Resting ECG	Often abnormal (myocardial infarction, ischemia or injury)	Normal
ECG during attack	Usually abnormal	Almost always normal
Cardiac arrhythmias	Common (almost every known type)	Rarely present (may show sinus tachycardia and extrasystoles)
Exercise ECG test	Often positive	Negative
Serum enzymes	Usually elevated in acute myocardial infarction	Normal
Commonly associated disorders	Hypertension, diabetes mellitus, hyperlipidemia, obesity	Various psychoneurotic disorders

51

TABLE 3.8. Characteristics of Coronary vs. Functional Chest Pain.

	CORONARY	FUNCTIONAL
Location	Mostly substernal but anywhere in the chest	Cardiac apex and around the nipple
Area	Diffuse	More localized
Quality	Squeezing, burning, pressure, tightness, heavy feeling	Dull-aching or knifelike, sharp, stabbing
Radiation	Both shoulders, arms, fingers, neck, cheeks, teeth, interscapular region	Left hemithorax, left shoulder or back
Duration	Often less than 5 minutes in angina pectoris	Often more than 10 minutes or continuous
Local tenderness	Usually absent	Often present
Rest	Pain often disappears or improves	Pain unchanged or becomes worse
Response to antianginal drugs	Good	No effect or doubtful
Response to morphine	Good	Doubtful or unchanged
Factors aggravating chest pain	Exercise, excitement, and other similar stress, cold weather, after meals, sexual intercourse	Emotional stress, anxiety, complete rest

Cardiac Arrhythmias
(Heart Rhythm Abnormalities)

In nearly 90 to 95 percent of patients with heart attack, some form of heart rhythm abnormalities is encountered, but many arrhythmias are relatively benign and self-limited (see Chapter 9). However, some of them are very serious and life-threatening. When an arrhythmia is too slow (less than 45 beats/min.) or too fast (faster than 180 beats/min.), it is potentially serious.

Arrhythmias are considered responsible for approximately 40 percent of the deaths among heart attack victims. The mechanism of sudden death is usually ventricular fibrillation (VF). VF is extremely rapid, irregular, and orderless, life-threatening rhythm abnormality, and the rhythm originates from the pumping chambers (Figure 3.5). There is little or no pumping action by the heart when VF occurs. Therefore, immediate application of electric shock is absolutely necessary.

FIGURE 3.5. Electrocardiograms showing frequent VPCs with short runs of ventricular tachycardia (indicated V—tracing A) followed by ventricular fibrillation (tracing B). Leads II-a to d in tracing A and lead II-a to c are continuous in each given tracing. Note an atrial premature beat (marked X).

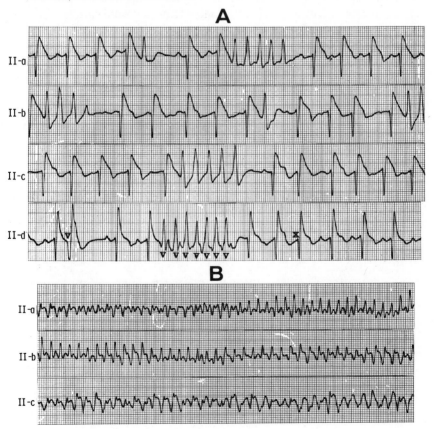

If the brain receives no blood as a result of VF for four minutes or longer, the patient often becomes a semiinvalid, even when heart function returns to normal. VF is frequently preceded by a slightly less serious arrhythmia—ventricular tachycardia (*tachy* means "rapid"; *cardia* means "heart"—Figure 3.5). Ventricular tachycardia is very rapid (rate: 160 to 250 beats/min.) and regular heart rhythm arising from the pumping chambers.

Abnormally slow heart rhythm is called "bradycardia" or "bradyarrhythmia" (*brady* means "slow"; *cardia* means "heart"; *arrhythmia* means "abnormal rhythm"). There are many types of slow heart rhythms, but clinically important and common arrhythmias include complete heart block and sick sinus syndrome (Figures 3.6 and 3.7). In most cases, implantation of an artificial pacemaker is indicated for very slow heart rhythm. Cardiac arrhythmias are discussed fully in Chapter 9.

Heart Failure

Heart failure (congestive heart failure—CHF) may be present at the onset of a heart attack or may develop following cardiac arrhythmias or pulmonary embolism. CHF means that the heart fails to pump blood adequately to meet demands because of weakened heart muscles from a damaged heart—heart attack. In other words, the left ventricle is unable to supply adequate blood to all parts of the body because of weakened pumping action in heart failure. Thus, heart failure causes fluid congestion and retention in various parts of the body, including the lungs, legs, and ankles. CHF is discussed fully in Chapter 6.

FIGURE 3.6. Permanent artificial pacemaker is implanted (see lead II-C) for complete A-V block (leads II-a and b). Note that the P waves (indicated by arrows) and the QRS complexes are independent throughout, and the ventricular rate is very slow (rate: 37 beats/min., leads II-a and b).

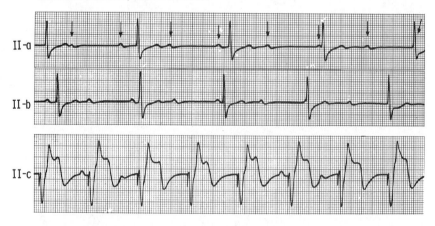

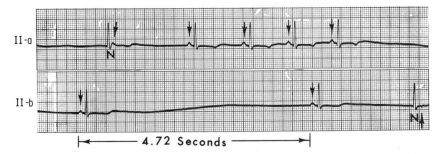

FIGURE 3.7. These ECG rhythm strips were obtained from a thirty-year-old woman who had received surgical correction for atrial septal defect ten years previously. Leads II-a and b are continuous. Downward arrows indicate the P waves of sinus origin. The tracing shows very unstable sinus activity (indicated by arrows) and an area of a long sinus arrest (4.72 seconds) and occasional A-V junctional escape beats (marked *N*) as a result of sick sinus syndrome. Note occasional retrograde (inverted) P waves (indicated by upward arrows). A permanent artificial pacemaker implantation was performed with good result.

Shock

Shock, likewise, may occur at the onset of a heart attack or may develop later following arrhythmias or pulmonary embolism. Shock often coexists with severe heart failure. Though shock may be due to various causes, including massive hemorrhage, infections, trauma, drug reactions, and so on, the term *cardiogenic shock* is used when shock is specifically a complication of heart attack. Cardiogenic shock is characterized by hypotension (systolic blood pressure less than 90 mmHg) with evidence of impaired blood circulation to the skin, kidneys, and central nervous system from the inability of the left ventricle to perform effectively as a pump in maintaining adequate cardiac output following a heart attack. Shock is discussed in Chapter 7.

Other Complications

Not uncommonly, tissue structures supporting the mitral valve (the heart valve between the left atrium and the left ventricle) may be damaged as a result of papillary muscle dysfunction or infarction, or chordae tendineae rupture. In this case, a physician can detect a heart murmur from mitral insufficiency (regurgitation). These complictions often lead to CHF, and cardiac surgery is indicated in some cases (see Chapter 25). Less commonly, perforation of the ventricular septum (the muscular wall between the right and left ventricles) may occur. In this circumstance, there is the sudden appearance of a loud, harsh, systolic murmur and thrill over the upper midportion or left side of the chest. Perforation of the ventricular septum also frequently causes CHF, and cardiac surgery is often required.

Ventricular aneurysm (bulging of a portion of the ventricle—explained previously) may occur, especially when the MI is huge and when there is an insufficient rest period following the attack. A ventricular aneurysm is more likely to be observed in patients with so-called silent MI, because no resting period was taken after the unrecognized heart attack. Ventricular aneurysm can readily be recognized with an ECG, echocardiogram, chest X-ray, and cardiac catheterizaion (see Chapter 24). Some of these patients develop refractory CHF and/or ventricular arrhythmias. Surgical excision of the aneurysm is necessary in these cases.

Rupture of the heart is uncommon, but if it occurs, it is usually in the first week after a heart attack. Rupture of the heart may be preceded by ventricular aneurysm, a finding comparable to an old, worn-out automobile tire's becoming a flat tire. Ruptured heart is invariably fatal.

Pulmonary embolism (blood clots in the lungs) occurs in 10 to 20 percent of patients following heart attack when anticoagulants (blood-thinning drugs) are not given. Cerebrovascular accidents (stroke) may result from a fall in BP (shock) or from embolism secondary to a mural thrombosis. Peripheral arterial embolism (e.g., blood clots in the leg artery) may also occur.

Post-MI syndrome (Dressler's syndrome) may occur two to eleven weeks after the onset of a heart attack. Post-MI syndrome is pleuropericarditis (a form of pericarditis), which is thought to be due to an autoimmune mechanism. The patient may experience a sharp chest pain that is often aggravated by deep breathing and by lying down flat. There may be low-grade fever, tachycardia, and evidence of pleural or pericardial effusion (fluid accumulation in the chest cavity or pericardial sac). At times, post-MI syndrome mimics recurrence or extension of heart attack, but in most cases, a physician can distinguish them by physical examination (often there is pericardial friction rub—scratch-quality noise through a stethoscope), ECG (diffuse S-T segment elevation), chest X-ray findings (globular-shaped heart may be seen only if there is a large pericardial effusion), and echocardiogram (primarily for confirmation of pericardial effusion). In most cases, this condition is self-limited. Some patients may require aspirin, indomethacin (Indocin), and corticosteroids (see Chapter 17).

The shoulder-hand syndrome is a rare, preventable complication caused by a long-standing disuse of the arms and shoulders following a heart attack. The patient may experience pain, stiffness, and limitation of motion of the shoulders and arms, generally on the left side. The skin of the hands may become swollen and discolored, with excessive or deficient sweating. Treatment consists of a rehabilitation program of physical therapy. Some individuals may require corticosteroids, but reassurance is the most important therapeutic approach. Prognosis is excellent. Recurrent MI or extension of the MI occurs in approximately 5 percent of patients during recovery from the initial heart attack.

Emotional problems of varying degrees may occur in some people with heart attack, especially in an early phase of the disease. Anxiety, restlessness, and fear of death are common during the early phases, and some patients develop profound depression and feelings of hopelessness during recovery. Occasionally, psychiatric consultation is required for persisting depression following a heart attack. Psychosocial problems after heart attack are discussed later in this chapter.

MEDICAL TREATMENT

It is unequivocally clear that all patients with heart attack are treated best in the CCU equipped with continuous monitoring (ECG as well as pressures in various heart chambers and blood vessels), CPR equipment (e.g., defibrillator), an artificial cardiac pacemaker, and specially trained nurses and physicians. Sudden death, which most commonly occurs in the first few hours of a heart attack as a result of VF, can be prevented most effectively in the CCU. When a mobile CCU is available, sudden death can be prevented even before the heart attack victim is transported to the hospital ER. The survival rate of heart attack victims has increased markedly in recent years, primarily because of the availability of a CCU in most hospitals. The survival rate at present is over 85 percent versus less than 75 percent before 1965, when the CCU was not available.

Monitoring and Common Tests

As soon as a heart attack is suspected, necessary emergency medications (pain-killers, drugs to stop rapid heart rhythm, and so forth) are given, and the administration of oxygen (either by mask or through a nasal tube) and the monitoring of the ECG and pressure in various heart chambers and large blood vessels connected with the heart are begun in the CCU.

An ECG (Figure 2.1) is continuously monitored via several electrodes (specially designed, small, and round—about the size of a quarter or half-dollar—paper or soft plastic pads with a metal center piece, like a small button) placed on the chest skin. Through these electrodes, any abnormality of the heart rhythm can be detected immediately through the ECG monitor, and proper treatment can be provided as needed. Physicians will determine the best therapeutic modality for a given heart rhythm abnormality. When the heart rhythm abnormality is extremely serious and urgent (e.g., VF), immediate application of the defibrillator can be performed by nurses, even without a physician's attendance.

For the determination of pressures within various heart chambers and large blood vessels, catheters are inserted into the heart and blood vessels with negligible risk. These catheters are inserted into the heart through the skin in various areas, including the neck, the arm, and the groin. This type of heart procedure is called "hemodynamic monitoring" (see Chapter 24); it is essential for patients with various complications, particularly CHF and/or cardiogenic shock. Hemodynamic monitoring is *not* absolutely required for every heart attack victim. The values obtained through the hemodynamic monitoring provide invaluable information for optimal management (see Chapter 24).

Rest

It is extremely important to emphasize that physical as well as mental (emotional) rest is absolutely necessary for any individual with a heart attack for at least two to three weeks. Heart rupture is most apt to occur during the first few weeks (particularly the first week) of the heart attack when there is inadequate rest. In addition, various serious complications (electric failure, CHF, and cardiogenic shock) will occur frequently unless there is a sufficient resting period. The mortality (death) rate, of course, will be greater with an inadequate resting period.

Remember that the heart has to continue to beat and pump blood in order to maintain adequate circulation to meet the demands of body functions in spite of the damage that has occurred in a heart attack. Even when there is only minimal physical movement, the heart has to pump harder in order to supply more oxygen and nutrients via increased blood circulation (Figures 2.2 and 3.1). In other words, the damaged heart muscle will have an extraordinary burden when an additional demand is made by any physical activity. This additional burden will lead to more damage to an already damaged heart muscle.

Analgesics (painkillers) should be give generously during the first few days of heart attack for chest pain. Likewise, sedatives (e.g., Valium) should be prescribed for anxiety and apprehension for the first few days. Adequate sleep is essential for all heart attack victims; therefore, sleeping pills may be necessary for some patients. Oxygen is also useful for the relief of dyspnea and chest pain.

As soon as the patient is examined in the ER, he or she will be transferred to the CCU. During the first three to four days in the CCU, *absolute* bed rest is recommended unless the heart attack is very mild and there are no significant complications. As a rule, patients should not be allowed to feed or care for themselves during the first few days. A bedpan or a bedside commode (toilet) is used during this period, depending upon the preference and convenience of the patient. A bedside toilet seems to require less effort than a bedpan for many patients. Some patients may require laxatives or stool softeners in order to avoid strenuous bowel movements. Special nursing care is highly desirable in the CCU. During the first few days, the patient will be spoon-fed and sponge-bathed by nursing staff in order to avoid any additional physical activity.

After a complete resting period of a few days in the CCU, the patient is usually transferred to a less intensive care area—called the "intermediate coronary care unit" (ICCU)—for further management. When an ICCU is not available, hospital beds with similar facilities are acceptable. The ICCU is equipped with similar, if not identical, facilities and medical as well as nursing personnel, so that continuous monitoring and care can be provided. The patient's condition must be good enough for him or her to be transferred to the ICCU. In other words, patients should be free of significant chest pain and/or major complications, and their condition should be very stable. This assessment will be made by the attending physician in view of clinical manifestations, ECG findings, and other laboratory results. By and large, it is not advisable to transfer the patient to the ICCU from the CCU when the resting heart rate is persistently faster than 100 beats/min. When the resting heart rate is rapid all the time, extension of heart damage or various complications should be suspected. Unless there is some complications, the patient may stay only an additional two to four days in the ICCU; then he or she will be transferred to an ordinary hospital room. Even in an ordinary hospital bed, continuous monitoring of the ECG is possible through remote control, portable ECG equipment using battery power, even when patients walk outside their rooms.

In general, patients are allowed to start minimal physical activities, such as moving the feet up and down, bending and stretching the knees, and moving the arms, as soon as critical period (the first few days) is over. Leg movements are helpful in preventing thrombophlebitis (inflammation of the leg veins with blood clots). Arm movements are useful in preventing stiffness or pain in the shoulders and arms (shoulder-hand syndrome). Pneumonia and pulmonary embolism can be prevented through physical activities.

Physical activities have to be increased slowly and progressively. In general, the patient is allowed to walk around very slowly and quietly within two weeks. After the resting period, most patients feel unusually tired and unsteady on their feet. This is the expected finding because the damaged heart has to heal completely, and the patient has to get back into condition. It may take several weeks to regain one's usual strength even after discharge from the hospital. In some medical centers, early ambulation after heart attack, even during the first week, has been practiced in hopes that recovery would be faster and have less problems, but this view is not uniformly accepted. During the second and third weeks, various rehabilitation programs are provided at various medical institutions that help to speed up reconditioning. Physical activities permissible after heart attack are discussed later (see Chapter 21).

A few days before discharge from the hospital, Holter monitor ECG is commonly performed to assess the presence or absence of heart rhythm abnormality. Through this test, proper medication can be prescribed according to the nature of the heart rhythm abnormality documented by the monitor. An exercise ECG test also is often performed just before discharge to evaluate functional capacity. Of course, the attending physician has to evaluate the patient's condition carefully before ordering the exercise ECG test to make certain that he or she is capable of performing the required exercise work loads.

It should be emphasized that the main purpose of resting (physical as well as mental) after a heart attack is to provide the best circumstances for speeding up the healing process in the damaged heart. The secondary benefit of resting is that it helps the formation of collateral (reserve) heart vessels for better blood circulation to compensate for the narrowed or blocked coronary artery(ies). By and large, it takes approximately four to six weeks for the complete healing process. The average length of the hospital stay is three weeks, but patients with mild heart attacks may be discharged within two weeks. Even after discharge, people must increase physical activity very slowly and gradually, particularly during the first several months. Vigorous or sudden physical exercise is extremely hazardous, and sexual intercourse must be prohibited during the first two months after heart attack (see Chapter 20).

Oxygen Therapy

As soon as the patient with suspected heart attack arrives in the ER, oxygen therapy is routinely begun through a plastic nasal tube or mask at most hospitals. Oxygen is administered because the damaged heart is unable to supply adequate oxygen because of its weakened pumping action. Therefore, oxygen is particularly valuable for the relief of dyspnea, chest pain, cyanosis (bluish-purplish skin from lack of adequate oxygen), and various complications associated with heart attack. In addition, oxygen is very effective in relieving anxiety, apprehension, and fear of death—medically as well as psychologically. Not only may the aforementioned symptoms be relieved, but the damaged heart also is able to pump more strongly because the heart muscle itself receives an oxygen-rich blood supply.

Oxygen may be given only for a short period of time, or it may be administered for many days or even weeks when the patient's condition is serious and there are various complications. Of course, oxygen may be administered in the ER, CCU, ICCU, and ordinary hospital room either continuously or intermittently, depending upon the patient's condition. Oxygen is also available in the ambulance or mobile CCU or in vehicles with similar facilities. In some cases, with chronic CHF or massive heart attack, oxygen therapy may be continued for many months or even indefinitely at home after discharge (a small oxygen tank with necessary equipment is available for home use) because of persisting symptoms, especially difficulty in breathing. In seriously ill patients, artificial respiration may be necessary because spontaneous respiration may not be possible. In this circumstance, a large plastic tube is placed in the patient's windpipe and is connected to an artificial respirator. Oxygen-rich air is thus pumped into the lungs at regular intervals to help the patient in breathing. An adequate supply of oxygen is administered by the artificial respirator until the patient is able to breathe spontaneously.

Medications

For heart attack victims, various medications are necessary for chest pain, heart rhythm abnormalities, and such complications as CHF, cardiogenic shock, and thromboembolic phenomena. In addition, sedatives (e.g., Valium), stool softeners, and laxatives are often needed. Detailed information regarding various medications is found in Chapter 17.

The first and most important therapeutic approach is to administer medications to control chest pain. The best painkiller is morphine sulfate, which is usually given intravenously in the dosage of 2 to 5 mg, slowly. Demerol hydrochloride (meperidine hydrochloride), which is considered the first cousin of morphine sulfate, is also often used in place of morphine. The usual dosage of Demerol is 50 to 100 mg, and it can be given either intravenously or intramuscularly.

Since various heart rhythm abnormalities are common in heart attack victims, one or more antiarrhythmic agents (drugs to suppress or prevent heart rhythm abnormalities) are often necessary during the first few days. Some patients may require antiarrhythmic agent(s) for weeks, months, or even indefinitely following a heart attack when clinically serious arrhythmias recur. Remember that the most common cause of sudden death after heart attack is heart rhythm abnormalities, especially VF. In clinically significant arrhythmias, the heart rhythm abnormality is either too fast (faster than 180 beats/min.) or too slow (slower than 40 beats/min.) or not present at all (cardiac arrest). In other words, the heart is unable to pump sufficient blood to meet demands when significant arrhythmias occur.

By and large, there are three ways to manage heart rhythm abnormalities. They include (1) medications, (2) direct-current (DC) shock (electric shock), and (3) artificial cardiac pacemaker. When heart rhythm is extremely rapid and in life-threatening situations, such as VF, immediate (preferably within thirty seconds) application of DC shock is the treatment of choice. An artificial cardiac pacemaker is essential in the treatment of various slow heart rhythms, especially heart block and sick sinus syndrome (Figures 3.6 and 3.7). Although there are many different antiarrhythmic agents available, lidocaine (Xylocaine) is the most important and most commonly used drug for heart attack victims. Lidocaine is indicated primarily for rhythm abnormalities arising from the ventricles (ventricular arrhythmias).

When the patient develops cardiac arrest (no heartbeat at all), immediate CPR is absolutely necessary (see Chapter 15). Depending upon the nature and cause of cardiac arrest, the patient may require defibrillator, various medications, and an artificial pacemaker. However, the most common underlying rhythm disorder responsible for cardiac arrest is VF.

Digitalis is commonly called the "heart pill" and is indicated primarily for the treatment of CHF (see Chapter 6). The main role of digitalis is to increase the strength of the heart muscle so that the pumping action of the ventricles will be enhanced. Various diuretics are indicated for patients with CHF in order to eliminate excess fluid accumulation by increasing the production of urine by the kidneys. There is a significant controversy among physicians regarding the use of anticoagulants (blood thinners) in patients with acute MI, and these drugs are much less commonly used at the present time than in the past. Many physicians do not use anticoagulants at all for mild heart attacks with no major complications. For the treatment of cardiogenic shock, sympathomimetic amines (e.g., norepinephrine and dopamine) are often necessary to increase abnormally low BP (hypotension).

According to the Persantine-Aspirin Reinfarction Study (PARIS) sponsored by the National Institute of Health, which dealt with 2,026 patients with previous heart attack(s), the efficacy of a combination of Persantine (dipyridamole) and aspirin or of aspirin alone was reported to be favorable in terms of mortality and the incidence of new heart attack, especially within six months after MI. An investigative drug, sulfinpyrazone (Anturane), was reported to be even more effectve in preventing sudden death in the early, high-risk period in patients with previous heart attack. Further investigations will be necessary to confirm these findings.

Direct-Current Shock

As indicated earlier, DC shock is often a life-saving measure for a variety of tachyar-rhythmias (rapid heart rhythms), especially VF. DC shock is discussed later (see Chapter 18).

Artificial Cardiac Pacemakers

Artificial cardiac pacemakers (Figure 3.8) are essential in the treatment of a variety of slow heart rhythms, primarily complete heart block and sick sinus syndrome (Figures 3.6 and 3.7). Artificial cardiac pacemakers are discussed later (see Chapter 16).

SURGICAL TREATMENT

Not only medical treatment but also surgical treatment is important for CAD (angina pectoris and MI) and its complications. Coronary artery bypass surgery (CABS–Figure 3.9) is, of course, the main surgical treatment for CAD, and it is the most common major surgery performed in the United States. Implantation of a permanent artificial pacemaker is also a very common surgical treatment for patients who develop very slow and unstable heart rhythm as a complication of heart attack (see Chapter 16). In addition, the use of the aortic balloon pump (discussed later in this chapter) is often a life-saving measure for intractable and severe CHF and cardiogenic shock. Surgical repairs of ventricular aneurysm (ventric-ular aneurysmectomy), ventricular septal defect, and papillary muscle dysfunction or chordae tendineae rupture are less common surgical procedures. Surgical repair for cardiac rupture is only rarely performed because cardiac rupture is invariably fatal. CABS and other surgical approaches are discussed in Chapter 25. Permanent

FIGURE 3.8. Artificial cardiac pacemaker in the body. (Medical illustration by Larry Stein.)

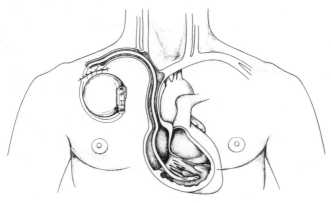

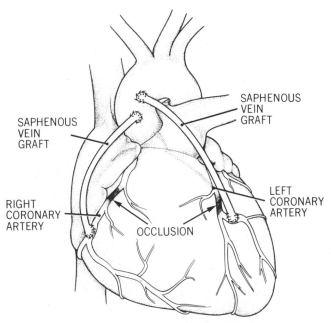

FIGURE 3.9. Coronary artery bypass surgery. (Medical illustration by Larry Stein.)

artificial pacemaker implanation is indicated in heart attack victims when slow heart rhythms (usually complete heart block and sick sinus syndrome) persist (Figures 3.6 and 3.7, 3.8, and 3.10; see Chapter 16).

FIGURE 3.10. Various artificial pacemaker pulse generators. (Reproduced with permission through the courtesy of Cardiac Pacemaker, Inc. [CPI] , St. Paul, Minn.)

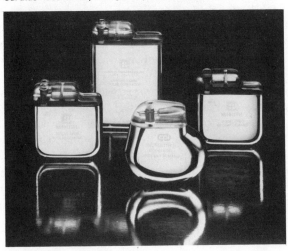

Aortic balloon counterpulsation (aortic balloon pump) is occasionally indicated in patients with serious cardiogenic shock (see Chapter 7) after a heart attack. The aortic balloon pump is a slender, sausage-shaped device (about a foot in length) that increases circulation in the heart while assisting the heart muscle in pumping blood. The balloon pump is inserted, under local anesthesia, into the aorta via an artery in the groin by a cardiac surgeon. This minor operation is often performed in the CCU or in a room with similar facilities.

The arotic balloon is rhythmically inflated and deflated electronically with helium or carbon dioxide gas during each heart cycle. The blood circulation through the narrowed coronary arteries is increased by inflation of the balloon, whereas deflation assists the left ventricular pumping chamber to deliver more blood to the entire body. Unfortunately, the long-term prognosis in patients who have been successfully treated with the aortic balloon pump for cardiogenic shock is still poor (approximately 10 percent survival after one year), primarily because of the extensive and far-advanced underlying CAD in most cases. The combined use of an aortic balloon pump and vasodilator therapy seems to have a better outcome, according to some physicians' experiences.

HOME CARE AFTER DISCHARGE FROM THE HOSPITAL

Before the patient is ready to be discharged from the hospital, an attending physician should give full instructions regarding the patient's activities, medications, a schedule for the next visit to the doctor's office with follow-up visits thereafter, diet, sexual activity, and other necessary precautions. Of course, the patient and his or her spouse may ask any necessary questions of the physician.

The speed of recovery varies considerably depending upon many factors, including the extent of the heart attack, the presence or absence and degree of major complications, the presence or absence of coexisting diseases and/or risk factors, the status of general health before the heart attack, and the age of the patient. For example, a previously healthy young individual who suffered a mild heart attack may recover completely within four to eight weeks. Conversely, recovery may take three to six months or even longer when the patient is elderly, when the individual has suffered a massive heart attack, or when there have been serious complications. It is natural for most patients to feel tired and weak for several weeks or even months after discharge from the hospital. Until the individual feels strong enough to increase various physical activities, he or she must have full physical and emotional rest to speed up the recovery. It may be necessary for the patient to take a nap whenever he or she feels like it, especially after meals or extraordinary physical activities. A good night's sleep is, of course, very important, and if necessary, mild sedatives or sleeping pills may be prescribed.

The first few months after discharge are the most important in the home care period for rapid recovery, and this is particularly true during the first few weeks. Every patient must follow the doctor's advice faithfully and must also use common sense in order to avoid unnecessary complications or adverse effects on the heart. Only the patient can judge his or her own physical limitations, an assessment made from individual feelings of well-being; no one can help the patient in this regard.

Regular Medical Checkups

Although it varies, most physicians would like to see their patients for a checkup two to three weeks after discharge from the hospital. Remember that the usual hospitalization ranges from two to four weeks (average: three weeks), including intensive care in the CCU and ICCU for one week, and less intensive care for recuperation in an ordinary hospital room for one to two weeks. During the first office visit after discharge, various laboratory tests (e.g., exercise ECG test, Holter monitor ECG, 12-lead ECG) may be performed, if necessary, in addition to a complete physical examination. Necessary medications may be prescribed, and other medical advice will be given. The follow-up medical visits thereafter occur, in general, at two- to three-month intervals for one year. After a one-year recovery period, most physicians see their patients every three to six months indefinitely.

Many physicians order an exercise ECG test periodically to assess patients' functional capacity using the standard exercise protocol. By doing so, each patient's physical limitations can be determined so that excessive physical activity can be prevented. The exercise ECG is especially important when the individual plans to engage in physical program or to return to work. Many physicians order the exercise ECG test one to two days before discharge. In addition, Holter monitor ECG is often performed periodically to detect any heart rhythm abnormality. When a rhythm abnormality is found, medication can be prescribed. Whenever a complication occurs or a new symptom (e.g., chest pain) is experienced, the patient must see a doctor immediately.

Home Environment

The home environment should be a pleasant atmosphere with comfortable temperature and ideal humidity. Preferably, the home should be air-conditioned during the summer season, and it should be well heated during the winter. If the house has two or more stories, the patient should go upstairs very slowly initially, with frequent rest as needed. It is important for the patient to stay on the first floor if the cardiac condition is so advanced that he or she is unable to go up the stairs without experiencing chest pain or shortness of breath. This is particularly true when the patient is elderly or has suffered major complications. If an electronically operated elevator is available, of course, it is the ideal solution. The ideal house is situated at sea level. When the elevation is higher than 3,000 feet, it is definitely hazardous to heart and lung function, especially when the heart is already damaged, as it is in heart attack victims. The individual with heart or lung disease is simply unable to tolerate high elevation because such atmosphere causes shortness of breath.

Warnings and Precautions for New Symptoms or Complications

As expected, most patients feel tired soon after discharge from the hospital. Many patients will be anxious, and some of them may be fearful of having another heart attack. Some patients may be depressed. However, these difficulties should fade gradually during the recovery phase after discharge. Many patients may experience minor chest discomfort from the shoulder-hand syndrome or miscellaneous causes, primarily because of the prolonged resting period at the hospital. These symptoms are expected after recovery from a heart attack and are entirely harmless. However, the physician should be notified immediately when a patient experiences significant chest pain similar to that of the first heart attack, severe shortness of breath, a feeling of impending fainting, palpitations, and so forth. There is no reason to wait until these symptoms subside. When the situation is urgent, the patient or a family member should call the medical emergency number 911 (Figures 3.2 and 3.3) or an ambulance to go to a nearby hospital ER. For chest pain, NG may be placed under the tongue and may be repeated while waiting for the ambulance to arrive.

It is an excellent idea for all family members of a heart attack victim to learn how to apply CPR (see Chapter 15). A simple course in CPR is available in many communities without charge, and it can be learned without much difficulty. Detailed information regarding CPR courses may be obtained from the local Heart Association or Medical Association. When lay people learn CPR, many lives, including those of family members who have suffered a heart attack, can be saved. A medical emergency number such as 911, an ambulance service, or similar emergency numbers should be visible around telephones throughout the house so that unnecessary delays can be avoided.

Remember that physical activity must be increased gradually according to the physician's advice, and all precautions must be clearly understood all the time in order to prevent needless complications, as well as the possibility of another heart attack or even sudden death. The patient has to perform appropriate daily activities according to medical guidance. Prescribed medications have to be taken faithfully unless side effects are observed. When any drug side effect is thought to be occurring, the attending physician must be notified without delay.

Psychosocial Aspects

It is natural to expect some degree of depression, helplessness, and hopelessness for most patients some time during the recovery period after discharge from the hospital. Psychosocial aspects are discussed later in this chapter.

Medications

Some patients, especially with massive heart attacks and various complications, must take one or more medications for many weeks, months, or even indefinitely, depending upon the clinical circumstances. Various medications are discussed in Chapter 17.

Artificial Cardiac Pacemakers

Following permanent pacemaker implanation, every patient has to follow necessary precautions and medical advice. Artificial pacemakers are fully discussed in Chapter 16.

Diets

Many patients require special diets (Tables 3.3, 3.9, and 3.10), following a heart attack to maintain ideal body weight (see Table 3.4), to reduce weight for obesity, to control hypertension, and to control other co-existing diseases, such as diabetes mellitus, or other risk factors, such as hyperlipidemia (a high content of cholesterol or triglycerides in the blood). Various special diets are fully discussed in Chapter 19.

Smoking

As repeatedly emphasized, cigarette smoking is one of the most serious and common risk factors for CAD. It is also important to know that smoking can be completely eliminated if the individual is properly informed and highly motivated. Smoking and the heart are discussed in Chapter 22.

Drinking Alcohol

Consumption of excessive amounts of alcohol is definitely harmful to the individual with a diseased heart. Alcohol and the heart are discussed in Chapter 23.

Physical Activities

It is extremely important to increase physical activities very slowly and gradually. Vigorous and sudden physical activity is most dangerous to individuals with known heart disease. Some younger and previously healthy individuals who recover from a mild heart attack may be able to regain their strength completely within two to four weeks after discharge. On the other hand, older patients and those with massive heart attacks may not be able to return to full activity even three to six months following discharge. The maximum exercise tolerance for various physical activities can be medically determined by evaluating a patient's functional capacity with the exercise ECG test (see Table 3.11, 3.12, and 3.13). Physical activities after a heart attack are discussed in detail in Chapter 21.

TABLE 3.9. 1800-Calorie Mild Sodium Restricted Food Exchange List.

MILK EXCHANGE LIST (Two [2] Exchange Units Per Day)	
Buttermilk, nonfat	2 fat exchange units and 1 cup
Milk, nonfat, dry (powder)	2 fat exchange units and 3 tablespoons
Milk, nonfat, dry (reconstituted)	2 fat exchange units and 1 cup
Milk, skim	2 fat exchange units and 1 cup
Milk, whole	1 cup
Milk, whole buttermilk	1 cup
Milk, whole (evaporated, reconstituted)	1 cup

Foods to avoid under the milk exchange list:
   Commercial foods such as ice cream, sherbert, milk shakes, chocolate milk, malted milk mixes, condensed milk.

BREAD EXCHANGE LIST (Seven [7] Exchange Units Per Day)	
Bread and Rolls	
Biscuit	1 medium
Bread	1 slice
Cornbread	1 cube (1 1/2″)
Griddle cakes	2 three-inch
Melba toast	4 pieces (3 1/2″ × 1 1/2″ × 1/8″)
Muffin	1 medium
Roll	1 medium
Cereals (cooked, lightly salted)	
Farina	1/2 cup
Grits	1/2 cup
Oatmeal	1/2 cup
Rolled wheat	1/2 cup
Wheat meal	1/2 cup
Cereals (dry)	
Shredded wheat	2/3 biscuit
Other dry cereal	3/4 cup
Other	
Barley	1 1/2 tablespoons (uncooked)
Cornmeal	2 tablespoons
Cornstarch	2 1/2 tablespoons
Crackers (unsalted tops)	5 two-inch-squares
Flour	2 1/2 tablespoons
Graham crackers	2
Macaroni	1/2 cup (cooked)
Matzo	1 five-inch square
Noodles	1/2 cup (cooked)
Popcorn (lightly salted)	1 1/2 cups
Rice, brown	1/2 cup (cooked)
Rice, white	1/2 cup (cooked)
Spaghetti	1/2 cup (cooked)
Tapioca	2 tablespoons (cooked)
Waffle	1 three-inch square section

Foods to avoid under the bread exchange list:
   Breads and rolls with salt toppings, any sugar-coated cereals, potato chips, pretzels, any heavily salted snack food.

TABLE 3.9 (continued).

FISH, MEAT, POULTRY EXCHANGE LIST (Five [5] Exchange Units Per Day)	
American cheddar cheese	1 ounce
Bass (fresh, frozen, or canned)	1 ounce (cooked)
Beef	1 ounce (cooked)
Bluefish (fresh, frozen, or canned)	1 ounce (cooked)
Brain	1 ounce (cooked)
Catfish (fresh, frozen, or canned)	1 ounce (cooked)
Chicken	1 ounce (cooked)
Clams (fresh, frozen, or canned)	1 ounce (cooked)
Cod (fresh, frozen, or canned)	1 ounce (cooked)
Cottage cheese (lightly salted)	1/4 cup
Crab (fresh, frozen, or canned)	1 ounce (cooked)
Duck	1 ounce (cooked)
Eels (fresh, frozen, or canned)	1 ounce (cooked)
Egg	1 medium
Flounder (fresh, frozen, or canned)	1 ounce (cooked)
Halibut (fresh, frozen, or canned)	1 ounce (cooked)
Kidney	1 ounce (cooked)
Lamb	1 ounce (cooked)
Liver (beef)	1 ounce (cooked)
Liver (calf)	1 ounce (cooked)
Liver (chicken)	1 ounce (cooked)
Liver (pork)	1 ounce (cooked)
Lobster (fresh, frozen, or canned)	1 ounce (cooked)
Oyster (fresh, frozen, or canned)	1 ounce (cooked)
Peanut Butter (low-sodium, dietetic)	2 tablespoons
Pork	1 ounce (cooked)
Quail	1 ounce (cooked)
Rabbit	1 ounce (cooked)
Rockfish (fresh, frozen, or canned)	1 ounce (cooked)
Salmon (fresh, frozen, or canned)	1 ounce (cooked)
Scallops (fresh, frozen, or canned)	1 ounce (cooked)
Shrimp (fresh, frozen, or canned)	1 ounce (cooked)
Sole (fresh, frozen, or canned)	1 ounce (cooked)
Swiss cheese	1 ounce
Tongue	1 ounce (cooked)
Trout (fresh, frozen, or canned)	1 ounce (cooked)
Tuna (fresh, frozen, or canned)	1 ounce (cooked)
Turkey	1 ounce (cooked)
Veal	1 ounce (cooked)

Foods to avoid under the meat, poultry, fish exchange list:
Anchovies, bacon, bologna, caviar, chipped beef, corned beef, frankfurters,
ham, salt koshered meats, luncheon meats, Roquefort cheese, salt pork,
sausage.

FAT EXCHANGE (Four [4] Exchange Units Per Day)	
Avacado	1/8 of four-inch
Butter	1 teaspoon (1 small pat)
Fat (for cooking)	1 teaspoon
French dressing	1 tablespoon
Margarine	1 teaspoon

TABLE 3.9 (continued).

Mayonnaise	1 teaspoon
Nuts (unsalted)	6 small
Oil (for cooking)	1 teaspoon
Sour heavy cream	1 tablespoon
Sour light cream	2 tablespoons
Sweet heavy cream	1 tablespoon
Sweet light cream	2 tablespoons

Foods to avoid under the fat exchange list:
Bacon, bacon fat, olives, salt pork, salted nuts, any other heavily salted snack foods.

VEGETABLE EXCHANGE LIST

GROUP A Vegetable Exchange List (at least one [1] exchange unit per day) plus 1 exchange unit from Group B and 1 exchange unit from Group C.

Artichoke	1/2 cup
Asparagus	1/2 cup
Beet greens	1/2 cup
Broccoli	1/2 cup
Brussels sprouts	1/2 cup
Cabbage	1/2 cup
Cauliflower	1/2 cup
Celery	1/2 cup
Chicory	1/2 cup
Cucumber	1/2 cup
Dandelion greens	1/2 cup
Eggplant	1/2 cup
Endive	1/2 cup
Escarole	1/2 cup
Green beans	1/2 cup
Green peppers	1/2 cup
Radishes	1/2 cup
Red peppers	1/2 cup
Spinach	1/2 cup
Summer squash	1/2 cup
Swiss chard	1/2 cup
Tomato juice	1/2 cup
Tomatoes	1/2 cup
Turnip greens	1/2 cup
Wax beans	1/2 cup
Yellow squash	1/2 cup
Zucchini	1/2 cup

GROUP B Vegetable Exchange List (one [1] exchange unit per day) plus 1 exchange unit from Group C and unlimited unit exchanges from Group A.

Acorn squash	1/2 cup
Beets	1/2 cup
Carrots	1/2 cup
Hubbard squash	1/2 cup
Onions	1/2 cup
Peas	1/2 cup

TABLE 3.9 (continued).

Pumpkin	1/2 cup
Rutabaga	1/2 cup
White turnip	1/2 cup
Winter squash	1/2 cup

GROUP C Vegetable Exchange List (one [1] exchange unit per day) plus 1 exchange unit from Group B and unlimited exchange units from Group A.

Baked beans (no pork)	1/4 cup
Corn	1/3 cup or 1/2 small ear
Cowpeas (dried)	1/2 cup (cooked)
Hominy	1/2 cup
Lentils (dried)	1/2 cup (cooked)
Lima beans (fresh, frozen, or dried)	1/2 cup (cooked)
Mashed potatoes	1/2 cup
Navy beans (fresh, frozen, or dried)	1/2 cup (cooked)
Parsnips	2/3 cup
Split green peas (dried)	1/2 cup (cooked)
Sweet potato	1/4 cup or 1/2 small
White potato	1 small
Yellow peas (dried)	1/2 cup (cooked)

Foods to avoid under the vegetable exchange list:
   Pickles, sauerkraut, or other vegetables prepared in brine or heavily salted.

FRUIT EXCHANGE LIST (Four [4] Exchange Units Per Day)	
Apple	1 small
Apple cider	1/3 cup
Apple juice	1/3 cup
Applesauce	1/2 cup
Apricots (dried)	4 halves
Apricots (fresh)	2 medium
Apricot nectar	1/4 cup
Banana	1/2 small
Blackberries	1 cup
Blueberries	2/3 cup
Cantaloupe	1/4 small
Cherries	10 large
Dates	2
Figs	1 medium
Pineapple juice	1/3 cup
Plums	2 medium
Prunes	2 medium
Prune Juice	1/4 cup
Raisins	2 tablespoons
Raspberries	1 cup
Strawberries	1 cup
Sweetened rhubarb	2 tablespoons
Sweetened cranberries	1 tablespoon
Sweetened cranberry juice	1/3 cup
Tangerine	1 large

71

TABLE 3.9 (continued).

Tangerine juice	1/2 cup
Watermelon	1 cup

Foods to avoid under the fruit exchange list:
All high calorie foods, such as canned fruit (in sugar syrup), crystallized fruit, frozen fruit (in sugar syrup), glazed fruit, sweetened fruit.

SEASONINGS (May Be Used as Instructed by a Physician or a Diet Counselor)

Allspice	Mustard (dry)
Almond extract	Mustard seed
Anise seed	Nutmeg
Basil	Onion
Bay leaf	Onion juice
Bouillion cube (low sodium, dietetic)	Onion powder
Caraway seed	Orange extract
Cardamon	Oregano
Catsup (dietetic)	Paprika
Celery leaves (dried)	Parsley
Celery leaves (fresh)	Parsley flakes
Celery seed	Pepper (black)
Chili powder	Pepper (fresh ground)
Chives	Pepper (fresh red)
Cinnamon	Pepper (red)
Cloves	Pepper (white)
Cocoa	Peppermint extract
Coconut	Pimiento peppers
Cumin	Poppy seed
Curry	Poultry seasoning
Dill	Purslane
Fennel	Rosemary
Garlic	Saffron
Garlic juice	Sage
Garlic powder	Salt (lightly used if permitted)
Ginger	Salt substitutes (if permitted)
Horseradish	Savory
Juniper	Sesame seeds
Lemon extract	Sorrel
Lemon juice	Sugar
Mase	Tarragon
Maple extract	Thyme
Marjoram	Turmeric
Meat extract (low-sodium, dietetic)	Vanilla extract
Meat tenderizers (low-sodium, dietetic)	Vinegar
Mint	Wine (if permitted)
	Walnut (extract)

Seasonings to be avoided:
Artificial sweeteners (unless recommended by physician), commercial bouillon in any form, catsup, celery salt (except when used as allowed seasoning), chili sauce, garlic salt (except when used as allowed seasoning), meat extracts (regular), meat sauces (regular), meat tenderizers (regular), mustard (prepared),

TABLE 3.9 (continued).

olives, onion salt (except when used as allowed seasoning), pickles, relishes, saccharin (unless recommended by physician), cooking wine, Worcestershire sauce.

BEVERAGES	
Alcoholic beverages	with physician's permission
Cocoa	made with milk allowance
Coffee (instant or regular)	
Coffee (substitute)	
Fruit juices	count as fruit units
Lemonade*	use sugar allowance
Milk	as allowed on milk list
Tea	

*If permitted a Free Choice selection, one unit is equivalent to 4 teaspoons of sugar.

TABLE 3.10. Recommended Diabetic Exchange Plan* (1800-Calorie Diabetic Diet).

*An individual diabetic diet plan (example, diet composition, energy content of diet, level of physical activity, and timing of meals) must be planned with a physician and/or a professional diet counselor.

Milk (Exchange List 1)—2 to 3 Exchanges Per Day

1% Fat fortified milk (omit 1/2 Fat Exchange)	1 cup
2% Fat fortified milk (omit 1 Fat Exchange)	1 cup
Buttermilk (from skim milk)	1 cup
Buttermilk (from whole milk)	1 cup
Nonfat milk	1 cup
Powdered, nonfat (dry, before adding liquid)	1/3 cup
Skim milk	1 cup
Skim milk (canned, evaporated)	1/2 cup
Whole milk (canned, evaporated, omit 2 Fat Exchanges)	1/2 cup
Whole milk (omit 2 Fat Exchanges)	1 cup
Yogurt (from 2% fortified milk, unflavored, plain, omit 1 Fat Exchange)	1 cup
Yogurt (from skim milk, unflavored, plain)	1 cup
Yogurt (from whole milk, unflavored, plain)	1 cup

Vegetable A (Exchange List 2-A)—1 Exchange Per Day

Asparagus (cooked)	1/2 cup
Baked beans, no pork (canned, omit 1 Bread Exchange)	1/2 cup
Bean sprouts (cooked)	1/2 cup
Beet greens (cooked)	1/2 cup
Beets (cooked)	1/2 cup
Broccoli (cooked)	1/2 cup
Brussels sprouts (cooked)	1/2 cup
Cabbage (cooked)	1/2 cup
Carrots (cooked)	1/2 cup
Cauliflower (cooked)	1/2 cup

TABLE 3.10 (continued).

Celery (cooked)	1/2 cup
Chard greens (cooked)	1/2 cup
Chicory (raw)	no limit
Chinese cabbage (raw)	no limit
Collard greens (cooked)	1/2 cup
Cucumbers (raw)	no limit
Dandelion greens (cooked)	1/2 cup
Dill pickles	no limit
Eggplant (cooked)	1/2 cup
Endive (raw)	no limit
Escarole (raw)	no limit
Green pepper (cooked)	1/2 cup
Green string beans (cooked)	1/2 cup
Kale greens (cooked)	1/2 cup
Lentils (cooked, omit 1 Bread Exchange)	1/2 cup
Lettuce (raw)	no limit
Mushrooms (cooked)	1/2 cup
Mustard greens (cooked)	1/2 cup
Okra (cooked)	1/2 cup
Onions (cooked)	1/2 cup
Parsley (raw)	no limit
Peas (cooked, omit 1 Bread Exchange)	1/2 cup
Radishes (raw)	no limit
Red pepper (cooked)	1/2 cup
Rhubarb (cooked)	1/2 cup
Rutabaga (cooked)	1/2 cup
Sauerkraut (cooked)	1/2 cup
Spinach greens (cooked)	1/2 cup
Summer squash (cooked)	1/2 cup
Tomato juice	1/2 cup
Tomatoes (raw)	1/2 cup
Turnip greens (cooked)	1/2 cup
Turnips (cooked)	1/2 cup
Vegetable juice cocktail	1/2 cup
Watercress (raw)	no limit
Yellow string beans (cooked)	1/2 cup
Zucchini (cooked)	1/2 cup

Vegetable B (Exchange List 2-B)—1 Exchange Per Day

Corn (cooked)	1/3 cup
Corn on the cob (cooked)	1 small
Green peas (canned, cooked)	1/2 cup
Green peas (frozen, cooked)	1/2 cup
Lima beans (cooked)	1/2 cup
Mashed potato (cooked)	1/2 cup
Parsnips (cooked)	2/3 cup
Pumpkin (cooked)	3/4 cup
Sweet potato (cooked)	1/4 cup
White potato (cooked)	1 small
Winter squash (cooked)	1/2 cup
Yam (cooked)	1/4 cup

TABLE 3.10 (continued).

Fruit (Exchange List 3)—3 to 6 Exchanges Per Day

Apple	1 small
Apple juice	1/3 cup
Applesauce (unsweetened)	1/2 cup
Apricots (dried)	4 halves
Apricots (fresh)	2 medium
Banana	1/2 small
Blackberries	1/2 cup
Blueberries	1/2 cup
Boysenberries	2/3 cup
Cantaloupe	1/4 small
Cherries	10 large
Cider	1/3 cup
Dates	2
Figs (dried)	1
Figs (fresh)	1
Grape juice	1/4 cup
Grapefruit	1/2
Grapefruit juice	1/2 cup
Grapes	12
Honeydew	1/8 medium
Mango	1/2 small
Nectarine	1 small
Orange	1 small
Orange juice	1/2 cup
Papaya	3/4 cup
Peach	1 medium
Pear	1 small
Persimmon	1 medium
Pineapple	1/2 cup
Pineapple juice	1/3 cup
Plums	2 medium
Prune juice	1/4 cup
Prunes	2 medium
Raisins	2 tablespoons
Raspberries	1/2 cup
Strawberries	3/4 cup
Tangerine	1 medium
Watermelon	1 cup

Bread (Exchange List 4)—7 to 8 Exchanges Per Day

Bread

Bagel (small)	1/2
Bread crumbs (dried)	3 tablespoons
English muffin (small)	1/2
Frankfurter roll	1/2
French bread	1 slice
Hamburger bun	1/2
Italian bread	1 slice
Pumpernickel bread	1 slice

TABLE 3.10 (continued).

Raisin bread	1 slice
Roll (plain bread)	1
Rye bread	1 slice
Tortilla (6″ diameter)	1
White bread	1 slice
Whole wheat bread	1 slice

Cereal

Barley (cooked)	1/2 cup
Bran flakes (uncooked)	1/2 cup
Cereal (cooked)	1/2 cup
Cereal (puffed, unfrosted, uncooked)	1 cup
Cornmeal (dry)	2 tablespoons
Flour	2 1/2 tablespoons
Grits (cooked)	1/2 cup
Macaroni (cooked)	1/2 cup
Noodles (cooked)	1/2 cup
Popcorn (popped, no fat, large kernel)	3 cups
Rice (cooked)	1/2 cup
Spaghetti (cooked)	1/2 cup
Unsweetened cereal (other ready-to-eat)	3/4 cup
Wheat germ	1/4 cup

Crackers

Arrowroot	3
Graham (2 1/2″ square)	2
Matzoh (4″ × 6″)	2
Oyster	20
Pretzels (3 1/8″ long × 1/8″ diameter)	25
Rye wafers (2″ × 3 1/2″)	3
Saltines	6
Soda (2 1/2″ square)	4

Desserts*

   *Only if allowed in the diet with the permission of physician or professional diet counselor.

Ice cream (omit 2 Fat Exchanges)	1/2 cup
Sponge cake (plain)	One 1/2″ cube

Meat (Exchange List 5)—7 to 8 Exchanges Per Day (trim off all visible fat)

American cheese	1 oz.
Baby beef (very lean, low fat)	1 oz.
Boiled ham (medium fat)	1 oz.
Boston butt (medium fat)	1 oz.
Canadian bacon (omit 1 Fat Exchange, medium fat)	1 oz.
Cheddar cheese	1 oz.
Chicken (no skin, low fat)	1 oz.
Chipped beef (low fat)	1 oz.
Chuck (low fat)	1 oz.

TABLE 3.10 (continued).

Clams	5 or 1 oz.
Cold cuts (4 1/2" square, 1/8" thick, medium fat)	1 slice
Corned beef (canned, medium fat)	1 oz.
Cornish hen (no skin, low fat)	1 oz.
Cottage cheese	1/4 cup
Crab (canned, packed in water)	1/4 cup
Cutlets (veal, low fat)	1 oz.
Egg	1
Fish (fresh)	1 oz.
Fish (frozen)	1 oz.
Flank steak (low fat)	1 oz.
Frankfurter (omit 2 Fat Exchanges, 8-9 per pound, medium fat)	1
Ground beef (15% fat, low fat)	1 oz.
Guinea hen (no skin, low fat)	1 oz.
Ham (low fat)	1 oz.
Leg (center shank, pork, low fat)	1 oz.
Leg of lamb (low fat)	1 oz.
Leg (veal, low fat)	1 oz.
Leg (whole rump, pork, low fat)	1 oz.
Lobster (canned, packed in water)	1/4 cup
Loin (all tenderloin cuts, medium fat)	1 oz.
Loin (chops, lamp, low fat)	1 oz.
Loin (roast, lamb, low fat)	1 oz.
Loin (veal, low fat)	1 oz.
Mackerel (canned, packed in water)	1/4 cup
Oysters	5 or 1 oz.
Peanut butter (omit 3 Fat Exchanges)	2 tablespoons
Pheasant (no skin, low fat)	1 oz.
Plate ribs (low fat)	1 oz.
Plate skirt steak (low fat)	1 oz.
Rib eye (medium fat)	1 oz.
Rib (lamb, low fat)	1 oz.
Rib (veal, low fat)	1 oz.
Round (bottom, low fat)	1 oz.
Round (ground commercial, medium fat)	1 oz.
Round (top, low fat)	1 oz.
Rump (all cuts, low fat)	1 oz.
Salmon (canned, packed in water)	1/4 cup
Sardines (drained, packed in water)	3
Scallops	5 or 1 oz.
Shank (lamb, low fat)	1 oz.
Shank (veal, low fat)	1 oz.
Shoulder-arm (picnic, medium fat)	1 oz.
Shoulder blade (medium fat)	1 oz.
Shoulder (lamb, low fat)	1 oz.
Shoulder (veal, low fat)	1 oz.
Shrimp	5 or 1 oz.
Sirloin (lamb, low fat)	1 oz.
Spare ribs (low fat)	1 oz.
Tenderloin (low fat)	1 oz.

TABLE 3.10 (continued).

Tripe (low fat)	1 oz.
Tuna (canned, packed in water)	1/4 cup
Turkey (no skin, low fat)	1 oz.

Fat (Exchange List 6)–3 to 7 Exchanges Per Day

    *Made with corn, cottonseed, safflower, soy, or sunflower oil only.
    **Fat content is primarily monounsaturated.
    ***If made with corn, cottonseed, safflower, soy, or sunflower oil.

Almonds**	10 whole
Avocado (4″ in diameter)**	1/8
Bacon (crisp)	1 strip
Bacon (fat)	1 teaspoon
Black olives**	5 small
Butter	1 teaspoon
Corn oil	1 teaspoon
Cottonseed oil	1 teaspoon
Cream cheese	1 tablespoon
Cream (heavy)	1 tablespoon
Cream (light)	2 tablespoons
Cream (sour)	2 tablespoons
French dressing***	1 tablespoon
Green olives**	5 small
Italian dressing***	1 tablespoon
Lard	1 teaspoon
Margarine (regular stick)	1 teaspoon
Margarine (soft)*	1 teaspoon
Margarine (stick)*	1 teaspoon
Margarine (tub)*	1 teaspoon
Mayonnaise	1 teaspoon
Nuts (all others)**	6 small
Olive oil**	1 teaspoon
Peanut oil**	1 teaspoon
Pecans**	2 large whole
Safflower oil	1 teaspoon
Salad dressing (mayonnaise type)***	2 teaspoons
Salt pork	3/4 inch cube
Soy oil	1 teaspoon
Spanish peanuts**	20 whole
Sunflower oil	1 teaspoon
Virginia peanuts**	10 whole
Walnuts	6 small

Soups

    *1/3 can of Soup (before milk or water is added) may be exchanged for:

Bouillon	no limit
Consommé	no limit
Clear broth	no limit
Beef*	1 slice bread and 1 oz. meat

TABLE 3.10 (continued).

Beef noodle*	1 slice bread
Black bean*	2 slices bread
Chicken gumbo*	1 slice bread
Chicken noodle*	1 slice bread
Chicken rice*	1 slice bread
Chicken vegetable*	1 slice bread and 1 teaspoon fat
Clam chowder*	1 slice bread and 1 teaspoon fat
Cream of asparagus*	1 slice bread
Cream of celery*	1 slice bread and 1 teaspoon fat
Cream of chicken*	1 slice bread and 1 teaspoon fat
Cream of mushroom*	1 slice bread and 2 teaspoons fat
Green pea*	2 1/2 slices bread
Minestrone*	1 slice bread and 1 teaspoon fat
Onion soup*	1 slice bread
Pepper pot*	1 slice bread and 1 oz. meat
Scotch broth*	1 slice bread and 1 teaspoon fat
Tomato*	1 slice bread and 1 teaspoon fat
Turkey noodle*	1 slice bread
Vegetable*	1 slice bread
Vegetable beef*	1 group B vegetable and 1 oz. meat
Vegetarian vegetable*	1 slice bread

Seasonings (no limit)

Cinnamon, celery salt, garlic, garlic salt, lemon, mushrooms (raw), mint, mustard, nutmeg, parsley, pepper, saccharin (and other sugarless sweeteners), spices, vanilla, and vinegar.

Other Foods (no limit)

Coffee or tea (without sugar or cream), fat free broth, bouillion, unflavored gelatin, rennet tablets, sour or dill pickles, cranberries (without sugar), rhubarb (without sugar).

TABLE 3.11. Energy Expenditure for Various Activities (For Average Adults—70 kg).

ORDINARY DAILY ACTIVITIES AND HOUSEWORK	
Energy Expenditure	Activities
1 MET	Resting on supine position, sitting, standing (relaxed), eating, conversation (ordinary), hand sewing.
1.5 METs	Sweeping floor, machine sewing.

TABLE 3.11 (continued).

2 METs	Dressing, undressing, washing hands or face, polishing furniture.
2.5 METs	Scrubbing (standing), washing small clothes, kneading dough, peeling potatoes.
3 METs	Making beds, cleaning windows, scrubbing floors, walking (2.5 mph).
3.5 METs	Ironing (standing), wringing by hand, hanging wash, mopping, showering.
4 METs	Sexual intercourse (with spouse), beating carpets, using bedpan.

OCCUPATIONAL ACTIVITIES

Energy Expenditure	Activities
1.5-2 METs	Desk (ordinary) work, watch repairing, typing, driving car, operating electric calculating machine.
2-3 METs	Repairing radio or TV, repairing car, bartending, janitorial work, sewing at machine, riding lawnmower.
3-4 METs	Bricklaying, plastering, tractor ploughing, cleaning windows, machine assembly, welding (moderate load), wheelbarrow (100-lb. load).
4-5METs	Carpentry (light), paperhanging, painting, masonry, horse plowing, raking leaves.
5-6 METs	Digging garden, shoveling (light earth), carpentry (heavy), binding sheaves.
6-7 METs	Snow shoveling, shoveling soil 10/min. (10 lbs.), mowing lawn by hand.
7-8 METs	Digging ditches, carrying heavy object (80 lbs.), sawing or splitting hardwood.
8-9 METs	Shoveling soil 10/min. (14 lbs.), tending of furnace.
10 or more METS	Shoveling soil 10/min. (16 lbs. or more).

RECREATIONAL ACTIVITIES

Energy Expenditure	Activities
1.5-2 METs	Walking (1 mph), playing cards, painting (sitting), motor-cycling, driving automobile.
2-3 METs	Walking (2 mph), bicycling (5 mph), billiards, volley ball, shuffleboard, driving powerboat, golf (power cart), skeet, horseback riding (walking), canoeing (2½ mph), playing piano or other musical instruments.
3-4 METs	Walking (3 mph), cycling (5.5-6 mph), horseshoe pitching, bowling, golf (pulling bag cart), sailing (small boat), badminton (social doubles), fly fishing (standing with waders), swimming (20 yards/min.), archery, horseback riding (slow trot), intense playing musical instruments.

TABLE 3.11 (continued).

4-5 METs	Walking (3½ mph), table tennis, cycling (8 mph), gardening, dancing (fox-trot), golf (carrying clubs), badminton (singles), tennis (doubles), calisthenics.
5-6 METs	Walking (4 mph), cycling (10 mph), horseback riding (fast trot), canoeing (4 mph), stream fishing (walking in light current in waders), ice or roller skating (9 mph).
6-7 METs	Walking (5 mph), cycling (11 mph), tennis (singles), badminton (competitive), square dancing, water skiing, skiing (light downhill), ski touring (2.5 mph—loose snow).
7-8 METs	Jogging (5 mph), cycling (12 mph), horseback riding (gallop), canoeing (5 mph), touch ball, paddelball, basketball, touch football, skiiing (steep downhill), ice hockey, mountain climbing.
8-9 METs	Running (5½ mph), cycling (13 mph), basketball (competitive), handball (social), squash racquets (social), ski touring (4 mph), fencing.
10 or more METs	Running: 6 mph (10 METs) 7 mph (11.5 METs) 8 mph (13.5 METs) 9 mph (15 METs) 10 mph (17 METs) Squash (competitive), handball (competitive), ski touring (5 or more mph)

TABLE 3.12. Chung's Protocol for Exercise (Treadmill) ECG Test.

Stage	Speed (m.p.h.)	Grade (%)	Duration (min.)	METs (units)	Total Time Elapsed (min.)
1	1.7	0	3	2	3
2	3.0	4	3	4-5	6
3	3.0	8	3	6	9
4	3.0	12	3	8	12
5	3.0	16	3	9	15
6	3.0	20	3	10	18
7	3.0	24	3	12-13	21
8[a]	3.0	28	3	14	24
9[a]	3.0	32	3	16	27

[a]Optional for physically active individuals.
Reproduced from Chung, E.K.: *Exercise Electrocardiography: Practical Approach,* Baltimore, Williams & Wilkins Co., 1979.

TABLE 3.13. Relationship Between New York Heart Association Functional Classification and Work Loads (METs).

1. Cardiac patient is able to perform exercise work loads:
   - *Functional Class I:*   6-10 METs
   - *Functional Class II:*   4-6 METs
   - *Functional Class III:*   2-3 METs
   - *Functional Class IV:*   1 MET

2. Healthy subject is able to perform exercise work loads:
   - *Healthy sedentary individuals:*   Beyond 10-11 METs
   - *Physically active individuals:*   Beyond 16 METs

Reproduced from Chung, E.K.: *Exercise Electrocardiography: Practical Approach,* Baltimore, Williams & Wilkins Co., 1979.

Sexual Activity

Opinions vary among physicians, but sexual activity may be resumed about seven to eight weeks after a heart attack in most cases. Sex and the heart are discussed fully in Chapter 20.

Driving an Automobile

Although driving an automobile seems to be a very simple activity for healthy people, particularly when the individual has been driving for many years, driving may cause significant stress and physical work loads that may be harmful during the early phase of recovery. It has been shown repeatedly that driving in heavy traffic for a long time frequently provokes a variety of heart rhythm disturbances even in apparently healthy people. When any heart rhythm abnormality occurs in patients with previous heart attack, of course, it will be more harmful to their already damaged heart.

By and large, driving an automobile is allowed ten to twelve weeks after a heart attack, providing the patient's condition is fully evaluated by a physician, preferably including an exercise ECG test. Needless to say, the individual must be free of any significant symptom and should be mentally alert. Patients taking tranquilizers and/or sedatives must consult the physician specifically regarding driving a car under the influence of such drugs.

It is advisable not to drive a car immediately after heavy meals and/or consumption of alcoholic beverages. The patient should avoid driving in heavy traffic, especially during rush hour. Initially, driving for a short duration is advisable so that the patient can determine his or her physical condition for more driving in the future. If any symptom (e.g., chest pain, shortness of breath, palpitation, dizziness) occurs, he or she should pull the car over to the side of the road for a rest, and medical assistance should be obtained if necessary. The physician should be notified of the incident, and the patient should await further medical advice before driving again. If possible, the automobile should be equipped with good climate control (air-conditioning and heating), power steering, and power brakes; and its general condition should be good. If the car breaks down, the patient should seek an assistant rather than attempting to repair it alone. This is especially true when the weather is very hot or cold and/or humid.

At the beginning, it is wise to drive a car with an assistant (another driver) sitting alongside, so that any emergency can be managed as needed. If the patient tends to become tense and nervous during driving, it is advisable to postpone driving further. If the individual must drive a vehicle without power steering or power brakes, he or she should wait at least twelve to fourteen weeks after a heart attack. Risks involved with driving vary greatly, depending upon such factors as the patient's general condition, age, driving skills and habits, degree of damage to the heart and recovery, duration of driving, and conditions of the automobile. If driving is related to a patient's occupation, the individual must discuss this with the physician in depth before attempting to drive.

Returning to Work

The nature of the patient's occupation will significantly influence when he or she is permitted to return to work; but in general, most people may be able to return to their previous jobs about two to three months after a heart attack (see Chapter 21).

Sports and Exercise Programs

Participating in mild exercise programs and sports is beneficial about two months after recovery from a heart attack, but certain sports are unquestionably harmful. Various sports and exercise prescriptions are discussed in detail in Chapter 21.

Taking Trips and Vacations

Before taking trips or vacations, a medical checkup is mandatory, and the nature of the trip and its destination should be clearly known by the physician. Riding as a passenger is, of course, safer than driving a car. A short trip in a well-equipped automobile may be allowed five to six weeks after a heart attack when medically suitable. When traveling for a long distance, the car should be stopped frequently (every one to two hours) so that the patient can get out and exercise his or her legs by walking around to prevent blood clots. This precaution may even be a good idea for apparently healthy people without heart disease, especially when they are older than fifty. When a trip is planned for business, ample time should be allowed to reach the destination on schedule in order to avoid unnecessary tension and anxiety. When taking a trip by airplane, the individual should get up frequently (every one to two hours) to stretch the legs and walk around a little again, to avoid blood clots in the legs. When any breathing difficulty is experienced, he or she should tell the stewardess immediately so that oxygen can be inhaled as needed. When an individual is anxious and nervous about traveling by air, he or she may take mild sedatives before boarding.

It is advisable to avoid long trips until at least three to six months after a heart attack. When a long trip is planned, however, a complete medical checkup is, of course, essential. It is advisable to carry a brief medical summary, including a recent ECG, all the time, so that any physician may quickly review the pertinent medical history if a given patient happens to require medical advice and care during a trip. When one has to take a trip away from home, it is advisable to obtain the phone number and address of a physician who can be reached at the destination. When a trip to a foreign country is planned, the patient should obtain a list of English-speaking physicians from the International Association of Medical Assistance to Travelers [Empire State Building, Suite 5620, 350 Fifth Avenue, New York, NY 10001, telephone number: (212) 279-6465]. With this, the patient can obtain necessary medical care when an emergency arises.

It is essential to take all prescribed medications faithfully and to follow all necessary precautions during a trip. For example, one should avoid excessive physical activities, emotional distress, overeating rich foods, excessive consumption of alcoholic beverages and smoking. Ample rest periods every day are extremely important. When a special diet is prescribed, the individual should not hesitate to request that diet on an airplane or ship. Commonly prescribed diets are usually available on most commercial flights and cruises. When sightseeing is scheduled, it is wise to ask for detailed plans, including the approximate distance to be walked, in advance. It is definitely harmful to walk too long immediately after meals and/or consumption of alcoholic beverages. Walking should be avoided when the weather is too cold or hot, and/or if the humidity is high. During a trip, the individual should not carry heavy burdens (at most, a small brief case). It is advisable not to visit a foreign country where modern medical facilities are not available, simply because adequate medical care may not be possible should an emergency occur. It also is not safe to take a trip to a mountainous area where the elevation is more than 3,000 feet above sea level. Many patients with heart conditions experience difficulty in breathing in such locales.

Chance of Having Another Heart Attack

It has been reported that patients who have suffered a heart attack previously have a slightly increased risk of having another heart attack, as compared with those who have never had one, but it is difficult to predict the future for each patient precisely. The probability of having a second heart attack depends upon various factors, including age, general health, extent of heart damage, the presence or absence and degree of major complications, response to medical as well as surgical therapy, the presence or absence of risk factors, and the speed of recovery. More importantly, aftercare by the patient following discharge from the hospital greatly influences his or her chances of having another heart attack. When an individual carefully and faithfully follows all necessary precautions and medical advice after a heart attack, the chance of having another attack is markedly reduced or even avoided. Of course, risk factors (see Table 3.1) should be reduced or even eliminated if possible. It is also important that the individual be under the care of a competent physician.

Although many people believe that the second heart attack is more serious than the first one and that it is invariably fatal, the second or even third (or fourth) heart attack may be milder than the first, and the individual may recover from it. It is not necessarily true, therefore, that a repeat heart attack is more serious and invariably fatal. There are many individuals who have survived repeated heart attacks and can enjoy productive lives for many years.

PREVENTION OF A HEART ATTACK

People who have never had a heart attack should stay in excellent health, should enjoy and carry out productive lives. And those who have recovered from a heart attack should try especially hard to prevent another one. Of course, prevention of heart attack is ideal, rather than having any heart problems at all. The best approach is to try one's best to control or even eliminate various risk factors. This is particularly true for someone who has already suffered a heart attack. With effort, motivation, and knowledge, most of the risk factors can be controlled well and can even be abolished. The best example is cigarette smoking, a risk factor that *can* be completely eliminated. Remember that risk factors have a cumulative effect (e.g., the combination of cigarette smoking and birth control pills). It is also important to emphasize that more than one risk factor often coexist. For instance, many obese individuals have high BP, hyperlipidemia, diabetes mellitus, and a sedentary life-style. In addition, many obese people smoke. When one risk factor (e.g., obesity) is well controlled, other coexisting risk factors are often spontaneously controlled or even eliminated. If someone has already suffered a heart attack, all necessary precautions and medical advice must be followed very carefully in order to prevent a second heart attack.

PSYCHOSOCIAL ASPECTS

Although heart attack victims react differently, most patients experience significant and intense emotional problems, at least for a short period of time. The initial reaction is commonly extreme fear, anxiety, and apprehension immediately following a heart attack. Later, many people feel considerable depression. On the other hand, some patients do not realize the serious nature of a heart attack, whereas others may try to hide their emotional difficulty. At times, some patients may become euphoric during the late state of recovery because the heart attack was not as bad as they had anticipated. As a result, some people may have a tendency to overdo physical activities beyond their physical limitations during the late recovery period. Many patients feel that their moods fluctuate up and down during the early recovery period, but eventually their emotional status returns to normal within days or weeks as they regain their strength and confidence. When emotional difficulty is severe and when it lasts longer than usual, various sedatives or tranquilizers may be prescribed. The best therapeutic approach to various psychosocial problems is to discuss the matter frankly with a physician directly, rather than hiding the problem. In serious cases, psychiatric consultation may be necessary.

Not only patients but also family members may experience significant psychosocial difficulties. The reason for this, obviously, is that the life-style of the patient must change considerably after a heart attack; and the entire family has to adjust their life-styles to the patient's. Psychosocial aspects of heart attack are discussed in the following order: (1) during the early phase, (2) during the late phase, and (3) among the family.

Psychosocial Aspects During the Early Phase

As expected, a majority of patients feel a fear of impending death as soon as they experience severe chest pain, marked weakness, profuse sweating, dizziness, near-syncope, palpitations, and irregular heart rhythm—warnings of a heart attack. When the diagnosis of a heart attack is announced by the physician, many patients experience emotional shock. During the first few days in the CCU, most patients continuously feel a fear of impending death associated with profound anxiety and apprehension because of uncertainty regarding their outcome. As soon as the stormy course is over, and as soon as the critical period (the first few days) in the CCU is past, most patients begin to regain their peace of mind. At this time, many people express their joy of survival after the heart attack, and they feel extremely fortunate because they realize that the probability of sudden death was very high. Some individuals may become euphoric as they are allowed to increase physical activity gradually after being transferred to the ICCU and the ordinary hospital room. Some people feel that the attack was not as bad as anticipated.

In patients with severe anxiety and apprehension, various types of sedatives and/or tranquilizers may be prescribed in conjunction with many other medications, including narcotics such as morphine or Demerol. When the patient is taking various medications, his or her mental status often becomes unclear and drowsy. Some patients may not remember exactly what happened during the first few days in the CCU, either because of severe heart damage itself and serious complications or because of various drug effects. Some people have difficulty sleeping, either because of serious symptoms, such as chest pain and dyspnea, or emotional problems (fear, anxiety, tension, and so on). Sedatives or sleeping pills are definitely beneficial under this circumstance because physical and emotional rest are absolutely essential during the early phase after a heart attack.

When fear, anxiety, and apprehension begin to subside, as the cardiac condition becomes stable, most patients cannot help experiencing considerable depression. This is primarily because many people feel that their future will be helpless, useless, and hopeless as a result of the damaged heart. Many people feel depressed because their lives will be as semiinvalids, even though they may recover from the heart attack. Some individuals get depressed because of repetitive occurrences of chest pain and generalized weakness. Fortunately, most patients progressively feel stronger physically and emotionally as heart function improves steadily during the second and third week. Intense emotional difficulties usually subside within a few days or, at the most, one week after the onset of heart attack unless new symptoms appear or the patient's condition becomes progressively worse. When discharge approaches at the end of the second or third week, however, many individuals again experience anxiety, apprehension, and some fear. The reason for this is that the patient will no longer be supervised and monitored by nurses and physicians at home. Consequently, some people are reluctant to go home after recovering from a heart attack.

Psychosocial Aspects During the Late Phase

Of course, it is a great joy for most patients to come home after recovering from a heart attack. On the other hand, some people become anxious, tense, and insecure because of the lack of close, daily medical attention at home. Many people fear having another heart attack even though they were lucky enough to survive the first. In addition, many people misbelieve that the second heart attack is more serious and often fatal. Fortunately, these emotional problems gradually subside as patients regain strength and confidence. Some individuals may experience a more profound depression after coming home because of various restrictions on their life-style. Others feel depressed because of general weakness resulting from long-standing bed rest and inactivity in addition to the damaged heart itself. Other people feel depression and anxiety because of minor and nonspecific chest discomfort that is often muscular or skeletal in origin and *not* from heart disease itself. By and large, many patients expect a complete recovery too soon; consequently, they are disappointed because their strength is not as good as expected. Remember that it takes weeks and sometimes six months to regain strength fully after a heart attack.

Some individuals may be so depressed that they may even withdraw from their family and close friends, and may become apathetic to everything because they feel there is no reason to live. It is common to lose libido (sexual desire) and to become irritable from depression rather than from heart disease itself. When the depression is profound and when it lasts too long, the problem should be discussed with the physician. When necessary, psychiatric consultation may be arranged by the family physician. Some patients feel boredom because of restricted physical and social activity. This is particularly true of people who had been very active before the heart attack. They have to try to find suitable things (such as reading books or magazines and doing handicraft) to enhance their lives under the circumstances. Some active people have a tendency to overdo physical activities against the doctor's advice. Of course, this is foolish and indirectly suicidal. Remember that overdoing is extremely hazardous to an already damaged heart.

Fortunately, all the psychosocial problems after a heart attack eventually go away as the patient regains strength and confidence and begins to learn how to live wisely within his or her limitations. It should be reemphasized that the well-being of the patient after recovering from a heart attack largely depends on the individual's motivation and faithfulness in following necessary precautions and medical advice.

Psychosocial Aspects Among the Family

Psychosocial aspects of family life are also very important, because necessary precautions and medical advice must be carefully followed by family members. This is particularly true for the spouse. Necessary adjustments of the life-style of the entire family are especially critical during the first week after discharge. All family members should be made familiar with the serious nature of the heart attack. The spouse should learn precisely how to cook foods suitable for the heart victim, as prescribed by the physician. Food should be discussed completely with the physician or dietitian in order to obtain full details of a given diet (see Chapter 19). Another very important psychosocial aspect is sexual activity (see Chapter 20).

Some family members, particularly the spouse of the patient, may feel guilty of having caused the heart attack in the first place. Others may hesitate to refuse any request by the patient because of fear of causing another heart attack. Overprotection by a family member or close friend may be harmful to the patient psychologically by causing him or her to feel incapable of performing daily activity. Whenever necessary, frank, open discussions between the family and the patient can be beneficial, from the psychosocial viewpoint, for the patient as well as the family. Well-coordinated teamwork between the family and patient is essential to maintaining a happy, harmonious, and productive life for the family and for the patient's health.

PROGNOSIS

As repeatedly emphasized, immediate medical attention is the key factor in surviving a heart attack. When proper medical treatment is provided, not only is the chance of survival great; but full recovery without serious complications is also more likely. When proper medical attention is delayed, brain damage is often permanent, especially from a serious heart rhythm abnormality such as VF. Once the patient is admitted to the CCU and as soon as he or she begins to experience symptoms, proper medical treatment with continuous monitoring will be provided, and the chance of full recovery will be very high.

The prognosis expected (outcome) of patients after a heart attack, however, is influenced by various factors, including the extent of damage, the presence or absence and degree of major complications, the age of the patient, the presence or absence and degree of known risk factors (see Table 3.1) and/or coexisting other diseases, the patient's general health before the heart attack, and, more importantly, the presence or absence and degree of delay until medical attention was provided.

The average mortality rate after a heart attack in the CCU of American hospitals is approximately 15 to 20 percent at the present time. This mortality rate is difficult to reduce any further in spite of continuous medical research because some patients have far-advanced CAD with massive cardiac damage that is often incompatible with life. In these cases, serious complications frequently occur. For example, the mortality rate of patients with heart attacks complicated by significant CHF is about 40 percent. Moreover, the mortality rate is extremely high (ranging from 80 to 85 percent) when heart attack is complicated by cardiogenic shock in spite of sophisticated medical and surgical treatment. In other words, the heart is so severely and extensively damaged that survival is impossible in some patients.

CABS is the most common major surgery performed today in the United States. It is unequivocally documented that the quality of life improves markedly in the majority of patients with CAD (angina pectoris and heart attack) who have CABS. The bypass surgery can also prolong the patient's life in many cases with advanced CAD (see Chapter 25).

Another very important factor that influences long-range prognosis is the degree of motivation and faithfulness the patient exhibits in following all necessary precautions and medical advice after discharge from the hospital. All known risk factors must be well controlled or even eliminated, when possible. Endless and in-depth understanding and cooperation by each family member, as well as by the patient, are extremely important for the patient's well-being after recovery from a heart attack.

It has been shown that sudden death and reinfarction in patients surviving a heart attack can be prevented considerably when certain medications are used. According to the Norwegian Multicenter Study Group (New England Journal of Medicine 304:801, 1981) dealing with 1,884 patients surviving acute MI, a reduction of 44.6 percent of the cumulated sudden death rate was observed when timolol maleate (Blocadren—a new beta-blocking agent), 10 mg twice daily was given, and the cumulated reinfarction rate was also reduced proportionately. The treatment was started seven to twenty-eight days after MI (945 taking timolol; 939 placebo), and the patients were followed for twelve to thirty-three months. Blocadren has been approved for clinical use by the U.S. Food and Drug Administration.

Other beta-blocking agents such as propranolol probably provide similar effects, and the beneficial effects of aspirin, Persantin, and sulfinpyrazone (Anturane) for the prevention of sudden death and another heart attack after recovering from the first MI have been described previously.

4

ANGINA

Chest pain is one of the most common symptoms in our daily lives, and it may be due to a variety of causes. In some instances, chest pain is totally functional—emotional, and not from any disease entity—while in other cases, it may be due to various serious diseases—cardiac as well as noncardiac. The term *angina* or *angina pectoris* is used when chest pain occurs as a manifestation of CAD—narrowing of the coronary artery (the artery that supplies blood to the heart muscle—see Figure 1.4). In medical terms, the narrowed coronary artery is called "coronary artery stenosis." When the narrowing is said to be significant, coronary artery stenosis covers more than 70 percent of the original diameter of the artery.

In ordinary terms, *angina* means that chest pain is produced by an extraordinary physical activity that overburdens heart function as a result of inadequate blood supply, secondary to the narrowed coronary artery. In other words, angina occurs when the demands for oxygen and blood exceed the supply that is limited by the narrowed coronary artery. The narrowing of the coronary artery is produced by a progressive and long-standing hardening of the artery—atherosclerosis. In medical terms, the condition of a heart muscle receiving inadequate blood supply is called "myocardial ischemia." Myocardial ischemia is a temporary and reversible phenomenon, and the ischemic heart muscle returns to normal as soon as adequate blood circulation is restored.

Many patients with angina can lead productive lives with good control of the problem when proper medical advice is carefully and faithfully followed. On the other hand, angina is often a precursor of heart attack when precautions and medical advice are not followed. Even in cases with advanced angina pectoris, most patients enjoy productive lives after successful CABS for many years.

CAUSES

The human heart has to pump regularly and constantly to bring nourishment and oxygen to all parts of the body. In order to perform this work, the heart itself must have a continuous and adequate blood supply through its own network of arteries—the coronary arteries (Figures 1.2 and 1.4). When there is inadequate blood circulation to the heart muscle to meet demands, the patient develops angina pectoris—usually due to narrowing of the coronary arteries (Figure 2.2). In most patients with angina pectoris, the coronary arteries are affected by atherosclerosis—hardening of the arteries. The process of atherosclerosis begins to develop very early in life, and most people have some degree of atherosclerosis by the time they reach middle age, although many have no symptoms until the narrowing of the coronary arteries becomes pronounced. The process of atherosclerosis speeds up very rapidly when various risk factors are present. Detailed descriptions of the underlying causes of angina pectoris and MI are found in Chapter 3.

SYMPTOMS (WHAT THE PATIENT MAY EXPERIENCE)

Exertional chest discomfort is a hallmark of typical angina in most cases. Although the term *angina* or *angina pectoris* automatically signifies the "pain in the chest" as a manifestation of CAD, in reality, angina is seldom expressed as chest pain. Rather, angina is commonly described as a viselike, constricting sensation, tightness, or pressurelike discomfort in the entire chest or only on the left side or midsection of the chest behind the breastbone. A unique feature of angina is that the exact location of the discomfort is difficult or almost impossible to pinpoint with one finger because it is rather diffuse in nature. Accordingly, most patients express angina with an open hand or fist to cover a large area of the chest.

In contrast to typical angina, some patients may experience chest discomfort with minimal physical activities, or it may even be totally unrelated to physical exertion. The angina may occur at rest or even while a patient is sleeping, especially while having a bad dream. Consequently, angina may wake the patient up in the middle of the night. This type of angina is called "variant angina" or "atypical angina." At times, another term *Prinzmetal's angina,* is used, because Dr. Prinzmetal described atypical angina in detail two decades ago.

92   Angina

In the mid-1970s, the term *coronary spasm* became popular among physicians because it was apparent that a spasm involving a segment of the coronary arteries may cause angina pectoris. It has been shown that coronary artery spasm predominantly affects the right coronary artery (about 80 percent); spasm involving the left coronary artery is much less common. The spasm may be segmental in a narrow or long single site, or it may affect multiple sites or even involve diffusely one or more coronary arteries. Coronary artery spasm may be present without any underlying fixed stenosis (narrowing), but, not uncommonly, spasm may coexist with significant fixed coronary artery stenosis. Coronary spasm seems to occur more frequently among young to middle-aged women who are heavy smokers and possibly regular users of birth control pills. Angina due to coronary spasm more commonly causes resting or nocturnal chest pain rather than conventional angina. Coronary spasm may occur spontaneously, or it may be provoked by various agents or maneuvers (this is discussed later).

One of the unique features of variant angina is a characteristic ECG change during chest pain (either spontaneous pain or pain provoked by various agents or maneuvers). Elevation of the S-T segment is observed during pain, and the ECG returns to normal as soon as the pain subsides (see Figure 4.1). This transient S-T segment elevation during chest pain is considered to be due to coronary spasm. It is important to remember that coronary spasm may result in a classical myocardial infarction (heart attack) and even death in the absence of fixed coronary artery stenosis (narrowing) or occlusion (blockage).

FIGURE 4.1. Electrocardiograms showing Prinzmetal's angina (variant or atypical angina). Note marked S-T segment elevation in many leads during chest pain (see tracing A) and normal ECG when the chest pain is subsided (see tracing B).

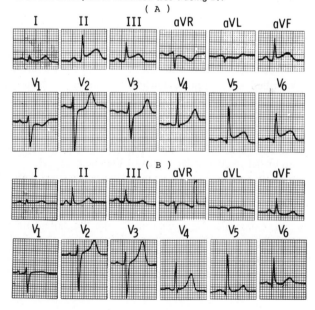

Detailed descriptions of unstable angina are in order, because this entity is extremely important to recognize. Unstable angina often proceeds to acute MI (heart attack), and sudden death may soon follow unless proper and immediate medical attention is provided. Unstable angina has many other names, including preinfarction angina, intermediate coronary syndrome, impending MI, coronary insufficiency, and crescendo angina, and it refers to a syndrome intermediate between conventional typical angina pectoris and acute MI. Unstable angina and crescendo angina are the most popular terms.

Unstable angina has received special attention in recent years because of the serious prognosis and unpredictability of sudden onset of acute MI in some patients with this problem. When unstable angina is suspected, the patient requires immediate hospitalization in the CCU in order for constant monitoring and proper medical treatment to be provided. Remember that various life-threatening cardiac arrhythmias are very common during the first few hours or days of acute MI and that sudden death is usually due to these heart rhythm abnormalities. All patients with unstable angina should be managed in the same manner as those with acute MI because heart attack is often preceded by unstable angina. When chest pain is not relieved by all available medical treatment for crescendo angina, CABS should be considered following coronary arteriography.

As described previously, most patients with typical angina experience exertional chest pain, and the pattern of chest discomfort is usually fixed in a given individual. In contrast to this, unstable angina or crescendo angina is characterized by chest pain of a different character, duration, radiation, and severity. Namely, chest pain in unstable angina may occur at rest or in the middle of the night, and it is easily produced by minimal physical activity that was not sufficient to cause chest pain in the past. The chest pain is usually crescendo in quality, and it may not subside readily with resting or sublingual NG. In many cases with unstable angina, acute MI is strongly suspected through the descriptions of symptoms, but the diagnosis of heart attack cannot be documented by diagnostic tests. Characteristic features of typical angina are found in Chapter 3.

PHYSICAL FINDINGS (WHAT PHYSICIANS MAY FIND IN A MEDICAL EXAMINATION)

As emphasized previously, the most important clue in diagnosing angina pectoris correctly is to recognize the characteristic features of chest discomfort induced by physical exercise and/or emotional excitement. There are various physical findings during a medical examination that are helpful in diagnosing angina pectoris, but none of them are pathognomonic of the disease. The cardiovascular examination may be entirely normal in approximately 25 to 40 percent of patients with proven angina pectoris. During an angina attack, however, a significant number of patients may show a considerable elevation in systolic as well as diastolic BP (transient hypertension), and in some patients a gallop rhythm (triple heart rhythm; see Chapter 8) may be audible through a stethoscope. Others may exhibit various types of abnormal heart rhythms, cardiomegaly (enlarged heart), heart murmurs (see Chapter 8), signs of CHF, hypertension, and signs of diabetes mellitus, obesity (overweight), or other risk factors. Again, none of these findings are diagnostic of angina, but they are supportive evidence when angina pectoris is strongly suspected clinically.

Carotid sinus stimulation (massaging the side of the neck near the Adam's apple below the chin) often causes anginal pain to subside more quickly than usual if the procedure slows the heart rate, and it is a particularly helpful maneuver in cases of atypical angina. During angina, many patients reveal rapid heart rate because of angina itself and also as a result of anxiety and fear.

DIAGNOSIS

In patients with typical angina pectoris, the diagnosis can readily be made by analyzing the characteristic descriptions of chest discomfort triggered by extraordinary physical activity (e.g., sudden or vigorous exercise, exposure to cold air, shoveling snow) and/or by emotional excitement (e.g., anger, fear, argument). On the other hand, atypical or variant angina may not be easy to diagnose with certainty by history alone. Various physical findings may be noted by physicians, but none of them are diagnostic. In nearly half the patients with proven angina pectoris, cardiovascular examination may be completely normal.

Immediate and good response to NG is very strong indirect evidence to support the diagnosis of angina pectoris, but a placebo effect (the effect of any drug or substance for emotional or psychological reasons) cannot be excluded. In addition, the diagnosis of angina is further supported by the presence of various risk factors, family history of CAD or hypertension, and previous history of heart attack or CABS. Remember that a significant number of patients suffer from angina even after recovering from a heart attack, and, of course, the prognosis under this circumstance is not favorable.

Various symptoms and physical findings of angina pectoris have been described in detail previously in this chapter. Although a correct diagnosis of angina pectoris is readily made on clinical grounds alone in many patients, documentation of the disease may often be necessary by utilizing various laboratory tests. Common diagnostic tests include a resting (12-lead) ECG, exercise (stress) ECG test, myocardial imaging, and coronary arteriogram. None of the blood tests are diagnostic of angina pectoris, but certain abnormalities (e.g., hyperlipidemia, hyperglycemia) indicative of risk factors are supportive evidence for the diagnosis. Likewise, evidence of diabetes mellitus (e.g., clinical history or the presence of sugar in the urine) also supports the diagnosis of angina. A routine chest X-ray again provides no definite information for the diagnosis of angina pectoris, but the presence of cardiomegaly and/or signs of CHF often favor this diagnosis.

Commonly used diagnostic tests for angina pectoris are now described in detail.

1. *Electrocardiogram (ECG).* A resting 12-lead ECG (a routine ECG recorded during resting state without chest pain) is normal in over 25 percent (even up to 75 percent in some reports) of cases with proven angina pectoris. A large number of angina patients have a normal ECG at rest because myocardium (heart muscle) may receive an adequate blood supply in spite of the narrowed coronary artery as long as the demands for oxygen and nourishment do not exceed the supply in a resting state. When demands exceed the supply, however, the ECG often shows abnormalities, including inverted T waves, peaking T waves, and depression or elevation of the S-T segment (Figures 4.1 and 4.2). In order to induce myocardial ischemia (transient change in the heart muscle because of inadequate blood supply through the narrowed coronary artery), an extraordinary physical exercise can be required of the patient with suspected angina pectoris utilizing a motor-driven treadmill or bicycle when the resting ECG is normal. Namely, the exercise (stress) ECG test (Figure 4.3) is performed by provoking myocardial ischemia, under direct medical supervision, in order to document angina pectoris. The exercise ECG test will show

FIGURE 4.2. Electrocardiogram showing inverted T waves in many leads, indicative of diffuse myocardial ischemia in a patient with advanced angina pectoris.

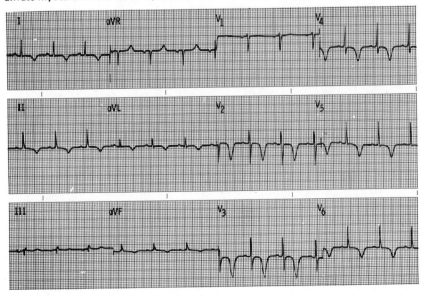

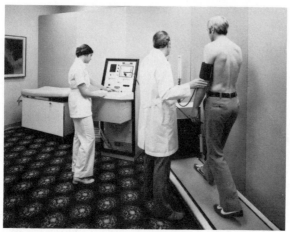

FIGURE 4.3. A scene of the exercise (treadmill) ECG testing. (Reproduced with permission through the courtesy of Quinton Instrument Company, Seattle, Wash.)

significant abnormality when the patient suffers from advanced angina pectoris (Figure 4.4). The exercise ECG test is discussed later in this chapter.

The ECG often demonstrates the S-T segment and/or T wave abnormalities during spontaneous chest pain (Figure 4.1), and normal ECG is restored as the pain subsides either spontaneously or by taking NG. In addition to the ischemic changes (abnormalities of the S-T segment and/or T waves), various other ECG abnormalities may be present on the resting ECG. Various cardiac arrhythmias (abnormal heart rhythms), A-V conduction disturbances, intraventricular blocks (e.g., left bundle branch block, right bundle branch block), and left ventricular hypertrophy (enlarged left pumping chamber) often coexist with the ischemic changes, but the ECG abnormalities other than the ischemic changes are *not* diagnostic of angina pectoris.

2. *Exercise (Stress) ECG Test.* The exercise (stress) ECG test (Figure 4.3) is one of the most common non-invasive diagnostic tests performed in cardiology at present. There are two major indications: (1) diagnosis of CAD, especially angina pectoris; and (2) assessment of functional capacity. Detailed descriptions of the exercise ECG test are found in Chapter 24.

3. *Myocardial Imaging (Radioisotope Studies).* Myocardial imaging involves the injection of radioactive materials (very small, safe amounts) into the body via the vein. After the injection, various organs including the heart will absorb a different amount of the chemicals (e.g., thallium-201) depending upon the nature of the organ and its status (normal versus abnormal or damaged tissues). Thus, a photograph or film of the heart will show different concentrations of radioisotope in healthy (normal) and damaged (diseased) heart muscle. Myocardial imaging is very useful as a noninvasive diagnostic tool when the result of the exercise ECG

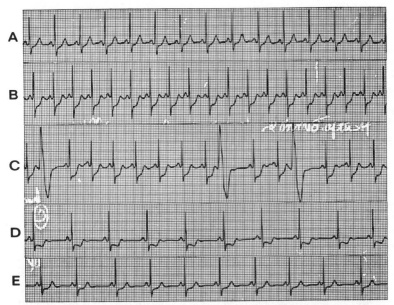

FIGURE 4.4. Exercise (treadmill) ECG test shows marked S-T segment depression with frequent VPCs provoked by exercise in a patient with coronary artery disease. Tracing A is a resting ECG that shows normal finding. Tracing B was taken during exercise, whereas tracings C to E were obtained after exercise.

test is equivocal or when the exercise ECG test is difficult to interpret because of preexisting electrocardiographic abnormalities (e.g., left bundle branch block) or various clinical situations (e.g., during digitalis or propranolol hydrochloride therapy) in which false positive or false negative exercise ECG test results are expected to occur. Myocardial imaging is also very valuable in patients who suffer from angina after recovering from MI. Myocardial imaging is discussed in Chapter 24.

   4. *Coronary Arteriography or Angiography.* In addition to the aforementioned noninvasive diagnostic tests, coronary angiography (or arteriography), which is an invasive test, is a confirmatory method to determine precisely the location and degree of stenosis (narrowing) or obstruction (blockade) of the coronary artery (see Figure 4.5). Coronary arteriography is a visualization of coronary artery circulation by means of an X-ray movie following injection of dye material via catheter (small plastic tube) into the heart. Coronary arteriography should *not* be performed only to diagnose angina in most cases. Coronary arteriography is usually recommended to anticipate CABS.

   Coronary artery spasm can be diagnosed during coronary arteriogram by demonstrating a focal spasm that may occur spontaneously or may be provoked by various agents or maneuvers. The provocative tests may be indicated if the clinical suspicion of coronary artery spasm is strong, but confirmation of the diagnosis is

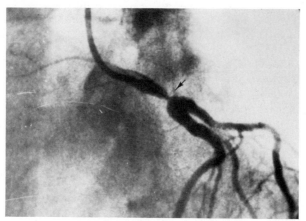

FIGURE 4.5. Coronary arteriogram showing marked stenosis (narrowing, indicated by an arrow).

necessary. The most commonly used provocative test is the intravenous administration of ergonovine maleate. After standard coronary arteriography and left ventriculography, ergonovine maleate is administered in a bolus intravenous injection of 0.05 mg, and the patient is observed for about three minutes. If chest pain and/or S-T segment elevation is noted, coronary arteriography is repeated. If there is still no spasm of the coronary artery, a second dose of 0.15 mg is administered, followed by observation for coronary artery spasm. When coronary artery spasm is provoked, it can be reversed by sublingual, intravenous, or intracoronary administration of NG. The diagnosis of coronary artery spasm is more confirmatory when there is a partial or complete regression of the coronary artery narrowing after administration of NG or other vasodilating agents. Demonstration of a focal spasm is the definite diagnostic criterion of coronary artery spasm, and diffuse but mild reduction in caliber of the coronary artery(ies) is *not* sufficient for the diagnosis. There are a few complications of this provocative test, including a slight elevation of the aortic blood pressure, mild and transient nausea, and ventricular arrhythmias. Metacholine is also used in a similar manner for the provocative test to diagnose coronary artery spasm.

Another commonly used provocative test is the cold pressor test to diagnose coronary artery spasm. The patient's hand is immersed in ice water for one minute, and coronary arteriography is repeated in selected oblique projections. In most patients with variant angina, coronary artery spasm is produced with this method. It should be noted, however, that a smaller percentage of patients with classical angina also may develop critical occlusive spasm of the coronary artery. Nevertheless, the cold pressor test is a safe and simple provocative test in demonstrating coronary artery spasm, and there is no significant complication associated with this test. It should be remembered that spasms may involve multiple sites of coronary artery(ies), and the spasm may also coexist with fixed coronary artery stenosis. Coronary arteriography is discussed in detail in Chapter 24.

5. *Other Diagnostic Tests.* Other cardiac tests, including echocardiography and Holter monitor ECG, are discussed in Chapter 24.

DIFFERENTIAL DIAGNOSIS (HOW TO DISTINGUISH BETWEEN ANGINA AND CHEST PAIN FROM OTHER CAUSES)

There is a variety of disorders that may produce chest discomfort resembling true angina. The differential diagnosis between true angina and other disorders is often difficult when dealing with patients with atypical clinical history or when there are two or more coexisting diseases. Nevertheless, in 80 to 90 percent of cases with typical angina, the diagnosis can be established without much difficulty. Several disorders that may produce chest pain similar to true angina are briefly discussed.

Functional disorders (psychophysiological cardiovascular reactions) are, at times, confused with true angina. Dull, aching chest pains, often described as "heart pain," usually last hours or days under these circumstances, and the pain may be aggravated by exertion but not promptly relieved by rest. Pain from functional disorders is frequently associated with emotional tension and fatigue, and the emotional problems make the functional chest pain worse. Functional chest pain may also be associated with hyperventilation, palpitations (without actual cardiac arrhythmias), and headache (see Tables 3.7 and 3.8). Continuous exhaustion is a common complaint. Remember that typical angina is usually triggered by extraordinary physical activity and that the chest pain is promptly (within a few minutes) relieved by rest and/or sublingual NG.

The "anterior chest wall syndrome," which is characterized by a sharply localized tenderness of intercostal muscles, may simulate true angina. The chest pain in anterior chest wall syndrome can be easily reproduced by local pressure. Remember that true angina is *not* associated with tenderness (pain on pressure). Sprain or inflammation of the chondrocostal junctions (called "Tietze's syndrome") may produce diffuse chest pain associated with local tenderness and warm, swollen, and red areas at the chondrocostal junctions. The chest pain of Tietze's syndrome is also reproducible with local pressure. Intercostal neuritis (e.g., herpes zoster, diabetes mellitus) may also produce chest pain similar to angina. Cervical or thoracic spine disorders (e.g., degenerative disk disease, postural strain, and various types of arthritis) involving the dorsal roots produces a sharp, severe chest pain that may be superficially confused with true angina. However, the pains due to these cervical or thoracic spine disorders are related to specific movements of the neck or spine, recumbency, and straining or lifting.

Various gastrointestinal disorders (e.g., peptic ulcer, gallbladder diseases, cardiospasm) may be confused with angina in some cases. In these disorders, symptoms are directly related to food intake rather than physical exertion. X-ray and fluoroscopic examination of the gastrointestinal tract and gallbladder will clarify the diagnosis of these disorders. Pain under these circumstances is usually relieved with proper diet and drug (e.g., antacids) therapy. Hiatal hernia, which is characterized by lower chest and upper abdominal pain following heavy meals, may simulate the clinical picture of true angina. The pain due to hiatal hernia usually occurs in recumbency or upon bending over, and it is relieved by bland diet, antacids, semi-Fowler position, and walking.

Degenerative and inflammatory processes of the left shoulder or cervical ribs may cause pain similar to angina, but the pain in these circumstances is usually precipitated by movement of the left arm and shoulder. Paresthesias are often present in the left arm. Likewise, rib fracture or other forms of trauma to the chest may cause chest pain similar to angina. Under these clinical circumstances, X-rays of the ribs, spine, and shoulders will clarify the diagnosis.

Spontaneous pneumothorax (collapse of lungs) also may be confused with angina, but the characteristic chest X-ray findings will confirm the diagnosis of pneumothorax. Pulmonary embolism (blood clots in the lungs) often causes a clinical picture that may closely simulate angina or acute MI. However, careful history taking, physical examination, and various diagnostic tests will clarify the differential diagnosis in most cases. Severe mitral stenosis or pulmonary hypertension resulting from chronic pulmonary (lung) diseases may produce chest pain similar to angina, but differential diagnosis is obvious in most cases from a careful clinical evaluation in conjunction with various laboratory studies. It should be reemphasized that a physician should be consulted immediately when any possibility of angina or impending myocardial infarction (heart attack) is raised.

TREATMENT

When an individual with known angina pectoris follows all necessary medical advice faithfully and intelligently, he or she may be able to enjoy a productive life for many years without much difficulty. It is important to understand the physical limitation that is determined by the exercise ECG tests utilizing the concept of METs (see Chapter 24). In other words, any physical activity that requires effort beyond a patient's capacity should be avoided. From their own experiences, most patients with angina should be able to learn how to avoid chest discomfort by limiting certain activities in conjunction with proper medical advice. All known risk factors should be well controlled or eliminated if possible.

The patient should not hesitate to take NG whenever necessary for chest pain. Other prescribed medications must also be taken regularly. When the physician determines that the angina is difficult or almost impossible to control with medications and necessary precautions, CABS should be considered in selected patients. Remember that the success or failure of medical treatment for angina largely depends upon the degree of understanding, willingness, faithfulness, and cooperation of the patient, under competent medical guidance. It is important to realize that the advanced case of angina (particularly crescendo angina) is often a precursor of acute heart attack. Likewise, a heart attack may not be avoided when a person with angina pectoris fails to follow the doctor's advice and to practice all necessary precautions. When angina is not relieved by rest and two or more tablets of sublingual NG, or when the intensity and duration of chest pain seem to be worse than before, the possibility of a heart attack or impending heart attack should be strongly considered. In this circumstance, of course, immediate medical attention should be sought, and the patient must be transported to a nearby ER as soon as possible (see Chapter 3).

Treatment of angina is divided into three major categories: (1) medical treatment, (2) surgical treatment, and (3) preventive measures.

Medical Treatment

The medical treatment can again be divided into two aspects: (a) treatment of acute attack and (b) long-term treatment for recurrent angina attacks.

Treatment of Acute Angina Attack

It is essential that the patient stops immediately whatever physical activity and/or emotional excitement caused the angina. Thus, the patient should stand still or sit or lie down—whichever position gives the most comfortable feeling—as soon as the chest pain begins and remain quiet until the attack has completely subsided. This is the natural reaction of most patients, but some of them try to overcome the chest discomfort by continuing or even increasing physical activity. Of course, the latter behavior is not only foolish but suicidal—it definitely must be avoided.

Sublingual NG is the drug of choice for an acute attack of angina, and it is effective within one or two minutes. One fresh tablet of NG (0.3 to 0.4 mg) should be placed under the tongue and allowed to dissolve. It is important *not* to swallow it whole or chew it. NG may be taken sublingually when an angina attack is anticipated, a few minutes before engaging in any physical activity and/or emotional excitement (e.g., sexual intercourse, long walks) as a preventative measure. Treatment of angina with NG was discussed in detail in Chapter 3.

In addition to NG, many other drugs are available for the treatment of angina. A crushed pearl of amyl nitrite is effective when inhaled through the nose. However, amyl nitrite often causes flushing of the face, pounding of the pulse, and sometimes dizziness and headache. These side effects can be minimized when the patient inhales it from a distance. Most patients can soon learn the optimal distance from which to inhale amyl nitrite for best effect. Isosorbide dinitrate (Isordil, Sorbitrate) and NG ointment may be used for acute angina attacks, but they do not act as rapidly as sublingual NG. A good point is that the efficacy of these is longer, and they can be used at four- to six-hour intervals during the day or at bedtime. Detailed discussions regarding isosorbide dinitrate and nitroglycerin ointment are found later (see the following section and Chapter 17).

Long-Term Treatment for Recurrent Angina Attacks

For long-term therapy, many patients require one or more antianginal drugs (e.g., propranolol, isosorbide dinitrate) for many months, years, or even indefinitely, in addition to short-acting sublingual NG. Application of NG ointment (2 percent) to the skin (about 2 to 3 in. in diameter), covered with plastic wrap, is often effective in preventing angina, especially at bedtime. Of course, it may be used during the day because the action of this agent usually lasts for four to eight hours.

A new transdermal NG pad is under investigation for the prevention and the treatment of angina pectoris. The laminated patches contain an NG reservoir microsealed in a polymer, and a semipermeable membrane is bonded to a flexible adhesive pad. Attached to the chest or upper arm, the patches release NG at a controlled rate through the skin into the systemic circulation. The NG patches are circular and vary in diameter from 10 to 25 cm, depending on the dosage. By sustaining constant blood plasma levels of NG around the clock for twenty-four hours, angina can be prevented and treated more effectively. The NG transdermal pads are scheduled to be approved by the U.S. Food and Drug Administration in early 1982.

When CHF is associated with angina pectoris, digitalis (heart pills) and diuretics (water pills) are also indicated. Propranolol is contraindicated for CHF. Likewise, various antiarrhythmic agents (drugs used for abnormal heart rhythms; see Chapter 9) are indicated when angina pectoris is complicated by any type of cardiac arrhythmias. Sedatives or mild tranquilizers may be beneficial when angina attack is precipitated or aggravated by emotional upset or anxiety. Of course, coexisting disorders that are closely related to angina and various risk factors for CAD, such as hypertension, hyperlipidemia, anemia, diabetes mellitus, obesity, and so on, must be controlled. Detailed descriptions regarding antianginal drugs appear in Chapter 17.

Surgical Treatment

CABS should be strongly considered (Figure 3.9) when angina is difficult to control with medications. Detailed descriptions of CABS are found in Chapter 25.

Prevention of Angina

Many episodes of anginal attack can be prevented when precautions are carefully followed and all necessary medications faithfully taken under the guidance of a competent physician. Any physical activity and/or emotional stress that may provoke an angina attack must be avoided. In certain unavoidable situations, a prophylactic NG should be taken sublingually a few minutes before a given activity (e.g., sexual intercourse) when angina attack is anticipated. Any physical activity beyond a patient's maximal physical capacity, as determined by the exercise ECG test, must be avoided. For instance, when an individual is able to perform the exercise work loads requiring 3 METs as the maximal effort as determined by the exercise ECG test (see Tables 3.12 and 3.13), he or she should avoid unquestionably any physical activity that requires more than 3 METs (see Table 3.11). The energy expenditures required by various daily business and other physical activities can be easily computed, and they can be expressed by utilizing the METs system (see Tables 3.11 to 3.13). The energy expenditures required in various physical activities are again readily compared with exercise work loads during the standard exercise ECG test (see Chapter 24).

All risk factors must be well controlled or eliminated if possible. For example, cigarette smoking is absolutely prohibited for patients with angina. Oral contraceptives should also be avoided. As repeatedly stressed, the combination of cigarette smoking and taking oral contraceptives is one of the worst risk factors for young women. These risk factors can easily be eliminated by those who are informed and highly motivated. Hypertension, hyperlipidemia, diabetes mellitus, and obesity must also be well controlled.

Every patient with angina pectoris must be examined by a competent physician on a regular basis (every one or two months to every three to six months, depending on the status of the disease), because the clinical picture of the disease may change from time to time. Exercise ECG test, coronary arteriogram, and other cardiac tests may be performed as needed, and the physician has to determine the indications of these tests during each visit. In addition, a regular medical checkup is important because it may be necessary to modify the therapeutic regimen from time to time, depending upon response to treatment and the progress of angina pectoris. Some patients may require CABS when the angina attack becomes refractory to medical treatment as described previously. Remember that the process of atherosclerosis is continuous and progressive.

Consumption of a large quantity of alcohol should be avoided (see Chapter 23), and even large meals are harmful to patients with advanced angina. In particular, any extraordinary physical activity should be avoided soon after (within one to two hours) heavy meals and/or alcohol consumption. For the same reason, physically demanding dancing (fast dancing) must also be avoided soon after meals and/or alcohol consumption. Any form of extraordinary outdoor activity is very hazardous to patients with angina during cold weather; in particular, shoveling snow is *absolutely* prohibited. Unnecessary emotional stress, anxiety, or anger must be avoided, and high-strung or anxious individuals have to learn how to relax and must try to change their characters in order to avoid emotional excitement. In other words, people with angina pectoris must learn how to take care of themselves wisely by modifying their life-style under medical guidance in order to avoid unnecessary burden to the heart. Thus, all patients with angina must eat proper diets (see Tables 3.3 and 3.9), maintain ideal weight (see Table 3.4), exercise regularly, and avoid vigorous or sudden physical activity and excessive fatigue. Proper diets and exercise are discussed later in detail (see Chapters 19 and 21). Remember that intelligent, faithful, and careful home care every day by the individual under a competent physician's guidance is the most important aspect of treatment for angina pectoris. Otherwise, it may lead to heart attack, and even sudden death may follow.

The prognosis (outcome) for patients with angina pectoris is greatly influenced by a variety of factors. They include the patient's age, the degree of coronary artery stenosis or obstruction (single-, double-, or triple-vessel disease), the site of stenosis or obstruction (proximal versus distal), the presence or absence of adequate collateral circulation (reserved vessels), and the presence or absence and degree of co-existing cardiac disorders or complications. More importantly, the prognosis is determined considerably by the patient's willingness, faithfulness, and cooperation in observing precautions and following medical advice.

Nevertheless, most medical studies report that the average mortality rate of angina pectoris over a period of five years is approximately 3 to 4 percent (ranging from 1 to 15 percent) per year. As mentioned earlier, diabetes mellitus, hypertension, cardiac hypertrophy (chamber enlargement), CHF, MI, and cardiac arrhythmias usually shorten life expectancy. Early onset of angina before age forty or a family history of premature cardiac death is, of course, unfavorable as far as prognosis is concerned.

Half of all patients die suddenly, and an additional third die following heart attack. CHF accounts for most of the remainder of the deaths. It should be re-emphasized that advanced angina pectoris is often a precursor of heart attack, but a heart attack and even sudden death may be prevented to a certain extent when the patient is able to maintain a desirable life-style intelligently according to the physician's advice and prescriptions. Remember that many patients with angina pectoris are able to enjoy productive lives for many years, as long as the heart can function properly by avoiding all unnecessary work loads, although atherosclerosis (the fundamental cause of angina) is a continuous and progressive disease process.

5

HIGH BLOOD PRESSURE

Every individual has a blood pressure (BP) to maintain adequate circulation to the entire body. BP in healthy people varies from day to day and even from moment to moment. It goes up when the individual engages in physical activity and/or emotional excitement, whereas it goes down when the person is in a resting state or sleeps. These BP changes are perfectly normal. BP is defined as the force of the blood against the arterial walls while the heart pumps blood constantly to all parts of the body. Arterial walls are elastic and muscular, and they stretch and contract according to cardiac pumping action. The machine that is designed to measure BP is called a "sphygmomanometer" in medical terms, but it is commonly called a "blood pressure cuff" or "blood pressure machine." The machine consists of a cuff, a rubber bulb, and a glass mercury tube or dial. The cuff is placed snugly around the arm just above the elbow, and it is inflated with air by squeezing the bulb repeatedly. As the cuff gets tighter, it compresses a large artery in the arm. This procedure temporarily shuts off the blood circulation through the arm artery, because the squeeze from the air pressure in the cuff is greater than the push of blood in the artery. At this moment, the mercury is high in the glass tube, and the numbers alongside the column of mercury (or in the dial) reveal the height of air pressure in the cuff. In the next step, air is let out of the cuff, and the mercury drops in the tube. A stethoscope is applied to the inner surface of the arm over the compressed artery just below the cuff. Blood begins to flow through the artery with each heartbeat as soon as the air pressure in the cuff is slightly lower than the BP in the artery. This rhythmic blood flow in the artery under the cuff produces a unique sound that can readily be heard through the stethoscope.

As soon as this sound appears, the height of the mercury is recorded—this is called "systolic pressure." Following measurement of the systolic pressure, air is let out of the cuff until the unique sound, corresponding to each heartbeat, disappears as the blood flows steadily through the artery. At this point, the height of the mercury reveals the least amount of pressure in the artery—called "diastolic pressure." The measurement of BP is relatively simple, and it can be done by any lay person with instructions and practice. Inexpensive BP machines are available for home use.

The four vital signs include BP, body temperature, respiration, and pulse or heart rate. By and large, BP is lower in children and young adults, while it goes up progressively as the individual gets older. Under the age of eighteen, normal BP ranges between 90/70 and 120/80 mmHg. After eighteen, a BP of 140/90 mmHg is considered the upper limits of normal.

As far as the regulatory mechanism of BP is concerned, BP is controlled by the "arterioles," which are the smallest twigs of the arterial tree branched off the aorta. Arterioles regulate BP by making it difficult or easy for the flow of blood to get through to the "capillaries," those blood vessels that actually deliver the blood and the nutrients to all parts of the body. When the arterioles clamp down, the blood cannot pass through them easily to the capillaries. In this circumstance, the heart must pump harder to push the blood through. Consequently, the BP in the arteries goes up. The BP will go down when the arterioles are relaxed (expanded). The manner in which arterioles regulate BP is somewhat comparable to the way a nozzle regulates water pressure in a garden hose. When the opening becomes narrower by turning the hose nozzle, the water pressure in the hose increases. With a larger opening, less pressure is required to force the water through the hose.

When the BP is abnormally elevated (above 140/90 mmHg in adults), it is called "hypertension" (*hyper* means "increased"; *tension* means "pressure"). Elevated diastolic pressure (pressure during dilatation or expansion of the ventricles) is more serious than elevated systolic pressure (pressure during contraction or the pumping phase of the ventricles), but most hypertensive patients have elevation of systolic as well as diastolic pressure. When the BP is abnormally elevated, the work loads of the heart and arteries are increased. In other words, the heart must pump harder with more force, and the arteries must carry blood under increased pressure. If high BP persists for a long time, the heart and the arteries are unable to function properly, and various complications occur. That is, hypertension often leads to increased risk of heart attack, angina pectoris, CHF, stroke, and renal (kidney) failure unless it is properly treated. Therefore, control of hypertension under constant medical supervision is essential.

It should be remembered that hypertension is one of the most common risk factors and that it often coexists with other risk factors such as obesity, hyperlipidemia, and diabetes mellitus. It has been shown that high BP is the primary and most common cause of CHF, particularly in the United States. Furthermore, there are many patients who have to live with kidney dialysis machines for their entire lives, who started out with moderate but uncontrolled hypertension, as did the hundreds of thousands who must live with the aftermath of a stroke, and numerous people die prematurely from heart attacks. Epidemiologic studies clearly indicate that the higher the BP, the greater the risk for heart attack, stroke, CHF, and kidney failure. Therefore, high BP remains a serious public health problem. The public should be adequately informed and educated, and the patient's endless cooperation is indispensable for control of hypertension under a competent physician's guidance.

It should be noted that one of every six American adults has high BP (at least 20 million people, and as high as 35 million people), but half of them are not aware of it. Even when BP is found to be elevated, many individuals do not seek medical attention, and many of them fail to take necessary medications regularly. According to some medical reports, almost 25 percent of black American adults are said to be hypertensive. In many patients, BP elevation occurs only intermittently during the early stage (called "labile hypertension"), and then eventually high BP persists. In most cases, hypertension is detected in persons between thirty and forty-five years of age. If either parent or any siblings have high BP, one's chance of having hypertension is at least doubled. Regular medical checkups are extremely important, even when an individual is considered healthy, because many hypertensive patients have no symptoms at all, and there may be nonspecific symptoms, such as dizziness or headache, so that the individual may not pay attention to the symptoms.

In 90 percent of cases with high BP, the exact cause is unknown—called "primary" or "essential" hypertension. In the remaining 10 percent, various causes responsible for the development of high BP can be found—called "secondary" hypertension. Nevertheless, no matter what the cause, control of high BP with diet (salt-restriction), weight reduction, and various antihypertensive drugs is associated with considerably reduced morbidity and mortality. In some patients, excessive salt intake causes high BP. In others, overweight and smoking speed up the development of hypertension and the risks of associated complications. Therefore, it is essential for all hypertensive individuals to avoid excessive salt intake and to maintain the ideal body weight (see Table 3.4). Smoking, of course, is unquestionably harmful to every aspect of health (see Chapters 3 and 22).

Twenty years ago, little could be done to interrupt the dead-end course from high BP other than restricting salt intake and controlling weight. Now, more than 80 percent of hypertensive cases can be well controlled with various antihypertensive medications. Diuretics ("water pills"), vasodilators (drugs to dilate blood vessels), and nerve blockers are the most commonly used medications to treat hypertension. With few exceptions, high BP cannot be cured, but it can be well controlled to prevent serious complications. Epidemiological study has documented that 10 percent of untreated hypertensive patients will die within five years; and if chest

X-ray and ECG show left ventricular hypertrophy (enlarged left pumping chamber), 89 percent will die within five years if they remain untreated. It is extremely important to take antihypertensive medication(s) indefinitely in most cases, unless advised otherwise by a physician for a specific reason.

CAUSES AND CLASSIFICATION

As described earlier, in nearly 90 percent of cases with high BP, no cause is found. In this case, various terms, including *essential hypertension, primary hypertension,* and *idiopathic hypertension,* have been used. When there is a clear-cut cause responsible for the production of high BP, the term *secondary hypertension* is used. Although it is not possible to document the direct cause of essential hypertension, it is obvious that hypertension results from a loss of regulatory mechanism(s) to maintain normal BP.

The kidneys or the adrenal glands (located just above the kidneys) may send substances (e.g., norepinephrine and epinephrine) into the bloodstream that start a chain of chemical events. These events result in hypertension. It is also known that any emotionally stimulating activity will temporarily increase BP in healthy people. For hypertensive individuals, however, emotional excitement (e.g., anger, frustration, argument) will raise BP even more. Therefore, it is very important for people who already have high BP to try to avoid any emotional trouble that may lead to an excessive rise in BP. Needless to say, most people are fully aware of the fact that with the pace and complexity of today's living, it is almost impossible to avoid various forms of stress. Thus, any individual with hypertension must take the required medication(s) regularly under a competent physician's guidance so that an excessive rise in BP due to emotional tension may be minimized.

Medical study has clearly documented that a tendency toward high BP is often inherited. In some individuals, excessive salt intake raises BP. Likewise, oral contraceptives also cause high BP in some women. It is, therefore, very important for young women who are hypertensive to tell their doctors if they are taking birth control pills.

Essential Hypertension (Primary Hypertension)

Although the term *essential* or *primary hypertension* means that no direct cause for high BP has been found, various factors that regulate BP are considered responsible. These include baroreceptor activity, cardiac output, systemic vascular resistance, blood volume, activity of the sympathetic and central nervous systems, and the "renin-angiotensin-aldosterone system." In other words, essential hypertension does not always have uniform pathophysiologic features, although an exact cause may not be identified. It has been shown that essential hypertension occurs in 10 to

15 percent of white adults and in 20 to 30 percent of black adults in the United States. The onset of essential hypertension is commonly between ages twenty-five and fifty-five, and the family history is often suggestive of hypertension and related complications (e.g., stroke, sudden death, CHF, heart attack at an early age). Hypertension occurs transiently in the early stage ("labile hypertension") of the disease, but eventually it becomes permanent.

Secondary Hypertension

When an identifiable cause or known disease can be found, the term *secondary hypertension* is used. Secondary hypertension is applicable in about only 10 percent of all cases of high BP. It is extremely important to emphasize that secondary hypertension is not necessarily "curable" through recognition and elimination of the cause of high BP in every case. For example, in cases of secondary hypertension associated with parenchymal disease of the kidneys (disease involving kidney tissue, such as glomerulonephritis and pyelonephritis), renal artery stenosis, and adrenal tumors, normal BP is restored only in a certain percentage of patients after correction of the problem. On the other hand, hypertension is often entirely curable after correction of coarctation of the aorta or removal of the pheochromocytoma (a tumor of the adrenal medulla or sympathetic paraganglia associated with headache, blurred vision, palpitation, and tachycardia). Hypertension induced by oral contraceptives is usually curable when the individual stops taking the pills, but it may persist for a few weeks or at times even months after discontinuation of oral contraceptives. Similarly, hypertension produced by excessive salt intake is often curable by eating a low-salt diet (see Table 3.9).

Renal Hypertension (High Blood Pressure Resulting from Diseases of the Kidneys or Narrowing of the Artery Supplying the Kidneys)

It is important to realize that long-standing high BP frequently leads to renal (kidney) failure, and that high BP is often a result of various diseases of the kidneys or renal artery stenosis (narrowing of the artery supplying blood to the kidneys). Therefore, it can be said that the relationship between high BP and kidney disease is definitely bidirectional.

Medical study has demonstrated that narrowing of one or both renal arteries is probably the most common cause of secondary hypertension. Renal artery stenosis is often due to atherosclerosis (the same process causing angina or heart attack), but it may result from fibromuscular hyperplasia or other disorders. Renal artery stenosis may be suspected in the following circumstances:

1. if the onset of hypertension is after age fifty;
2. if there are epigastric or renal artery bruits (abnormal sound audible through a stethoscope placed on the abdomen);

3. if there is evidence of atherosclerosis elsewhere (e.g., history of angina, heart attack, or stroke);

4. if there are variations in the size and appearance of the kidneys by X-ray, time of appearance of contrast media, or delayed hyperconcentration of contrast material in the involved kidney on the intravenous urogram (see Chapter 24);

5. if there are increased amounts (relative to the other kidney) of renin (a form of chemical substance closely related to the production of hypertension) activity in renal vein blood;

6. if there is abnormal excretion of radioactive materials as shown by renal scan (isotope study of the kidneys); or

7. if atherosclerosis or fibromuscular hyperplasia is demonstrated by renal artery angiogram.

When hypertension is a direct result of renal artery stenosis, this type of secondary hypertension is often curable by correcting the lesion. It should be noted, however, that some patients with secondary hypertension due to renal artery stenosis may not be cured even after surgical correction of the lesion. Another form of renal hypertension is high BP produced by parenchymal diseases of the kidneys. In particular, chronic glomerulonephritis and pyelonephritis (forms of infectious and inflammatory processes involving kidneys) frequently lead to secondary hypertension. Polycystic kidney disease (a form of congenital kidney deformity) and congenital or acquired obstructive hydronephrosis occasionally produce renal hypertension. In addition, hypertension may result from acute glomerulonephritis. Unfortunately, renal hypertension secondary to parenchymal diseases of the kidneys may not be curable even after treatment of the underlying kidney disease.

Endocrine Disorders

Pheochromocytoma (a small, well-encapsulated, lobular, vascular tumor of chromaffin tissue of the adrenal medulla or sympathetic paraganglia) causes persisting or intermittent hypertension by virtue of releasing norepinephrine and epinephrine into the blood circulation. High BP often occurs with a paroxysm in this disorder, and it is commonly associated with a pounding headache, blurred vision, palpitations, and tachycardia. High BP is usually cured by removing the pheochromocytoma.

In addition, hypertension may be due to other endocrine disorders, such as Cushing's disease (or syndrome) and primary aldosteronism. Cushing's disease or syndrome is characterized by "moon face"; "buffalo hump"; obesity with protuberant abdomen and thin extremities; a plethoric appearance; abnormal menstruation; impotence; weakness; backache; headache; skin infections; hirsutism (abnormal hair growth) on the face, upper trunk, arms, and legs; purple striae; easy bruising; psychosis; and glycosuria (sugar in the urine) associated with hypertension as a result of hyperplasia or tumor of the adrenal cortex with or without a small tumor of the pituitary gland. Primary aldosteronism is characterized by hypertension, muscular weakness, paresthesias (abnormal sensations of the skin,

such as burning or prickling) with frank tetanic manifestations, headache, polyuria (excessive urination—especially during the night), and polydipsia (excessive
thirst persisting for long periods of time) associated with various electrolyte imbalances, particularly hypokalemia (reduced potassium content in the blood) as
a result of aldosterone excess secondary to tumor(s) or hyperplasia of the adrenal
cortex (tumors are usually too small to be seen on X-ray).

Coarctation of the Aorta

Congenital constriction of the arch of the aorta produces high BP in the arms
and carotid arteries (arteries running along the neck), but BP in the legs is normal
in this condition. The hypertension due to coarctation of the aorta is thought to be
a direct result of the mechanical constriction, which leads the left ventricle to eject
blood into a "short chamber," although renal mechanism may play a role, at least
in part, in producing hypertension in this congenital defect. Hypertension is often
curable after surgical correction.

Miscellaneous Conditions

Hypertension of varying severity is observed in patients with *preeclampsia-
eclampsia (toxemia of pregnancy)*. The term *preeclampsia* denotes the nonconvulsive
form, whereas *eclampsia* designates a more advanced form with the development of
convulsions and coma. Preeclampsia-eclampsia usually occurs in the last trimester
of pregnancy and the first few months after childbirth. Approximately 10 to 20
percent of pregnant women develop preeclampsia-eclampsia in America, and
primigravidas (women with their first pregnancy) are most commonly affected.
Uncontrolled preeclampsia-eclampsia leads to a permanent disability and may be
fatal. About 5 percent of cases with preeclampsia progress to eclampsia, and 10 to
15 percent of women with eclampsia die. The exact cause of preeclampsia-eclampsia
is not yet clearly understood, but malnutrition is considered to play a role.

Preeclampsia is characterized by persistent hypertension or a sudden elevation of BP, and by generalized edema and proteinuria (protein in the urine) associated
with headache, vertigo, malaise, nervous irritability, nausea, vomiting, pain in the
abdomen, partial or complete blindness, and liver enlargement with tenderness.
The symptoms of eclampsia are those of a severe and advanced form of preeclampsia. Therefore, eclampsia is characterized by marked hypertension associated with
generalized tonic-clonic convulsions, coma followed by amnesia (loss of memory)
and confusion, severe proteinuria, stertorous breathing, frothing at the mouth,
twitching of various muscle groups (e.g., face and arms), nystagmus (an involuntary,
rapid movement of the eyeball, which may be horizontal, vertical, rotatory, or
mixed), and oliguria (reduction in the amount of urine) or anuria (no urine at all).
In this condition, marked hypertension usually precedes a convulsion, and it is
followed by hypotension (low blood pressure) thereafter during coma or vascular
collapse. It is often fatal unless prompt and vigorous treatment is provided.

Hypertension may also develop following the use of oral contraceptives,
with increased intracranial pressure (increased pressure in the brain) due to a

tumor or hematoma in the brain and in the late stage of polyarteritis nodosa (inflammatory damage to blood vessels with obscure etiology), systemic lupus erythematosus (an inflammatory autoimmune disorder that may affect multiple organ systems), and scleroderma (a chronic disorder characterized by diffuse fibrosis of the skin and internal organs with unknown cause).

Malignant Hypertension

The term *malignant hypertension* is used when the diastolic pressure goes beyond 130 mmHg. Any form of sustained hypertension (either primary or secondary) may abruptly become accelerated, leading to malignant hypertension. Without proper treatment, there is rapidly progressive renal failure, CHF, and stroke. Markedly elevated BP results in severe headaches, acute visual disturbances (difficulty in vision), and gross hematuria (blood in the urine) associated with papilledema, hemorrhages, and exudates in the retina (swollen optic disk with blurred margin and hemorrhage in the eyeground—inside of the eyes). The mortality rate approaches 80 percent in one year and nearly 100 percent within two years if no treatment is given for malignant hypertension. Prompt treatment to lower the BP is extremely urgent. Otherwise, CHF and/or kidney failure may occur very rapidly, and fatal outcome may not be avoidable in many cases with malignant hypertension.

CLINICAL FINDINGS

Most patients with mild high BP have no unusual symptoms. Therefore, it is impossible to ascertain the presence of hypertension unless BP is actually measured. Even if there are symptoms, most patients do not pay attention because they are nonspecific. Nevertheless, there are three very common symptoms associated with hypertension: (1) headache, (2) fatigue, and (3) epistaxis (nose bleeding). When any of these symptoms is present singly or in combination, BP must be checked immediately by a physician. Headache due to hypertension often occurs early in the morning, and it usually subsides during the day. But any type of headache may occur in hypertension, and it may simulate migraine in some cases. Other symptoms may include dizziness, fullness in the head, palpitations, pounding in the chest, rapid or irregular heartbeats, shortness of breath, and tinnitus (ringing in the ears).

Remember that hypertension is the most common cause of cardiomegaly (enlarged heart), particularly hypertrophy of the left pumping chamber. Progressive left ventricular hypertrophy eventually leads to CHF. Thus, without a doubt, the most common cause of CHF today is hypertension. When the patient develops CHF, various symptoms (e.g., shortness of breath, swelling of the legs and ankles) may be observed. Hypertrophy of the left ventricle can be detected by physical examination, and it is readily confirmed by ECG, chest X-ray, and echocardiogram. In addition, the left atrium (left upper chamber) is often enlarged, and a fourth heart sound (due to contraction of the atria) may become audible. A loud second aortic sound (heart sound due to closure of the aortic valve) is also often present in hypertensive patients. Advanced CHF often leads to acute pulmonary edema, and it is frequently followed by death. Of course, many patients with long-standing hypertension develop CAD at an early age because hypertension is one of the major risk factors.

As part of a physical examination for hypertensive patients, the tiny blood vessels inside the eyes (eyeground) are carefully checked by physicians. These tiny arteries in the retinas (inside the eyes) can readily be seen through an opthalmoscope (a magnifying glass with a small light operated by battery). In hypertensive patients, retinal arteries will show minimal narrowing and irregularity during the early stage. These early retinal changes will be followed by more marked narrowing with atriovenous nicking and flame-shaped or circular hemorrhages and fluffy "cotton-wool" exudates as hypertension advances further. In far-advanced hypertension—malignant hypertension—papilledema (blurred margin with elevated or swollen optic disk) eventually develops. Papilledema is a hallmark of malignant hypertension.

When the kidney begins to show abnormal function in hypertensive patients, the earliest sign is nocturia (frequent urination at night). Eventually, many patients with long-standing hypertension or hypertension associated with parenchymal diseases of the kidneys will develop renal failure. Renal failure produces various symptoms and signs resulting from abnormal kidney function. They may include anorexia, nausea, vomiting, lethargy, proteinuria, hematuria, anemia, weakness, peripheral edema, and high BP associated with a variety of abnormal kidney tests (e.g., elevation of blood urea nitrogen, creatinine, and potassium). Of course, many patients with advanced renal failure will die.

The diagnosis of renal artery stenosis is strongly suggested when there is a bruit (an abnormal, high-pitched sound generated by blood flow through a narrowed kidney artery) in the abdomen. Under this circumstance, renal artery stenosis is most likely responsible for the production of hypertension when the bruits are well localized and of both systolic and diastolic timing. These bruits may also be heard over the flank areas. The bruits are usually most audible with the diaphragm of a stethoscope. When hypertension is due to polycystic kidneys, they are usually large and readily palpable.

When brain function is impaired by severe hypertension, a variety of symptoms and signs may be observed. For example, malignant hypertension causes severe headaches, confusion, coma, convulsions, blurred vision, nausea, vomiting, and many other abnormal neurologic signs. Various findings (e.g., weakness or complete paralysis of one side of the body or extremities, difficulty in speech, semi- or total unconsciousness) may be observed when hypertensive patients develop stroke. When abnormal brain function is produced directly as a result of severe hypertension, the term *hypertensive encephalopathy* is used.

The diagnosis of coarctation of the aorta (defined previously) is almost certain when femoral arterial pulsations (pulses in the groin) are very weak (in comparison with radial pulses) or absent in young individuals. Supportive findings for the diagnosis include a basal systolic murmur transmitted to the interscapular area and palpable collateral arteries along the inferior rib margins and especially around the scapular borders. Various symptoms and signs in secondary hypertension due to endocrine disorders have been described previously.

DIAGNOSIS

As emphasized previously in this chapter, the diagnosis of hypertension is made only when BP is measured to be higher than normal. By definition, BP higher than 140/90 mmHg is termed "hypertension," but one high BP reading is *not* sufficient to designate hypertension. It is recommended, therefore, that BP be measured on at least three different occasions after about twenty minutes or more in a resting state. Namely, the diagnosis of hypertension can be entertained when BP has been found to be elevated on three separate occasions. It should be stressed again that there is no way to diagnose hypertension unless BP is actually measured. Moreover, many patients with hypertension have no symptoms and feel perfectly healthy as long as there is no major complication. In other words, hypertension itself is perfectly compatible with normal life, but associated complications are major concerns.

Hypertension is clinically suspected when one or more common symptoms (headache, fatigue, epistaxis) are present. As far as secondary hypertension is concerned, a variety of clinical symptoms and physical findings can provide useful clues to a specific underlying disorder (discussed previously).

Recently, the Joint National Committee on Detection, Evaluation and Treatment of High BP has recommended a simple approach to diagnostic evaluation of the hypertensive patient, and has indicated that in the majority of patients, secondary causes for hypertension may be ruled out by a careful history and physical examination and a minimal workup. This author fully concurs with the recommendation of the Joint National Committee, and believes that minimal workup is indicated for approximately 90 percent of all patients with hypertension.

Blood and Urine Tests

Routine baseline tests should include hematocrit, hemoglobin, white cell counts, urinalysis, and automated blood chemistry (e.g., electrolytes, glucose, creatinine, blood urea nitrogen or BUN, cholesterol, triglycerides, uric acid). In addition, most physicians also recommend an ECG and chest X-ray as part of the routine laboratory tests, although they are not absolutely essential for every patient with hypertension. No other tests beyond these are indicated for the majority of patients with essential hypertension unless there is a significant degree of renovascular damage and/or any evidence of secondary hypertension. As stressed earlier, the special tests are indicated only when any form of secondary hypertension is suspected clinically. Routine urinalysis may reveal a low fixed specific gravity compatible with renal parenchymal disease, which is the most common form of secondary hypertension. In other words, renal parenchymal disease can be diagnosed or ruled out by a simple urine test.

For all intents and purposes, primary aldosteronism can be ruled out when serum potassium is normal. On the other hand, the excretion of more than 50 mEq of potassium per twenty-four hours suggests a variety of diseases associated with potassium wastage (including primary aldosteronism, Cushing's syndrome or disease, renal disease), providing that the causes of secondary aldosteronism are excluded (e.g., vomiting, diarrhea, chronic laxative ingestion, and oral contraceptive therapy). Similarly, the diagnosis of renal failure is ruled out in most cases when the BUN or serum creatinine is normal. In renal failure (uremia), the BUN and serum creatinine are usually elevated, and there is also some degree of anemia in most cases.

Proteinuria, casts, red blood cells, and white blood cells in the urine specimen usually indicate various kidney diseases. Bacteria growth in a fresh urine specimen by means of urine culture signifies pyelonephritis, and in this case, white cell casts are occasionally found. As far as the excretion of protein in the urine for twenty-four hours is concerned, the exact amount of excretion provides invaluable information for the workup in hypertensive patients. The normal kidneys excrete not more than 0.2 g of protein in twenty-four hours, while excretion between 0.2 and 0.4 g is compatible with any type or severity of hypertension. Renal parenchymal disease is indicated when protein excretion is more than 0.4 to 0.5 g for twenty-four hours. Chronic pyelonephritis should be strongly considered if the protein excretion is beyond 2.0 to 3.0 g per twenty-four hours. Quantitative determination of urinary excretion of 17-hydroxycorticosteroids (elevation of this chemical substance diagnostic of Cushing's disease or syndrome) is indicated when Cushing's disease or syndrome is clinically suspected. Likewise, quantitative determination of urinary excretion of catecholamines and vanillylmandelic acid (VMA—elevation of this chemical substance diagnostic of pheochromocytoma) is justified when pheochromocytoma is clinically suspected.

Since thiazide diuretics frequently cause hyperglycemia and hyperuricemia, it is wise to have tests for baseline serum uric acid concentrations and blood sugar prior to the initiation of antihypertensive therapy. It is also important to remember that many hypertensive patients have diabetes mellitus. Although it is not critical to be tested for serum triglycerides and cholesterol level as far as the diagnostic workup for hypertension is concerned, these serum lipid values provide very important information for the therapeutic approach. The reason for this is, obviously, that many hypertensive patients have elevated serum cholesterol and/or triglycerides, which are very serious risk factors for CAD, and they directly and indirectly influence the morbidity and mortality of the patient.

Some physicians advocate that a plasma renin profile (a substance closely related to the mechanism of hypertension) be obtained as a part of the evaluation of almost all hypertensive patients, but this view is not uniformly accepted. Nevertheless, the renin assay may be valuable when there is suspicion of a low-renin disease, such as primary aldosteronism (based on the finding of low plasma potassium), or of a high-renin form of disease, such as renovascular hypertension (based on the presence of an abdominal bruit upon physical examination).

Chest X-Ray

Chest X-ray finding per se does not provide any diagnostic information in hypertensive patients except for secondary hypertension due to coarctation of the aorta. Characteristic features of the chest X-ray findings in coarctation of the aorta include rib notching (as a result of collateral circulation that causes indentation in the lower edge of the ribs) and the small aorta knob. On the other hand, a chest X-ray is an important diagnostic tool for recognizing cardiac involvement from hypertension. For example, the presence or absence, and degree, of enlargement of the left atrium and left ventricle, which is the most common complication of hypertension, can be clearly assessed by chest X-ray finding. In addition, pulmonary congestion and pulmonary edema as a manifestation of CHF will be demonstrated in the X-ray film.

Electrocardiogram

Again, the electrocardiogram is *not* a diagnostic tool for hypertension, but it provides valuable information regarding cardiac complications from hypertension. ECG is fully discussed in Chapter 24.

Intravenous Urograms (Pyelograms)

Intravenous urograms (X-ray films taken consecutively with certain intervals on both kidney areas following intravenous injection of contrast material) will disclose valuable information regarding various abnormalities of the kidneys. Namely, intravenous pyelograms (urograms) will demonstrate the relative size of both kidneys, the relative rate of appearance and disappearance of the contrast material, the displacement of the kidneys and obstruction, as well as congenital deformity such as polycystic kidneys.

For instance, the presence of calyceal clubbing, contour irregularity, or scarring should suggest chronic pyelonephritis (infection of the kidneys by microorganisms). Asymmetry, delayed appearance, and pelvic hyperconcentration of the contrast material should suggest main or branch stenosis of the renal artery. Of course, a definite diagnostic tool for renal artery stenosis is a renal arteriogram. It should be noted that the right kidney is normally 0.5 cm shorter than the left kidney.

Renal Arteriogram

In order to confirm the exact site, nature, and degree of renal artery stenosis, a renal arteriogram is performed. In this study, the contrast medium is introduced via a femoral (groin) vessel at a level at or just below the orifices of the renal arteries, with a technique similar to that of cardiac catheterization (see Chapter 24). Renal arteriography is particularly essential when the surgical approach for renal artery stenosis is planned. When a renal arterial lesion is identified, and if renin is secreted from the diseased kidney in a concentration equal to or greater than 1.5 times that of the unaffected (normal) kidney, corrective surgery may be considered. On the other hand, the patient with renal artery stenosis, associated with atherosclerosis involving the heart and/or brain, may not be considered for corrective surgery until kidney function becomes markedly impaired or medical antihypertensive therapy is ineffective. The reason for this is that the mortality rate is considerably high when atherosclerosis involves many arteries and organs diffusely; therefore, the surgical approach is only considered as a last resort. Since the fibrosing disease of the renal arteries does not progress rapidly, renal artery stenosis due to this lesion may be treated first with medications. If hypertension becomes resistant to medical treatment, or if renal artery stenosis is progressive under this circumstance, however, surgical approach should be considered.

Other Special Tests

Other special tests (e.g., differential radioisotope excretion studies, differential urinary function studies on each kidney) are available as a part of hypertensive workup, but these tests are not commonly used.

COMPLICATIONS

As described previously, hypertension per se is compatible with normal life, but associated major complications definitely influence morbidity and mortality. Namely, untreated and long-standing hypertension is frequently associated with serious complications that involve three vital organs—heart, brain, and kidneys. Consequently, many hypertensive patients develop hypertensive heart disease, angina pectoris, MI, CHF, hypertensive encephalopathy, stroke, and renal failure, singly or in combination.

Effects on the Heart

Unquestionably, high BP adds to the work load of the heart and arteries. The heart, forced to work harder than normal over a long period, tends to enlarge. A slightly enlarged heart may be able to function well, but a markedly enlarged one has a difficult time keeping up with the demands put on it. In other words, the hypertrophied left ventricle is unable to increase its mass continually, and gradually collagen deposits accumulate. Eventually, CHF is produced as an end result when the work load goes beyond the capacity of the enlarged heart. In addition, other effects of hypertension are imposed on the heart, and in particular, the process of atherosclerosis speeds up. This premature atherosclerosis of the coronary arteries leads to angina pectoris and heart attack even when patients are in their late thirties or early forties. Remember that hypertension is one of the major and most common risk factors. Of course, cardiac function further deteriorates rapidly when CHF is superimposed on angina pectoris or heart attack in hypertensive patients.

It has been shown that 10 percent of untreated hypertensive patients will die within five years even if the ECG and chest X-ray fail to reveal cardiomegaly. When left ventricular hypertrophy is demonstrated on the ECG and chest X-ray, 89 percent will die within five years unless hypertension is well treated.

Before hypertensive patients develop overt CHF, there is a period of stable hyperfunction of the ventricle (hyperdynamic circulation). During the hyperfunction stage, many hypertensive patients demonstrate an active apical heartbeat (forceful heartbeat at the apex), tachycardia, and an ejection-type systolic murmur at the base of the heart (see Chapter 8). This hyperdynamic circulation is often designated "hyperkinetic heart syndrome," which is common in young people with mild essential hypertension. Thus, many young hypertensive individuals experience palpitations and rapid heart rhythm. Although the exact underlying reasons for the production of hyperkinetic heart syndrome are not fully understood, a total body autoregulation to increased cardiac output is considered responsible for this response to high blood pressure.

Eventually, patients with left ventricular hypertrophy demonstrate reduced cardiac output (amounts of blood pumped by the left ventricle) as a result of impaired contractile force in the heart. When cardiac performance diminishes progressively and the reserve capability of the heart becomes exhausted, CHF is the ultimate outcome. The term *hypertensive heart disease* is commonly used when the heart disease is directly caused by high BP.

Effects on the Kidneys

As emphasized previously in this chapter, high BP and kidney disease have a close bidirectional relationship. During an initial stage, thickening of the small arterial and arteriolar walls develops with progression of high BP, especially when it is untreated. This kidney damage results in the changes of nephrosclerosis when the renal vessels are involved. Eventually, clinical manifestations of renal damage will be expressed by nocturia (urination at night), polyuria (frequent urination), reduced renal concentrating ability, and proteinuria. As the renal failure progresses, the patient complains of weakness, general malaise, easy fatigue, insomnia (difficulty in sleeping), slight shortness of breath, anorexia (loss of appetite), bad taste in the mouth, and intractable nausea, especially in the morning. The patient looks pale because of anemia and becomes increasingly lethargic. There may be hiccups and uncontrollable twitching of the limbs as renal function deteriorates, especially when acidosis and azotemia become more pronounced.

If renal failure is untreated, progressive anemia and bleeding into the skin, mucous membranes, and gastrointestinal tract herald the final illness. The skin becomes dry with a sallow tint, and the breath becomes uriniferous (odor of urine on the breath). Vision is often impaired as hemorrhages and exudates appear in the fundi (inside the eyes). The urinary output becomes progressively reduced as renal failure is far-advanced. Pericarditis and/or pleurisy (see Chapter 13) may appear within a few weeks of death. Disorientation and coma usually precede the final outcome of the fatal illness. It has been reported that approximately 10 percent of the deaths secondary to hypertension result from renal failure.

Effects on the Brain

Markedly elevated BP may be associated with nausea, vomiting, and headache that progresses to coma, and is accompanied by clinical signs of neurological deficits. This clinical syndrome is termed "hypertensive encephalopathy." When severe hypertension is immediately controlled with medications (see Table 5.1), the patient promptly awakens from the coma, with disappearance of various clinical manifestations resulting from abnormal function of the nervous system. When proper treatment is not given early enough, however, the syndrome proceeds to stroke, chronic encephalopathy, or malignant hypertension. Under these circumstances, reversibility is much slower, and many patients may ultimately die.

In general, the possibility of stroke is increased in hypertensive patients. Blood vessel damage in the brain may be due to blood clots in the brain artery(ies), or it may be cerebral (brain) hemorrhage. Blood clots in the artery of the brain are comparable to those in the coronary artery that cause heart attack. Brain hemorrhage is, as a rule, fatal. When BP is well controlled, however, this stroke risk is dramatically reduced.

Accelerated and Malignant Hypertension

Accelerated and malignant hypertension has been discussed previously.

Aortic Dissection

Dissecting aortic aneurysm (dissection of the inner layer of the aorta) is not uncommonly observed in hypertensive patients. If untreated, dissecting aneurysm may lead to rupture, and it is often fatal. When high BP is well controlled, however,

TABLE 5.1. The Major Antihypertensive Drugs and Doses.

Agent	Usual Initiating Dose	Maximum Daily Dose
Diuretics (these agents are compiled in equivalent forms so that one agent is the same as another)		
Chlorothiazide	500 mg. b.i.d.	1000 mg.
Hydrochlorothiazide	50 mg. b.i.d.	100 mg.
Furosemide	40 mg. b.i.d.	As high as 2.0 g.
Spironolactone	25 mg. q.i.d.	100 mg.
Smooth muscle relaxants		
Hydralazine	10 mg. q.i.d.	200 mg.
Nitroprusside	60 μg./ml.	
Rauwolfia derivatives		
Reserpine (typical of this group)	0.25 mg. q.d. (oral)	0.25 mg.
Reserpine (parenteral)	0.5 mg. (to see if unusual response)	2.5 to 5.0 mg. q. 6 H
Adrenergic inhibitors		
Methyldopa	250 mg. t.i.d. or q.i.d.	4.0 g.
Guanethidine	10 mg. q.d.	150-250 mg.
Clonidine	0.1 mg. b.i.d.	2.4 mg.
Trimethaphan	1 mg./ml., IV	
Receptor antagonist		
Alpha-		
Phentolamine	5 mg., IV	10 mg. or by infusion
Dibenzylene	5 mg. b.i.d.	As necessary; see text
Beta-		
Propranolol	10 mg. q.i.d.	160 mg. q.i.d. (see text for precautions and contraindications)

Reproduced with permission from Chung, E.K.: *Quick Reference to Cardiovascular Disease.* Philadelphia, J.B. Lippincott Co., 1977.

severe pain in the chest and back from the dissection is often relieved, and the dissecting process will usually cease as the BP is reduced.

TREATMENT

Epidemiologic studies clearly indicate that the higher the BP, the greater the risk. There are, however, significant controversies among physicians as to the criteria for placing a patient on a specific medication, treatment of elderly hypertensives, values of sedatives or tranquilizers, an exact role of diet therapy, and so on. Nevertheless, treatment of hypertension should include proper diet therapy, proper weight control, antihypertensive medications, surgical approach for certain secondary hypertensions, and management for complications. It is extremely important to stress that the therapeutic approach to hypertension should be individualized according to the BP level, the presence or absence and degree of associated cardiovascular risks, and the patient's age and sex. In general, BP of 140/90 mmHg in men younger than forty is comparable to BP of 145/95 mmHg in men older than forty or to BP of 160/95 mmHg in women of all ages.

General Measures

It is very important to emphasize that the best therapeutic approach can be achieved only when there is full understanding and cooperation between the patient and the physician. The patient's part is just as important as the physician's. Once the diagnosis of hypertension is made, each patient must follow the doctor's instructions closely about taking medications, proper diet, control of body weight, and adjustment of life-style.

The patient must take prescribed medications exactly as the physician has instructed. It is very important for the patient not to stop the medications simply because he or she feels well. When any unusual drug side effect occurs, the patient should report this to the physician immediately. All hypertensive patients also must be seen by physicians regularly (every one to two months or every three to six months, depending on clinical circumstances) indefinitely. The physician can thus make any needed changes in the treatment program for hypertension and its complications. Remember that high BP is a lifetime illness in most cases, and the patient needs constant medical care and advice. Adequate rest and sufficient sleep are essential for all hypertensive individuals. Adequate relaxation is an important general health measure, and unnecessary stress must be avoided as much as possible. Mild sedatives or tranquilizers are beneficial if a hypertensive patient is anxious and easily excitable. Cigarette smoking is unquestionably harmful to all hypertensive patients, and excessive consumption of alcohol should also be avoided. In addition, proper physical exercise is, of course, advisable.

For established mild hypertension (BP above 140/90 mmHg and up to 160/105 mmHg) in young adults and middle-aged patients, the treatment may begin with modest sodium restriction to a level of 4 to 6 g/day of sodium chloride, weight reduction in the presence of obesity, increasing physical activity involving isotonic exercise and the relief of stress if possible. If this nondrug therapy is ineffective, antihypertensive medications (see Table 5.1) should be considered.

If the blood pressure is significantly elevated, however, as with a diastolic level above 110 mmHg, or in the presence of other serious risk factors, antihypertensive drug therapy should be instituted immediately with an intermediate to long-acting diuretic (see Table 5.1). The second drug commonly prescribed is an adrenergic blocking agent when the diuretic alone is inadequate to control hypertension.

Although some physicians do not treat elderly patients with only systolic hypertension, it definitely carries an increased risk. Therefore, systolic hypertension above 170 to 180 mmHg should be treated. The best approach is to attempt to lower the BP by using intermittent diuretics. When this approach is ineffective, a daily diuretic is given. If systolic hypertension persists in spite of daily diuretic therapy, the second drug (such as alpha methyldopa, reserpine, or a beta blocker; see Table 5.1) may be added. Unfortunately, the therapeutic result for elderly patients with systolic hypertension is often disappointing. It is important not to reduce BP too vigorously in elderly patients. The patient should be protected from weakness, dizziness, or even fainting as a result of postural hypotension (sudden reduction of BP on standing or sitting) produced by too aggressive antihypertensive therapy.

As far as the therapeutic approach to hypertensive children is concerned, dietary treatment is very important, particularly as it relates to weight loss or prevention of obesity. It has been shown that the association between excessive weight and fixed hypertension is strong in children. Caloric intake should be reduced, as should salt consumption. It is essential to prevent salt abuse in all hypertensive children. Most children and adolescents with borderline to mild hypertension will not require medication. When high diastolic pressure persists above 90 mmHg in children below twelve years, after the aforementioned measures, antihypertensive drug therapy should be considered. The same therapeutic approach is applied for persisting diastolic hypertension above 100 mmHg for older children, above twelve years of age. Of course, the possible underlying disorder responsible for secondary hypertension (e.g., coarctation of the aorta) should always be considered for children with persisting hypertension.

Diet Therapy

There are two major purposes for dietary therapy. One of these is to restrict sodium intake, and the other is to reduce animal fat intake. Diet therapy is discussed in detail in Chapter 19.

Medications

There are many types of medication available to reduce high BP, and some drugs can eliminate extra fluid and salt from the body. Fortunately, in most cases of primary (essential) hypertension and even in some of secondary hypertension, various antihypertensive medications will lower BP. However, it is necessary to go through a trial period before a medicine or combination of medicines is found to work best and to cause the fewest side effects, because every individual responds to medication in very different ways. Remember that high BP is a lifetime illness and that every patient needs constant medical care. Once a medication is prescribed for hypertension, the patient should take that drug indefinitely. No one should discontinue any antihypertensive drug without consulting the physician. Patients with high BP should go to see their doctor regularly so that changes in medication can be made if necessary and other necessary medical advice can be provided. When constant and proper medical care is not provided, serious and life-threatening complications may develop, and it may be too late to reverse the clinical situation. Death may be unavoidable in this circumstance.

Antihypertensive drug therapy is indicated when nondrug therapy (e.g., low-salt diet, weight reduction) is ineffective for mild hypertension. Likewise, antihypertensive drugs may be instituted immediately if the BP is significantly elevated, as with a diastolic level about 110 mmHg, or in the presence of other serious cardiovascular risks. In almost all patients, drug therapy should be started with an intermediate to long-acting diuretic. When diuretic therapy is ineffective, a second drug (e.g., propranolol, methyldopa, or reserpine) may be added. In general, the standard "stepped care" treatment approach is commonly utilized for antihypertensive drug therapy (see Table 5.2). Major antihypertensive drugs and doses are summarized in Tables 5.1 and 5.2.

For long-term therapy, all medications for hypertension are tablet forms (occasionally capsules) that are taken by mouth. In some patients, supplementary potassium may be necessary during antihypertensive drug therapy because some medications (e.g., diuretics) cause excessive excretion of potassium ion. Fortunately, potassium loss from diuretic therapy is not significant in most cases, and the generous intake of fruit juice (e.g., orange juice) is sufficient to supplement the potassium loss. For severe hypertension (e.g., malignant hypertension), medications are administered intravenously (discussed later).

Special diagnostic tests (discussed previously) for some forms of secondary hypertension may be necessary when various combinations of antihypertensive drugs are ineffective in reducing high BP.

TABLE 5.2. Standard "Stepped Care" Treatment Approach.*

Therapy Stage	Drug	Daily Dose Range
One	Thiazide congeners (e.g., hydrochlorothiazide) plus	50-100 mg.
Two	Rauwolfia derivatives (e.g., reserpine) or	0.25-0.50 mg.
	Methyldopa or	500-3000 mg.
	Propranolol plus	60-320 mg.
Three	Hydralazine or plus	75-200 mg.
Four	Methyldopa or Guanethidine or Clonidine	500-3000 mg. 10-200 mg. 0.4-3.6 mg.

*The physician adds additional antihypertensive therapy to the maximal dose of previous level of therapy when arterial pressure fails to become reduced to normotensive levels (less than 140/90 mm. Hg).
Reproduced with permission from Chung, E.K.: *Quick Reference to Cardiovascular Diseases.* Philadelphia, J.B. Lippincott Co., 1977.

Treatment for Secondary Hypertension

In certain forms of secondary hypertension, high BP may be cured by eliminating its directly underlying causes. For secondary hypertension, the surgical approach is often a successful cure for high BP. Excision of the coarctation of the aorta or repair of the renal artery stenosis is usually effective. Likewise, removal of a tumor is often successful in curing hypertension (e.g., cortical or medullary adrenal tumors, pheochromocytomas, aldosterone-producing tumors).

When hypertension is not cured by the surgical approach under these circumstances, antihypertensive drug therapy as outlined previously should be instituted. Likewise, the drug therapy is indicated if the surgical approach is contraindicated as technically impossible or otherwise. Fortunately, antihypertensive drug therapy is often effective in some patients with secondary hypertension even when the underlying disorder responsible for the production of high BP is not eliminated.

Treatment for Hypertensive Emergencies

When BP is markedly elevated, the clinical situation becomes extremely serious, and various life-threatening conditions (e.g., acute hypertensive encephalopathy, acute CHF, intracranial hemorrhage, acute coronary insufficiency, acute dissecting aortic aneurysm, and malignant and accelerated hypertension) occur singly or in combination. In these clinical circumstances, the term *hypertensive emergencies* is used, and immediate reduction of BP is indicated. For treatment of hypertensive emergencies, various rapid-acting and moderately rapid-acting antihypertensive drugs have to be administered intravenously (sometimes intramuscularly). Several parenteral agents are available, but no single agent can be classified as the drug of choice. Nevertheless, an outline for preferred drugs for the treatment of various clinical circumstances in hypertensive emergencies is shown in Table 5.3. The usual dosage and major side effects of commonly used drugs for hypertensive emergencies are summarized in Table 5.4. Among these drugs, diazoxide (Hyperstat), sodium nitroprusside (Nipride), and trimethaphan (Arfonad) are the most commonly used, rapid-acting antihypertensive agents. Reserpine (Serpasil), hydralazine (Apresoline), and methyldopa (Aldomet) are commonly used moderately rapid-acting antihypertensive agents. As soon as the BP elevation is no longer at a critical level and the clinical condition becomes stable, oral antihypertensive drugs can be instituted so that intravenous drugs may gradually be stopped as clinical circumstances permit.

Before the initiation of therapy for hypertensive emergencies, baseline chest X-ray, ECG, determination of serum electrolytes, renal function studies, and routine blood tests (blood counts, hemoglobin, and so on) should be obtained. In addition, constant and careful monitoring, particularly of BP level, is essential during parenteral antihypertensive drug therapy. Otherwise, excessive reduction of BP may be produced by a potent agent, and it may be fatal.

124

TABLE 5.3. Outline for Parenteral Drug Treatment of Hypertensive Emergencies.

Emergency	Preferred Drugs	Drugs to Avoid or Use with Caution
Acute hypertensive encephalopathy	Diazoxide Sodium nitroprusside	Reserpine Methyldopa
Acute ventricular failure	Sodium nitroprusside Trimethaphan Pentolinium	Hydralazine
Intracranial hemorrhage	Sodium nitroprusside Trimethaphan Pentolinium	Reserpine Methyldopa
Acute coronary insufficiency	Sodium nitroprusside Reserpine	Hydralazine
Acute dissecting aortic aneurysm	Trimethaphan	Hydralazine Diazoxide
Malignant and accelerated hypertension	Diazoxide Sodium nitroprusside Reserpine Trimethaphan Pentolinium	
Excess circulating catecholamines	Phentolamine Sodium nitroprusside	All others

Reproduced with permission from Chung, E.K.: *Cardiac Emergency Care*, Second Edition. Philadelphia, Lea & Febiger Publishers, 1980.

Treatment of Complications

All patients with *hypertensive encephalopathy* should be treated in an intensive care unit where changes in BP, state of consciousness, convulsive activity, and airway obstruction can be monitored closely and treated expeditiously. As outlined previously, antihypertensive drug therapy should be administered parenterally for rapid reduction of high BP. The agents of choice in most instances are diazoxide (Hyperstat) or sodium nitroprusside (Nipride), but hydralazine (Apresoline) may be particularly effective in controlling hypertensive encephalopathy associated with acute glomerulonephritis or toxemia of pregnancy (see Tables 5.3 and 5.4).

In *acute CHF* (see also Chapter 6), prompt BP reduction is generally more important than digitalis, although digitalis is also beneficial in conjunction with the use of parenteral antihypertensive drug therapy. Sodium nitroprusside (Nipride) or trimethaphan (Arfonad) is particularly useful in the management of hypertensive

TABLE 5.4. Drugs Commonly Used in Hypertensive Emergencies.

Drug	Route	Usual Dosage	Onset of Action	Major Side Effects
Vasodilators				
Diazoxide (Hyperstat)	IV rapidly	300 mg	3-5 min	Hyperglycemia, flushing, nausea, vomiting
Sodium nitroprusside (Nipride)	IV drip	50-150 mg/L	Immediate	Nausea, vomiting, muscle twitching, possible thiocyanate toxicity
Hydralazine (Apresoline)	IM or IV	10-50 mg	IV:10 min IM:30 min	Palpitation, tachycardia, flushing, headache, angina
Sympathetic Inhibitors				
Trimethaphan (Arfonad)	IV drip	1000 mg/L	Immediate	Urinary retention, ileus, dry mouth, loss of accommodation
Phentolamine (Regitine)	IM or IV	5-15 mg	Immediate	Flushing, tachycardia
Reserpine (Serpasil)	IM or IV	1-5 mg	1-3 hr	Drowsiness, stupor
Methyldopa (Aldomet)	IV	250-1000 mg	2-6 hr	Drowsiness, liver abnormalities
Duretics				
Furosemide (Lasix)	IM or IV	40-80 mg	1-5 min	Cramps, hypokalemia
Ethacrynic acid (Edecrin)	IV	50-100 mg	1-5 min	Cramps, hypokalemia

Reproduced with permission from Chung, E.K.: *Cardiac Emergency Care*, Second Edition. Philadelphia, Lea & Febiger Publishers, 1980.

emergency associated with acute CHF. Potent diuretics (e.g., furosemide [Lasix]) should also be employed, because they tend to enhance the BP reduction and to exert favorable anticongestive effects as well. Markedly elevated BP may be complicated by *brain (subarachnoid or intracerebral) hemorrhage.* BP reduction is generally indicated in this clinical circumstance, and the agents of choice are sodium nitroprusside (Nipride) or trimethaphan (Arfonad). Neurologic consultation should also be obtained, especially in subarachnoid hemorrhage, in which surgical treatment may be more important than antihypertensive drug therapy.

It has repeatedly been emphasized that the risk of *angina or heart attack* is much greater in hypertensive patients than in normotensive people. When acute coronary insufficiency is associated with marked BP elevation, sodium nitroprusside (Nipride) is very useful. In addition, parenteral reserpine (Serpasil) is also valuable because of its gradual antihypertensive effect, as well as its sedative action. Hypertension is the most common precursor of *acute aortic dissection,* and this condition can often be stabilized by antihypertensive drug therapy. Rapid reduction of elevated BP is indicated either to prevent further dissection until surgery can be performed or as the definitive, permanent measure to prevent extension of the dissection. Intravenous administration of trimethaphan (Arfonad) is commonly used in this condition. Unless surgery is imminent, it is also advisable to begin immediately long-term drug therapy including a diuretic and antihypertensive agent (e.g., propranolol or guanethidine) that decreases myocardial contractility.

Malignant and accelerated hypertension represents a semiemergency in which BP reduction is required within days rather than within minutes or hours. Prompt BP reduction may at times be achieved with oral antihypertensive drug therapy. However, for rapid control of hypertension, parenteral antihypertensive drug therapy is preferable for at least the first several days. Commonly used agents include diazoxide, sodium nitroprusside, reserpine, trimethaphan, and pentolinium (see Tables 5.3 and 5.4).

Hypertensive crises associated with excess circulating catecholamines should be suspected in patients with markedly elevated BP associated with headache, palpitations, excessive sweating, tachycardia, facial pallor, and tremor of the hands. This condition may be caused by pheochromocytoma, abrupt withdrawal of clonidine, or ingestion of monoamine oxidase inhibitors plus tyramine-containing foods. Under these circumstances, phentolamine or sodiun nitroprusside are the pharmacologic antagonists of choice to control high BP. In addition, propranolol may be administered intravenously in order to control any associated tachyarrhythmias.

In the presence of *renal failure,* hypertension is quite dependent on blood volume. If the BP is not reduced by vigorous use of antihypertensive drugs including furosemide, propranolol, or repeated injections of diazoxide, renal dialysis should be employed. In most cases, the BP will be reduced as the patient achieves a dry weight state. On rare occasions, bilateral nephrectomy (removal of both kidneys) may be necessary to control severe hypertension.

Although many individuals with slight elevation of BP may be able to live a normal or near-normal span, most patients with untreated hypertensive cardiovascular disease die of complications within twenty years. Before modern antihypertensive agents were available, approximately 70 percent of patients died of CHF or CAD, 15 percent of brain hemorrhage, and 10 percent of renal failure. In the past decade, the mortality rate in all hypertensive patients has declined considerably, primarily because of the availability of effective antihypertensive agents (see Tables 5.1 to 5.4), and it is not more than 40 percent even in advanced cases. Today, serious complications directly from high BP occur very rarely in the well-treated patient population. Likewise, the incidence of brain hemorrhage and of dissecting aneurysm of the aorta has decreased markedly.

Another important reason for the improved mortality rate is the better understanding and faithful cooperation of many patients. Remember that inadequate medical treatment has practically the same result as no treatment at all. Therefore, it is extremely important that every patient be highly motivated and fully educated to be aware of the serious nature of life-threatening complications of high BP. Otherwise, a constant and lifelong program of medical treatment is virtually impossible.

One important fact regarding the efficacy of treatment and mortality in hypertensive patients is that the benefits of antihypertensive drug therapy are much more pronounced in younger individuals, before atherosclerosis takes place. The efficacy of medical treatment is much less obvious in older patients who have other risk factors for atherosclerosis, such as hyperlipidemia, diabetes mellitus, obesity, and so forth (see Table 3.1). Therefore, high BP must be treated while the patient is still young, before other risk factors are present.

6

HEART FAILURE

Heart failure or congestive heart failure (CHF) means that the heart is unable to pump enough blood to meet the body's demands. It is important to emphasize that CHF is a final expression of deteriorating function of the heart; it is by no means a complete diagnosis of heart disease. Deteriorating cardiac function is primarily due to two major mechanisms: (1) impairment of myocardial contractile force (e.g., heart attack, cardiomyopathy), and (2) mechanical abnormality (e.g., valvular heart diseases—narrowing or leaking of heart valves and various congenital heart diseases). However, in many cases, both mechanical abnormality as well as the impairment of myocardial contractile force are responsible for the production of CHF. Numerous underlying heart diseases (e.g., CAD, hypertensive heart disease, rheumatic heart disease, congenital heart disease, cardiomyopathy) may cause CHF. Therefore, CHF is *not* the primary diagnosis of heart disease; rather, it is the expression of the end result of abnormal cardiac function of differing degrees resulting from a variety of underlying diseases.

There are many ways to classify CHF. For example, it may be placed in two major categories: (1) left ventricular failure and (2) right ventricular failure, depending upon the underlying cardiac disease and the resultant involvement of a particular cardiac chamber. In many cases with advanced CHF, both ventricles are involved; in this circumstance, the term *biventricular failure* is used. In many cases, CHF starts with left ventricular failure only, but right ventricular failure often follows as cardiac function deteriorates, so that the end result is biventricular failure. It can be said, therefore, that the most common cause of right ventricular failure is left ventricular failure in most cases with advanced heart disease.

Congestive heart failure is also classified according to functional capacity. For instance, the *New York Heart Association Functional Classification* provides an extremely useful guideline for categorizing patients with CHF:

Class   I: Patients with documented heart disease (any type) who are completely symptom free.

Class II: Slight limitation of physical activity because symptoms (e.g., shortness of breath, chest pain) occur only with more than ordinary physical activity.

Class III: Marked limitation of physical activity because symptoms occur even with ordinary physical activity (e.g., eating meals).

Class IV: Severe limitation of physical activity because symptoms occur even at rest (e.g., in a sitting or lying position).

Of course, the functional class may change from time to time, even in the same individual, depending upon progress of the underlying heart disease and responses to treatment. For example, the patient with functional III or IV CHF on admission to the hospital may be discharged with a functional I or II condition when cardiac function improves markedly after treatment. On the other hand, functional I or II patients may progressively change to functional III or even IV when the underlying heart disease rapidly deteriorates and when response to treatment is poor.

Clinical manifestations (symptoms and physical signs) are principally related to the resultant dysfunction of other vital organs (e.g., lungs, kidneys, and liver). Namely, CHF is commonly manifested by pulmonary congestion, pulmonary edema, pleural effusion, enlargement and tenderness of the liver from congestion, ascites, and various abnormalities in kidney function. For best therapeutic results with CHF, it is essential that a physician have a firm knowledge of pathophysiology, and a specific underlying heart disease must be identified. With patients with refractory and advanced CHF, identification of surgically correctable cardiac lesions is extremely important. In addition, various contributing factors (e.g., excessive salt intake, thyroid disease, anemia, abnormal heart rhythms) must be identified and corrected. When medications are used, it is vital to prevent a variety of side effects and toxicity of drugs, and electrolyte imbalance and drug toxicity must be corrected immediately.

CAUSES (ETIOLOGY)

There are numerous underlying disorders, and the causes may be divided into two major categories: (1) cardiac diseases and (2) extracardiac diseases. Without question, hypertension is the most common underlying disease.

Cardiac Diseases

Cardiac diseases can be further divided into two categories: (1) impairment of the contractile force and (2) mechanical abnormalities.

Impairment of the Contractile Force

The typical example of contractile impairment is heart attack in which the left ventricular myocardium becomes necrotic and is replaced by useless and noncontracting fibrous tissues (like scar tissues). Other examples include cardiomyopathy (heart muscle disease—see Chapter 12), hypertensive heart disease, and myocarditis (inflammatory or infectious process of the heart muscle—see Chapter 13).

Mechanical Abnormalities

Mechanical abnormalities may include a variety of valvular heart diseases (see Chapter 11), congenital cardiac defects (see Chapter 10), ventricular aneurysm, and constrictive pericarditis or cardiac tamponade (see Chapter 13).

In many cases, however, mechanical abnormalities and impairment of myocardial contractility coexist. For instance, most patients with CHF resulting from acquired valvular heart diseases and adult congenital heart diseases develop significant abnormalities of myocardial contractile function consequent to the mechanical abnormality. In addition, CHF may be triggered or aggravated by a variety of cardiac arrhythmias (see Chapter 9) in the presence of mechanical abnormalities and/or impairment of cardiac contractile force. Rapid heart rate itself often precipitates or aggravates CHF; and a loss of atrial contribution to ventricular filling in the presence of atrial fibrillation or A-V dissociation (see Chapter 9) and disordered synchrony of ventricular contraction also aggravates CHF. Likewise, markedly slow heart rhythm results in inadequate cardiac output, and it may precipitate or aggravate CHF.

Extracardiac Diseases

A variety of extracardiac or noncardiac diseases may cause CHF. That is, cardiac function may be significantly altered by various systemic diseases. In other words, high-output heart failure will be produced by a variety of systemic diseases, including hyperthyroidism (thyrotoxicosis—hyperfunction of thyroid gland), arteriovenous fistula (abnormal communication between an artery and a vein from various causes, such as trauma), and anemia. In these cases, a cardiac abnormality may not be apparent, but the heart is unable to meet the excessively increased systemic demands. The term *high-output state* of the heart is somewhat comparable to an excessive fuel flow in an automobile engine, so that the engine is running fast all the time. Extracardiac CHF may also be due to mechanical disorders. For example, inadequate venous return to the heart with subsequent extracardiac CHF may result from obstruction by a tumor of the inferior or superior vena cava (the largest vein connected to the heart—see Figures 1.1 and 1.2).

When dealing with chronic and known CHF, cardiac function is frequently deteriorated, and the preexisting CHF becomes markedly aggravated primarily when any patient fails to follow necessary medical advice. For example, CHF gets worse (1) when the patient fails to take medication(s) regularly; (2) when the patient engages in activity beyond physical limitations; (3) when the patient ingests excessive salt; (4) when the patient develops drug toxicity, such as digitalis intoxication; and, finally, (5) when the underlying cardiac disease is more advanced or a new heart disease or complication is superimposed.

CLINICAL FINDINGS (SYMPTOMS AND SIGNS)

Although the speed of progression of symptoms varies depending upon the underlying disease process, the majority of patients develop remarkably similar, if not identical, complaints and symptoms during the course of CHF. Of course, symptoms vary depending upon which ventricle is predominantly involved. The earliest symptom or complaint of left ventricular failure is dyspnea, and this indicates elevated pulmonary venous pressures. Difficulty in breathing may be observed only during physical effort in the early stage (called "exertional dyspnea"), but it gradually gets worse as cardiac function deteriorates. Thus, in later stages, dyspnea occurs even at rest, and the patient often experiences a shortness of breath at night (called "paroxysmal nocturnal dyspnea"—or "PND"). Consequently, the dyspnea frequently wakes the patient during the night. The term *orthopnea* is applied when dyspnea is so marked that the patient is unable to breathe except in an upright position. Fatigue is a late symptom, and it indicates inadequately compensated reduction of cardiac output. In addition, left ventricular failure may be manifested by nocturia, diaphoresis, cough, hemoptysis (spitting up blood), and cachexia (generalized ill health and malnutrition with marked weight loss). Remember that the principal manifestations of left ventricular failure are due to pulmonary congestion. When left ventricular failure is far advanced, acute pulmonary edema is produced, and the outcome is often fatal unless it is recognized early and treated promptly.

On physical examination, the patient with marked dyspnea is very apparent. Common physical findings of left ventricular failure include tachycardia (rapid heart rate), tachypnea (rapid breathing), cool skin, diaphoresis, cyanosis (purplish skin color), moist rales, and wheezing (bubbling or squeaking sounds in the lungs from difficult air passage because of excessive congestion) in the chest (through a stethoscope), signs of cardiomegaly, and gallop heart rhythms. On precordial palpation, the apical impulse is enlarged, and it is displaced to the left. There may be pansystolic (or holosystolic) murmur (the murmur occupying the entire systolic phase of the cardiac cycle) of functional mitral insufficiency as a result of dilatation of the mitral valve ring in advanced left ventricular failure. In some patients with severe left ventricular failure, there may be pleural effusion (fluid accumulation in the thoracic cavity) and/or pericardial effusion (fluid accumulation around the heart—in the pericardial sac).

Right ventricular failure is manifested by elevated venous pressure (e.g., engorgement of neck veins), hepatomegaly (enlarged liver) with tenderness, jaundice (yellowish skin), and edema of extremities. In advanced cases, there may be splenomegaly (enlarged spleen), ascites (fluid accumulation in the abdominal cavity), and anasarca (generalized massive edema involving all parts of the body, including genitalia, the chest wall, and even the face). These manifestations of right ventricular failure are principally related to resultant dysfunction of the liver. There may be a pansystolic murmur of functional tricuspid insufficiency (regurgitation) as a result of dilatation of the tricuspid valve ring. In biventricular failure, of course, there will be combined manifestations of left and right ventricular failure. In advanced and refractory heart failure, both ventricles are usually diseased. Needless to say, various symptoms and physical findings of the underlying heart diseases and/or systemic diseases (e.g., anemia, hyperthyroidism) will be observed in addition to the manifestations of CHF.

DIAGNOSIS

The diagnosis of CHF is relatively easy to establish when there are characteristic clinical findings, as already described. However, the diagnosis is *not* always simple in every case when clinical manifestations of the underlying heart disease are predominant and CHF is incipient or mild. Likewise, the diagnosis becomes less apparent when other complications (cardiac as well as noncardiac) and/or other disorders (e.g., various lung diseases) coexist. Various laboratory tests are available to assist the diagnosis, but none of them are specific for the documentation of CHF. Detailed descriptions of various diagnostic tests are found in Chapter 24.

Routine Laboratory Tests

Routine blood and urine tests may be entirely within normal limits, especially in the mild form. Electrolyte imbalance may be present, depending upon the duration and severity of CHF and previous diuretic therapy. Hyponatremia (reduced sodium content in the blood) and reduced urinary sodium concentrations may be present. Blood counts are usually normal unless there is preexisting anemia. Serum enzymes will be elevated when there is sufficient congestion and dysfunction of the liver; otherwise, they are within normal limits. Other liver function tests will also be abnormal when liver function is significantly impaired. Of course, serum enzymes will be markedly elevated when CHF is secondary to acute MI. When there is significant renal dysfunction from reduced renal blood flow in advanced CHF, blood urea nitrogen (BUN) will be elevated, and other kidney function tests will also be abnormal. Other abnormal laboratory test results (e.g., elevated blood sugar, increased contents of serum cholesterol and/or triglycerides) may be present depending upon the coexistence and severity of other disorders (e.g., diabetes mellitus, hyperlipidemia) that are closely linked to CAD, hypertension, and CHF.

Chest X-Ray

Chest X-ray is useful primarily to detect any abnormality in the heart and lung field. Heart size is commonly enlarged either because of dilatation of the chambers from CHF itself or because of preexisting hypertrophy from various underlying heart diseases.

Various abnormalities in the lung fields are frequently observed in patients with long-standing or advanced CHF primarily as a result of pulmonary congestion and even pulmonary edema. Common chest X-ray findings include increased pulmonary vascular markings consisting of bilateral prominence of the superior pulmonary veins, dilatation of the central right and left pulmonary arteries, interstitial density of the central lung markings, interlobar fluid, and Kerley-B lines (horizontal thin lines at the lower lung fields). In far-advanced cases, pleural effusion (fluid accumulation in the thorax) may be present. In acute pulmonary edema, the entire lung field becomes so hazy and ill defined that pulmonary markings cannot be identified because of excessive fluid accumulation in the lungs. Pericardial effusion, which is a common manifestation of severe and advanced CHF, produces a diffusely enlarged heart shadow (see Chapter 13).

Electrocardiography

There are no ECG findings that are specific for the diagnosis of CHF. Rather, various ECG abnormalities are produced primarily as a result of underlying heart diseases. In addition, a variety of cardiac arrhythmias are frequently associated with CHF because cardiac arrhythmias may trigger the development of CHF and because they are often produced by CHF. Therefore, there is a bidirectional relationship between cardiac arrhythmias and congestive heart failure. Low voltage of the ECG complexes (reduced amplitude of ECG deflections) is common in advanced congestive heart failure.

Echocardiography and Myocardial Imaging

Both echocardiography and myocardial imaging are discussed in Chapter 24.

Cardiac Catheterization and Coronary Arteriography

Cardiac catheterization is *not* routinely performed for patients with CHF, but it is often necessary to confirm the underlying heart lesion, especially when dealing with refractory CHF and when any form of heart surgery (e.g., surgical repair of congenital cardiac defect, CABS) is attempted.

Miscellaneous Tests

Prolongation of the *arm-to-tongue circulation time* is highly suggestive of a depressed cardiac output, which is commonly found in CHF. The circulation time is measured from when a chemical substance (called Decholin, 3 to 5 ml) is injected into the arm vein until the patient experiences a bitter taste on the tongue. In normal people, the arm-to-tongue circulation time is between ten and sixteen seconds, but if the circulation time is above sixteen seconds, the test result is considered abnormal.

Measurement of venous pressure is often helpful in diagnosing CHF, because the venous pressure is usually elevated in this circumstance. As far as the technique of venous pressure measurement is concerned, the arm is abducted to about 60°, and the antecubital fossa (inner surface of the elbow joint) is supported at the level of midchest. The arm vein is punctured with a large (18-gauge) needle so that there is a brisk backflow of blood. A 10-ml flushing syringe and heparin-saline-filled manometer tube are connected to the needle by a three-way stopcock. The manometer is then turned on to monitor the venous pressure now represented by the height of the saline column above the selected reference level. Normal peripheral venous pressure ranges from 2 to 12 cm of water, and pressure above these values is considered abnormal.

DIFFERENTIAL DIAGNOSIS

The diagnosis is usually straightforward when the underlying heart disease is obvious and when various symptoms and physical signs are characteristic of CHF. However, various primary diseases involving lungs, kidneys, and liver may closely mimic CHF in some cases. For example, pneumonia or acute bronchitis may resemble CHF because of abnormal chest X-ray findings, pulmonary rales, dyspnea, and cough. However, clinical and laboratory confirmation of infection and response to antibiotic (e.g., penicillin) therapy will distinguish from CHF. High fever, sputum production, and leukocytosis (increased white blood cell counts) are hallmarks of pneumonia, but these findings are absent in CHF.

In some patients with pulmonary embolism (blood clots in the lungs), the clinical picture and, at times, chest X-ray findings superficially resemble CHF, but

135

differential diagnosis is usually made in most cases. In careful examination, there is usually a source of a blood clot (commonly in the lower extremities–thrombophlebitis) in a patient with pulmonary embolism, and hemoptysis (spitting up blood) is relatively common in this disease. Lung scan usually confirms the diagnosis of pulmonary embolism. In a lung scan, a radioactive compound is injected into the circulation of the lungs, and areas of the lungs containing blood clots are thus revealed.

Chronic pulmonary diseases (e.g., pulmonary emphysema) at times mimic CHF; however, patients with pulmonary diseases usually have no paroxysmal nocturnal dyspnea (this is most common in CHF). In addition, pulmonary asthma may resemble acute CHF because wheezing and severe dyspnea occur in both conditions. The mechanisms involved in both entities are entirely different, however. An asthma attack is usually triggered by bronchospasms from an allergic reaction, whereas wheezing and dyspnea in CHF are due to congestion and edema in the lungs from weakened heart function. In fact, the term *cardiac asthma* has been used to describe severe wheezing from acute CHF, because the finding closely simulates pulmonary asthma in many cases. Needless to say, a patient with pulmonary asthma fails to show any evidence of heart disease. Various pulmonary function tests, clinical history, physical findings, chest X-ray findings, and cardiac catheterization will distinguish between cardiac failure and lung diseases in difficult cases.

At times, various kidney diseases and renal failure may mimic CHF because advanced renal diseases frequently cause generalized edema. However, various kidney function tests and urinalysis will determine the diagnosis of a specific kidney disease. Elevated venous pressure, which is very common in heart failure, usually does not occur in a pure kidney disease. Of course, there is no evidence of heart disease in patients with pure kidney disease. Primary liver diseases may result in an enlarged liver, ascites, and elevated serum enzymes similar to those present in passive liver congestion due to CHF. The term *cardiac cirrhosis* has been used to describe the enlarged liver from long-standing congestion secondary to chronic CHF. One should not confuse this with liver cirrhosis (better known as alcoholic liver cirrhosis) from excessive consumption of alcohol over a long period of time. Remember also that the heart may be damaged by alcohol by an individual who drinks too much for a long time (causing alcoholic cardiomyopathy–see Chapter 12). The primary liver disease and CHF are usually distinguished by a clinical history, physical findings, and laboratory tests.

TREATMENT

The objectives of treatment for CHF are to eliminate or correct the underlying cause, increase the force and efficiency of myocardial pumping action, and reduce the abnormal retention of sodium (salt) and water. Since the diagnosis of CHF is by no means a complete description of heart disease, the underlying disorder must be identified. For the best therapeutic approach, simultaneous treatment of underlying heart diseases is essential. For the same reason, underlying noncardiac and systemic diseases (e.g., anemia, hyperthyroidism) responsible for the production of CHF must be treated simultaneously.

A specific search should be made for surgically correctable cardiac lesions (e.g., various forms of congenital lesions, valvular heart diseases), especially when CHF fails to respond to conventional medical therapy. In some CHF cases, particularly those due to congenital or valvular lesions, the surgical treatment may cure the underlying heart disease as well as CHF altogether. Other forms of curable CHF may be due to nutritional deficiencies (e.g., beriberi heart disease resulting from vitamin B deficiency) or dysfunction of the thyroid gland (e.g., thyrotoxicosis or hyperthyroidism resulting from hyperfunction and myxedema or hypothyroidism resulting from hypofunction). Under these circumstances, no further medical therapy may be indicated after surgical correction of the cardiac lesion or correction of noncardiac disorders. However, long-term medical treatment is necessary for most patients with CHF, and many individuals require constant care.

It is extremely important to recognize that the patient shares a significant responsibility in the management of CHF, because the treatment is long-term in most cases and because it involves certain degrees of restriction on diet and physical activity in addition to faithful usage of various medications, especially digitalis (the "heart pill") and diuretics (the "water pill") under a competent physician's guidance. The prescribed medications must be taken even when the patient feels well. Remember that most people with CHF may feel well simply because of the action of various essential medications.

Various contributing factors should be carefully sought, especially in patients with chronic CHF when the clinical picture has suddenly deteriorated. In most cases, CHF is triggered or aggravated by omission of necessary medications, excessive intake of salt, excessive activity beyond physical limitations, or any combination of the above. Otherwise, any cardiac arrhythmia, worsening of the underlying heart disease, or development of new heart diseases or noncardiac diseases frequently cause new CHF or aggravate preexisting chronic CHF. From the preceding observation, it is very important that all patients be properly educated and highly motivated so that they may be able to share the important responsibility to achieve best therapeutic results. Unfortunately, every important medication used to treat CHF can cause various side effects and toxicity. This is also one of the most important reasons why every patient must be followed constantly by a competent physician.

Rest

Physical as well as emotional rest is one of the most important aspects of treatment of CHF regardless of its underlying disorder. When an adequate resting period is not provided, good results are impossible to achieve regardless of how well other therapeutic regimens are followed. Depending upon the severity of CHF and the nature of the underlying heart disease, some patients may require complete bed rest, whereas others may just need to sit in a chair. It has been clearly documented that rest alone reduces the work load on the heart and promotes diuresis. Complete bed rest is essential in patients with acute advanced CHF, especially when the underlying disorder is any form of active heart disease (e.g., heart attack). Adequate rest should be maintained until heart function returns to normal with a gradual increment in physical activity. If necessary, mild sedatives or sleeping pills may be required to promote a comfortable resting period for some patients. The duration of the resting state varies depending upon the severity of CHF and the nature of the underlying heart disease, but rest should be continued as long as necessary to permit the heart to regain reserve strength. On the other hand, unnecessary prolongation of the resting period should be avoided, because generalized debility of the patient may be produced under this circumstance.

In addition, many patients with heart disease are prone to develop phlebitis (inflammation of veins) or thrombophlebitis (blood clot formation in the inflamed veins), especially in the lower extremities, after prolonged bed rest. Therefore, passive or active leg exercises should be performed frequently in order to prevent thrombophlebitis. An elastic stocking may also be useful. In patients with chronic or long-standing CHF, excessive activity beyond their physical limitations should be avoided. Detailed descriptions of physical activities in cardiac patients are found in Chapter 21.

Diet

The degree of sodium restriction depends upon the severity of CHF and the ease with which it can be controlled by other means. Nevertheless, sodium restriction (to some degree) is mandatory for every patient with CHF, even during diuretic therapy. In many patients with mild CHF, control of physical activities with careful diet therapy is sufficient to improve cardiac function without drugs. Detailed descriptions of diet therapy are found in Chapter 19.

Digitalis ("Heart Pill")

Digitalis (better known as the "heart pill") is one of the oldest and most commonly used drugs in medicine. The inotropic action of digitalis causes an increase in myocardial contractility, leading to stronger and more effective pumping action in the ventricles. This is why digitalis is very valuable in the treatment of CHF, particularly with low-output failure consequent to myocardial dysfunction. Various methods of digitalization are summarized in Table 6.1, and digitalis is discussed fully in Chapter 17.

TABLE 6.1. Methods of Digitalization.

	Very Rapid Digitalization (Within 12 Hr)	Rapid Digitalization (Within 24 Hr)	Moderately Rapid Digitalization (Within 2-3 Days)	Slow Digitalization (Within 5-8 Days)	Digitalization With Daily Oral Maintenance Dosage
Digoxin	0.5-1 mg IV initially, then 0.25-0.5 mg q̄ 2-4 hr as needed	1-1.5 mg by mouth initially, then 0.5 mg q̄ 6 hr until digitalized	0.5 mg t.i.d. by mouth for 2-3 days until digitalized	0.25 mg t.i.d. by mouth for 5-8 days until digitalized	0.25 mg daily by mouth
Deslanoside	0.8-1.6 mg IV initially, then 0.4 mg q̄ 2-4 hr as needed	—	—	—	—
Ouabain	0.25-0.5 mg IV initially, then 0.1 mg q̄ ½ hr as needed	—	—	—	—
Digitoxin	—	0.8 mg by mouth initially, then 0.2 mg q̄ 6 hr until digitalized	0.2 mg t.i.d. by mouth for 2-3 days until digitalized	0.1 mg t.i.d. by mouth for 5-8 days until digitalized	0.1 mg daily by mouth
Digitalis leaf	—	0.8 g by mouth initially, then 0.2 g q̄ 6 hr until digitalized	0.2 g t.i.d. by mouth for 2-3 days until digitalized	0.1 g t.i.d. by mouth for 5-8 days until digitalized	0.1 g daily by mouth

Reproduced from Chung, E.K.: *Cardiac Emergency Care*, Second Edition, Philadelphia, Lea & Febiger Pub., 1980.

Diuretics ("Water Pills")

Various diuretics (better known as "water pills") are extremely useful in the treatment of CHF. The type, dosage, and route of administration depend on the severity and duration of CHF, previous diuretic therapy, and the status of serum electrolytes. In mild cases, oral diuretic therapy is sufficient without digitalis in most cases, in conjunction with a proper rest and diet program. In advanced cases, both diuretics and digitalis are indicated along with the restricted diet program and adequate rest. When CHF is far advanced or very acute (such as in acute pulmonary edema), rapid-acting diuretics must be administered intravenously. Otherwise, oral diuretics (e.g., thiazides) are used in mild cases, and they are suitable for long-term therapy.

Furosemide (Lasix) and Ethacrynic Acid (Edecrin)

Furosemide (Lasix) and ethacrynic acid (Edecrin) are available as oral tablets and also in liquid form for intravenous route. For urgent clinical situations, Lasix can be given intravenously (at times intramuscularly) in dosages of 20 to 40 mg in average adults; the second dose may be given after two hours as needed. Similarly, Edecrin can be given intravenously in a dosage of 50 mg (0.5 to 1.0 mg/kg of body weight) in average adult patients. Intramuscular or subcutaneous injection of Edecrin must be avoided because the drug often causes severe local pain or irritation of the injection site. Lasix is preferable because of fewer side effects. These parenteral diuretics possess the rapid onset of action within thirty minutes. Potassium replacement is required during administration of these drugs.

When the clinical situation is not urgent, these diuretics can be given orally. The usual doses of Lasix by mouth range from 20 to 80 mg daily, whereas Edecrin can be given orally in dosages ranging from 25 to 100 mg daily. Again, supplementary oral potassium is advised. Lasix is also a very valuable antihypertensive drug, so this agent is ideal when congestive heart failure is due to hypertension.

Thiazide Diuretics

Thiazide diuretics (available in tablets) are probably most commonly used, particularly for long-term diuretic therapy, and they are given by mouth. The usual dosages of chlorothiazide (e.g., Diuril) range from 250 to 1,000 mg daily. Hydrochlorothiazide (e.g., Hydrodiuril, Esidrix) can be given in doses between 25 and 100 mg daily, but it may be increased up to 200 mg per day, if necessary, under careful medical supervision. Again, supplementary potassium is recommended, particularly when large doses are prescribed. Periodic determination of serum potassium is necessary so that proper potassium replacement can be carried out during diuretic therapy. At times, hyperkalemia (increased potassium value in the body) may be produced by excessive administration of potassium. Of course, hyperkalemia is also harmful to the body, particularly to heart function. Many physicians start with a small dose (e.g., 25 to 50 mg of hydrochlorothiazide daily), and the drug is often given intermittently (e.g., 25 or 50 mg every other day or every third day) during the early stage of treatment for mild CHF, especially in elderly people.

One of the common side effects of thiazide therapy is gout (painful swelling of the toes), but discontinuation of the drug is usually sufficient to cure thiazide-induced gout. Remember that hypokalemia (reduced potassium value in the body) induced by thiazides may cause digitalis intoxication when digitalis and thiazide are given together, because hypokalemia predisposes to digitalis toxicity (see Chapter 17).

In addition to having potent diuretic effects, thiazide diuretics are the most important and most popular antihypertensive agents. Therefore, various thiazide diuretics are the ideal drugs for treating CHF when it is due to or associated with hypertension. In fact, thiazide diuretics are probably one of the most commonly prescribed drugs today.

Potassium-Sparing Diuretics

Potassium-sparing diuretics such as spironolactone (Aldactone) or triamterene (Dyrenium) can be used in conjunction with a thiazide to neutralize the potassium-wasting effect of the latter. The initial dosage of Aldactone is 25 mg four times daily, and 50 to 100 mg are recommended as a daily dosage. Aldactone is an aldosterone-antagonist, and it may cause hyperkalemia, drowsiness, hypotension (low blood pressure), and breast tenderness. Onset of the clinical effect of the drug may be delayed for one week. Aldactone is an expensive drug compared to other drugs, and it is *not* recommended for patients with renal failure. The drug may also be used with ethacrynic acid or furosemide. Dyrenium may be given in place of Aldactone, and the usual dosage ranges from 100 to 200 mg per day.

Mercurial Diuretics

Mercurial diuretics are slightly more potent than the thiazide diuretics but are less commonly used today because they must be administered parenterally. The best known mercurial diuretic is mercaptomerin (Thiomerin), which can be injected intramuscularly or subcutaneously. The drug may be administered daily in a dosage of 0.1 to 1 ml, or it may be given intermittently. The effect of the drug occurs in approximately two hours and lasts ten to twelve hours. It is rather inconvenient to administer mercurial diuretics, and there are many other superior drugs available on the market. Consequently, mercurial diuretics are seldom used today.

Oxygen

Oxygen is very useful when a patient suffers from dyspnea as a result of inadequate oxygen supply from CHF.

Vasodilators

Various vasodilators (drugs that dilate the blood vessels) are highly recommended when patients with advanced CHF respond very poorly to conventional management. Detailed descriptions of vasodilators are found in Chapter 17.

Other Drugs

Prophylactic use of an *anticoagulant* (an agent that prevents blood clots, such as heparin or Coumadin) is recommended in order to reduce the high risk of pulmonary emboli (blood clots in the lungs) when there is long-standing edema in the legs, elevation of systemic venous pressure, or when prolonged bed rest is anticipated. In addition, prophylactic anticoagulation is indicated in patients with previous episodes of blood clot formation in any part of the body.

Morphine sulfate is a very important and effective agent in treating acute pulmonary edema or acute CHF. Morphine induces a central sympatholysis with beneficial relief of anxiety, decrease in tachypnea (rapid breathing), and decline in peripheral vascular resistance, resulting in less venous return to the heart. The usual dose of morphine sulfate ranges from 4 to 5 mg intravenously, and its onset of action is within ten to fifteen minutes after injection. The same dosage may be repeated as needed.

Aminophylline relieves bronchospasm and, through its inotropic effect on the heart, increases cardiac output. Aminophylline is particularly useful for acute pulmonary edema or acute CHF. This agent should be administered with caution, however, because serious and life-threatening ventricular tachyarrhythmias may be induced by rapid injection of aminophylline. Aminophylline in a dosage of 500 mg is usually administered by a slow intravenous drip over twenty to thirty minutes.

When hypertension is the underlying disorder, it should be treated with various *antihypertensive agents* (see Table 5.1), as described previously (see Chapter 5). Likewise, various *antiarrhythmic agents* (drugs that are effective in treating a variety of abnormal rapid heart rhythms) must also be used when CHF is associated with or triggered by any form of cardiac arrhythmias (see Chapter 9 and Table 6.2).

Other *inotropic agents* (drugs that produce more effective pumping action of the heart), such as isoproterenol (Isuprel), dopamine, and dobutamine, may be used in place of digitalis (heart pill) when digitalis is contraindicated, or is difficult to administer because of serious side effects, especially in the postoperative period after open heart surgery or following heart attack.

Mechanical Measures

Tourniquets, applied sufficiently tight to block venous return but not tight enough to interfere with arterial blood flow, may be applied to three extremities and rotated every fifteen minutes. Tourniquets that are designed to inflate and deflate BP cuffs automatically are available for this purpose. Rotating the tourniquets is often sufficient in treating pulmonary edema and is superior to *phlebotomy* (removal of blood). If the response is inadequate, however, phlebotomy (e.g., the withdrawal of 500 ml blood) may be used, and it is often effective in some cases. Patients with chronic CHF, an increase in blood volume, and an enlarged heart who develop pulmonary edema may benefit by rotating the tourniquets and/or phlebotomy. On the other hand, the application of tourniquets or phlebotomy may precipitate hypotension (low blood pressure) when acute pulmonary edema develops in a patient with a normal blood volume and normal (or near-normal) heart size in some cases. This type of complication is often encountered in patients with recent heart attack. When the blood volume is altered, it is essential that the BP, urine output, and BUN (blood urea nitrogen) be monitored very carefully. At the present time, rotating tourniquets and phlebotomy are less often required because rapid-acting and very effective potent diuretics (e.g., furosemide) are readily available.

Paracentesis of fluid (removal of fluid via a large needle) in the chest and abdomen should be undertaken if respiration is disturbed by fluid accumulation and if diuretic therapy is not readily effective. When there is fluid accumulation in the pericardium (called "pericardial effusion"), *pericardiocentesis* (removal of pericardial fluid via a large needle) is indicated.

Surgical Approach

Any surgically correctable cardiac lesion(s) must be looked for carefully when dealing with refractory CHF. The underlying congenital cardiac defect or significant valvular lesion is often responsible for the development of CHF. Under these circumstances, surgical correction of the lesion may cure the CHF entirely. Similarly, CABS may be extremely effective when dealing with advanced CHF due to surgically correctable CAD (see Chapter 25).

Miscellaneous

A cardioverter (direct-current shock) is indicated when tachyarrhythmias (very rapid heart rhythms) are not readily treated with various antiarrhythmic agents (see Table 6.2 and Chapter 18). Likewise, an artificial cardiac pacemaker is indicated when significant bradyarrhythmias (slow heart rhythms) are associated with CHF (see Chapter 16).

Remember that any coexisting or underlying cardiac, as well as noncardiac, disorder must be treated simultaneously. For example, in right ventricular failure due to chronic pulmonary emphysema, the underlying lung disease must be treated even more aggressively than the CHF itself. Similarly, when dealing with CHF secondary to thyrotoxicosis (hyperthyroidism), the underlying thyroid disease must be diligently treated. Otherwise, it is impossible for the best therapeutic result to be achieved.

PROGNOSIS

The prognosis of CHF largely depends on various factors, including the patient's age, nature and severity of underlying heart disease, the degree of cardiac enlargement, the extent of myocardial damage, and the nature and severity of coexisting

TABLE 6.2. Common Antiarrhythmic Drugs.

Drug	Full Dosage	Maintenance Dosage	Onset of Action	Maximum Effect	Duration of Action	Indications	SIDE EFFECTS AND TOXICITY	
							Dosage-Dependent	Dosage-Independent
Digoxin (Lanoxin)	0.5-1 mg IV initially, then 0.25-0.5 mg q̄ 2 hr as needed (total: 1-2.5 mg)	0.125-0.75 mg (average: 0.25 mg) daily (PO)	10-30 min	2-3 hr	3-6 days	SV tachyarrhythmias (AF, AFl, AT, AV JT)	Almost all known arrhythmias, aggravation of CHF, anorexia, nausea, vomiting, color vision, headache, dizziness, confusion	Allergic manifestations (urticaria, eosinophilia) idiosyncrasy, thrombocytopenia, GI hemorrhage and necrosis
Deslanoside (Cedilanid-D)	0.8-1.6 mg IV initially, then 0.4 mg q̄ 2 hr as needed (total: 1.2-2 mg)	—	10-30 min	2-3 hr	3-6 days	As above	As above	As above
Oubain (G-Strophanthin)	0.25-0.5 mg IV initially, then 0.1 mg q̄ ½ hr as need (total: 0.5-1.2 mg)	—	3-10 min	30 min-1 hr	12 hr-3 days	As above	As above	As above
Lidocaine (Xylocaine)	75-100 mg direct IV q̄ 10-20 min as needed (total: 750 mg) or 200-250 mg IM q̄ 10-20 min as needed	1-5 mg/min IV infusion	At once	At once	Minutes	Primary: V tachyarrhythmias Secondary: SV tachyarrhythmias	Dizziness, drowsiness, confusion, muscle twitching, disorientation, euphoria, cardiac and respiratory depression, convulsion, hypotension, AV and IV block	—
Procainamide Pronestyl	1-2 g/200 cc 5% D/W IV drip, 100 mg q̄ 2-4 min (1 g in 30 min-1 hr) (total: 2g) or 1 g PO initially, then 0.5 g q̄ 2-3 hr (total 3.5 g)	0.25-0.5 g q̄ 3 hr (PO)	At once / Rapid	Minutes / 1-2 hr	6 hr / 6-8 hr	Primary: V tachyarrhythmias Secondary: SV tachyarrhythmias	AV and IV block, ventricular arrhythmias, LE, nausea, vomiting, lymphadenopathy, hypotension, confusion	Allergic manifestations (eosinophilia, urticaria), agranulocytosis

Drug	Dosage	Oral maintenance	Onset of action	Maximum effect	Duration	Indications	Side effects
Quinidine gluconate	0.8 g/200 cc 5% D/W IV drip, 25 mg/min or 0.4-0.6 g IM initially then 0.4 g q̄ 2-4 hr (total: 2.6g)	—	10-15 min	Not immediate / 30-90 min	6-8 hr	Primary: SV tachyarrhythmias. Secondary: V tachyarrhythmias	AV, IV block, nausea, vomiting, photophobia, diplopia, headache, tinnitus, diarrhea, ventricular arrhythmias; Respiratory depression, hypotension, convulsion, rashes (mascular or papular), thrombocytopenic purpura, thrombocytopenia, hemolytic anemia
Quinidine sulfate	Oral route (see text)	0.3-0.4 g q̄ 6 hr (PO)	—	2-3 hr	6-8 hr	—	—
Disopyramide phosphate (Norpace)	300 mg (PO) initially, then 150 mg q̄ 6 hr	100-150 mg q̄ 6 hr (PO)	30 min-3 hr	2 hr	6-7 hr	Ventricular arrhythmias	Urinary retention, frequency, urgency, abdominal pain, nausea, anorexia, constipation, blurred vision, dryness of nose, eyes, and throat, dry mouth, headache, rash, edema, weight gain, IV block, prolonged Q-T interval and sinus node depression; —
Diphenyl-hydantoin (Dilantin)	125-250 mg IV q̄ 10-20 min as needed (total: 750 mg/hr)	100-200 mg q̄ 6 hr (PO)	At once	Minutes	4-8 hr	Primary: Digitalis-induced arrhythmias. Secondary: Nondigitalis-induced arrhythmias (ventricular)	Cardiac depression, hypotension, AV, SA block, sinus bradycardia, ataxia, tremor, gingival hyperplasia; Allergic manifestations (urticaria, purpura, eosinophilia)
Propranolol (Inderal)	1-3 mg IV initially, then second dose may be repeated after 2 min. Additional medication should not be given less than 4 hr (total: 10 mg)	10-30 mg q̄ 6 hr (PO)	At once	Minutes	3-6 hr	Various tachyarrhythmias	SA, AV block, CHF, nausea, vomiting, diarrhea, asthma, cardiogenic shock; Erythematous rashes, paresthesias of hands and fever

IV: intravenous injection; IM: intramuscular injection; q̄: every; D/W: dextrose in water; PO: orally; IV block: intraventricular block; LE: lupus erythematosus; CHF: congestive heart failure; GI: gastrointestinal; AF: atrial fibrillation; AFL: atrial flutter; AT: atrial tachycardia; AV JT: AV junctional tachycardia; SV tachyarrhythmias: supraventricular tachyarrhythmias; V tachyarrhythmias: ventricular tachyarrhythmias.

Reproduced from Chung, E.K.: Cardiac Emergency Care, Second Edition, Philadelphia, Lea & Febiger, 1980.

cardiac as well as noncardiac diseases. Without treatment, the prognosis in CHF is poor, with a five-year mortality rate of approximately 50 percent.

The availability of potent diuretics, effective antihypertensive agents, surgical correction of congenital cardiac defects or valvular lesions, and CABS significantly improves the prognosis. Nevertheless, the prognosis is still unfavorable in patients with CHF due to cardiomyopathy (heart muscle disease; see Chapter 12), heart attack, and any advanced cardiac condition not correctable by surgery. Of course, early recognition and elimination of various precipitating factors that trigger CHF or make the preexisting CHF worse will definitely improve the prognosis.

Fortunately, the majority of patients with CHF will improve with modern medical treatment. In patients with refractory CHF, vigorous efforts should be made to detect a surgically correctable cardiac lesion.

7

SHOCK FROM
HEART ATTACK

In a broad sense, the term *cardiogenic shock* includes the clinical syndrome accompanying various cardiovascular disorders associated with hypotension (low blood pressure) with evidence of impaired blood circulation to the skin, kidneys, and central nervous system. The most common cause of cardiogenic shock is, without question, acute MI, but shock may also be due to serious cardiac arrhythmias, myocarditis, cardiomyopathy, cardiac tamponade, pulmonary embolism, and advanced CHF due to various heart diseases. On the other hand, *cardiogenic shock* is commonly used in medical literature to describe specifically shock following acute MI. In this book, the author uses the latter definition. The definition of cardiogenic shock is a BP of less than 90 mmHg or a systolic fall greater than 80 mmHg in a patient with previously known hypertension. It should be pointed out that the diagnosis of cardiogenic shock is applicable only when there is unequivocal clinical evidence of acute MI in conjunction with serum enzyme elevation and the ECG changes. Cardiogenic shock is the most serious complication of acute MI, and its high mortality rate still exceeds 75 to 80 percent, despite modern and sophisticated therapy. In addition, many patients with cardiogenic shock suffer from other major complications such as serious cardiac arrhythmias and CHF. These coexisting complications further lead to grave outcome with a higher mortality rate.

Various other medical conditions may also produce a shock state, and they include external loss of fluid (e.g., hemorrhage, burns, vomiting, diarrhea), internal loss of fluid (e.g., peritonitis, hematoma), gram-negative bacteremia neurogenic disturbances (e.g., fright, pain, emotional shock), anaphylaxis (e.g., penicillin shock), and use of vasodilator drugs. It is also important to remember that some healthy individuals may have lower than usual BP without any disease. For example, systolic BP around 90 mmHg is not uncommon in children or young adults (even in some older people), especially when they are tall and slender in build. Of course, this low blood pressure in apparently healthy people is a perfectly normal finding.

CAUSES (ETIOLOGY)

Cardiogenic shock results from significant destruction of the left ventricular myocardium (muscle mass of the left pumping chamber). It has been shown that the destruction of 40 to 50 percent of the total mass of the left ventricular myocardium is usually necessary to produce cardiogenic shock. Destruction of myocardium is usually due to acute MI. The myocardial destruction produces impairment of the mechanical performance (pumping action) of the left ventricle so that cardiac output and BP are markedly reduced.

In addition to massive destruction of the myocardium, many patients with cardiogenic shock reveal severe triple-vessel disease or left main coronary artery lesion. By and large, MI produces transmural necrosis (*necrosis* means "dead tissue") that involves the entire thickness of the ventricular wall (called "transmural MI"). On the other hand, cardiogenic shock may be produced by extensive subendocardial infarction that involves only the subendocardium (inner layer) of the left ventricle. Of course, reduction of the cardiac output and BP as a result of cardiogenic shock leads to progressive deterioration of cardiac function because of marked reduction in coronary blood flow.

CLINICAL FINDINGS (SYMPTOMS AND SIGNS)

Clinical findings are combined manifestations of cardiogenic shock and acute MI. Namely, there is a history of recent severe chest pain associated with ECG evidence of acute MI, in conjunction with various manifestations of reduced organ perfusion as a result of cardiogenic shock. Clinically, the patient is restless with altered sensorium (e.g., disoriented to time, place, and the like, with unclear mental state) as a result of reduced blood flow to the central nervous system, and the skin is pale, cyanotic (blue or purplish color), cool, and moist. Urine output is reduced as a result of impaired blood flow to the kidneys, and it is generally less than 20 ml/hour. If the patient has a history of chronic CHF, neck vein distension, liver enlargement, and peripheral (e.g., ankle) edema can be detected. Heart sounds are often weak and distant because of markedly reduced pumping action of the left ventricle. When the patient has acute CHF and pulmonary edema, moist rales (bubbling sounds) are audible in the chest. In addition, atrial and ventricular gallops or a summation gallop (triple or quadruple heart sounds) are often audible in this circumstance.

When the patient suffers from other complications (e.g., rupture of papillary muscle or the ventricular septum), there will be a harsh pansystolic heart murmur (a heart murmur audible throughout the systolic or pumping phase of the ventricle). The heart size may be normal or enlarged. Peripheral pulses (e.g., pulse on the wrist) are generally diminished, thready, or even not palpable at all in advanced cases. The heart rhythm or pulse may be grossly irregular, very rapid, or very slow depending upon the type of cardiac arrhythmias. Every patient with cardiogenic shock has low BP (below 90 mmHg), and in advanced cases, BP may be so low that it may not be measurable with the BP cuff. Body temperature is usually normal, but respiratory rate may be normal or increased. Of course, various manifestations of acute MI are present (see Chapter 3) in all patients with cardiogenic shock.

DIAGNOSIS

The diagnosis of cardiogenic shock is established without any difficulty in most cases from the characteristic clinical manifestations, as already described. In addition, acute MI is diagnosed on the basis of clinical background in conjunction with typical ECG abnormalities and serum enzyme studies. It must be certain, however, that hypotension is *not* drug induced. Remember that morphine sulfate and various other analgesics ("painkillers") frequently produce low BP. It is also important to distinguish cardiogenic shock from shock due to a variety of other disorders (e.g., hemorrhage, trauma—discussed later).

As far as laboratory studies are concerned, routine blood and urine tests may be perfectly normal in cardiogenic shock. Of course, ECG reveals the characteristic abnormalities of acute MI (see Figure 3.4 and Chapter 3). In addition, serum enzymes are usually elevated, although they may be normal in a very early stage of acute MI. Various cardiac arrhythmias are also commonly associated with acute MI and cardiogenic shock. Low amplitude of ECG complexes is extremely common in patients with cardiogenic shock because of markedly reduced pumping action in the left ventricle. Cardiomegaly is often present in patients with cardiogenic shock, and it is detected by physical examination, chest X-ray, and ECG. Pulmonary congestion, pulmonary edema, or even pleural effusion (fluid accumulation in the chest cavity) can be detected on the chest X-ray when the patient suffers from CHF. Arterial blood gas determinations often reveal hypoxemia (reduced contents of oxygen), normal CO_2, and acidosis of varying degrees. Evaluation of kidney function will be valuable not only for detection of preexisting renal impairment but also for the establishment of a baseline for comparison during management of cardiogenic shock. Many patients exhibit various signs of impaired kidney function as a result of reduced blood circulation to the kidneys. Remember that urine outflow is, by and large, less than 20 ml/hour in most patients with cardiogenic shock.

DIFFERENTIAL DIAGNOSIS

As emphasized previously, a shock state may be due to various disorders other than acute MI. Thus, other mechanisms possibly responsible for the production of shock should be considered carefully unless clinical and ECG manifestations of cardiogenic shock and acute MI are unquestionably evident. Remember that shock due to any underlying disorder produces a reduction of coronary blood flow, particularly in patients with known CAD, and hypotension itself can cause myocardial damage.

Cardiogenic shock should be distinguished from a shock state from a variety of other clinical circumstances.

Hypovolemic Shock

Hypovolemic shock may be produced by massive blood loss, and a common site of bleeding is the gastrointestinal tract with peptic ulcer disease. Internal bleeding can develop from trauma, and the bleeding site may not be obvious soon after trauma. In this circumstance, the initial clinical picture may be of shock syndrome.

Dissection of the aorta (a tear in the inner layer of the aorta) usually produces intense chest or back pain similar to acute MI. Blood loss from a dissecting aorta can accumulate in the mediastinum (behind the breastbone), the pleural space, or the retroperitoneal space (behind the abdominal cavity), leading to shock syndrome. On rare occasions, the dissection may extend into the pericardium and produce cardiac tamponade (see Chapter 13). Of course, massive bleeding from any site regardless of cause can produce hypovolemic shock.

Pulmonary Embolism

Pulmonary embolism (blood clots in the lungs) can produce shock with obstruction of pulmonary blood flow. The clinical picture closely mimics acute MI, but various laboratory tests (ECG, chest X-ray, serum enzyme studies, and lung scan) usually distinguish these two life-threatening conditions. In most cases, a source of the blood clots can be identified (commonly thrombophlebitis—inflamed veins of the lower extremities) in patients with pulmonary embolism.

Anaphylactic Shock

Anaphylactic shock can develop after medications are received orally or intravenously as a result of idiosyncrasy (abnormal and unusual body reaction to drugs). A typical example is penicillin shock, but any type of drug may cause anaphylactic shock for an individual who shows an unusually sensitive reaction. Similarly, anaphylactic shock may also be produced by injection of substances for a variety of diagnostic procedures.

Bacteremia

Bacteremia is the invasion of bacteria into the bloodstream as a result of severe infection. Shock syndrome may be produced by gram-negative bacteremia, and this clinical condition is usually associated with chills and fever. Bacteremia is often induced by urinary tract manipulation or surgical procedure. Of course, identification of the bacteria that are responsible for the production of bacteremia is essential.

Neurogenic Shock

The term *neurogenic shock* is used to describe the shock syndrome due to action of the nervous system producing vasodilation. Neurogenic shock can develop from intense pain, trauma, fright, or any unusual emotional shock. It is important for physicians to remember, however, that considerable blood loss should seriously be considered under any traumatic circumstance (e.g., automobile accidents) when they are dealing with neurogenic shock associated with trauma.

COMPLICATIONS

As stressed previously, cardiogenic shock is the most serious complication of acute MI, and the mortality rate is extremely high (75 to 80 percent) despite modern medical treatment. In addition, cardiogenic shock is frequently associated with other serious complications of heart attack, including CHF, cardiac arrhythmias, and a ruptured papillary muscle or ventricular septum. Furthermore, cardiogenic shock itself can cause other serious complications.

Renal (Kidney) Failure

When cardiogenic shock is present for prolonged periods, the patient may develop renal failure secondary to acute tubular necrosis as a result of poor blood circulation to the kidneys.

151

Cerebrovascular Accidents

Cerebrovascular accidents ("stroke") may be produced by reduction of blood circulation to the brain, especially in patients with a previous history of cerebrovascular disease.

Gastrointestinal Disorders

Prolonged shock may lead to gastrointestinal disorders such as ischemia of the bowel with necrosis and bleeding as a result of inadequate blood circulation to the gastrointestinal system.

Cardiovascular Disorders

Although cardiogenic shock is the most serious complication of acute MI, cardiogenic shock itself frequently leads, in turn, to the development of various other complications, such as cardiac arrhythmias, CHF, and pulmonary edema as a result of reduction in coronary blood flow. For the same reason, CAD is aggravated further when there is prolonged cardiogenic shock. Therefore, it can be said that there is a bidirectional relationship between CAD and cardiogenic shock.

MANAGEMENT

As soon as the diagnosis of cardiogenic shock is made, the initial management of the patient requires the rapid establishment of an intravenous route for the administration of various drugs. The general therapeutic approach to cardiogenic shock is outlined in Table 7.1; various drugs commonly used to treat cardiogenic shock are summarized in Table 7.2. Various vasoactive medications are available (see Table 7.2), but levarterenol (Levophed), dopamine, and metaraminol (Aramine) have proved most reliable in raising BP and restoring vital organ perfusion. The filling pressure of the left ventricle should be raised, and an effective blood volume should be established for the maximum effect of the vasopressor medications. The Swan-Ganz catheter can provide this important information in patients with cardiogenic shock. By and large, systolic BP should be maintained at at least 90 mmHg with infusion of a vasopressor (a drug that raises BP). In addition to the prompt administration of vasopressors, the insertion of a Foley catheter (a small plastic catheter that is inserted into the bladder via the urethra) is essential so that the exact amount of urinary output can be measured. In general, most patients are able to maintain respiratory (breathing) control in cardiogenic shock, even though the arterial blood gases are significantly altered. When the patient is unable to breathe spontaneously, however, artificial respiration (intubation with ventilatory support) should be performed.

TABLE 7.1. Rules for the Treatment of Cardiogenic Shock.

Maintain adequate oxygenation (monitor the arterial blood gases).

Correct tachyarrhythmia ($>$140 beats per min) or bradyarrhythmia ($<$60 beats per min).

Measure the arterial pressure directly and keep the systolic pressure above 90 mm Hg.

Measure the pulmonary wedge pressure and keep it between 15 and 20 mm Hg.

Correct acidosis (monitor the arterial blood gases).

Use albumin if necessary to adjust the pulmonary wedge pressure.

Use sodium nitroprusside (20-200 μg/min) if the systolic arterial pressure $>$100 mm Hg.

Use dopamine or dobutamine (10-15 μg/kg/min) if the systolic pressure $<$100 Hg. Add sodium nitroprusside if necessary.

Use norepinephrine if the arterial pressure cannot be maintained.

Consider mechanical support or emergency surgery in refractory cases.

Reproduced from Chung, E.K.: *Cardiac Emergency Care,* Second Edition, Philadelphia, Lea & Febiger, 1980.

When there are other complications such as pulmonary edema, CHF, and cardiac arrhythmias—a common occurrence—they should, of course, be treated simultaneously (see Chapters 6 and 9). Metabolic acidosis often develops in patients with cardiogenic shock, and infusion of sodium bicarbonate should be carried out in order to restore acid-base balance. The development of catheterization techniques and facilities for hemodynamic monitoring has provided very important informa-

TABLE 7.2. Drugs Commonly Used to Treat Shock.

Drug	Dosage
Vasodilator drugs	
Sodium nitroprusside (Nipride)	20-200 μg/min IV
Hydralazine (Apresoline)	10-50 mg IM
Phentolamine (Regitine)	0.5-2 mg/min
Inotropic drugs	
Dopamine (Intropin)	10-30 μg/kg/min
Dobutamine (Dobutrex)	5-15 μg/kg/min
Inotropic-vasodilator drug	
Isoproterenol (Isuprel)	1-5 μg/min
Inotropic-vasoconstrictor drugs	
Norepinephrine (Levophed)	5-30 μg/min
Metaraminol (Aramine)	100-1000 μg/min
Diuretic drugs	
Furosemide (Lasix)	20-200 mg IV

Reproduced from Chung, E.K.: *Cardiac Emergency Care,* Second Edition, Philadelphia, Lea & Febiger, 1980.

tion on cardiac performance in patients with cardiogenic shock. It has been demonstrated that the pulmonary artery end-diastolic pressure accurately reflects the left ventricular end-diastolic pressure in patients with cardiogenic shock. These hemodynamic measurements can provide valuable information on the prognosis of the patient and can also establish a monitoring system for the best selection and proper regulation of various medications (see Table 7.2). In addition, the diagnosis of other complications, such as ruptured ventricular septum or mitral regurgitation, can be confirmed by the Swan-Ganz catheter.

When the aforementioned medical therapy is not satisfactory, insertion of the intraaortic balloon (described briefly in Chapter 3) can restore BP by means of diastolic augmentation of cardiac output and coronary blood flow. It should be noted, however, that counterpulsation with the intraaortic balloon pump is only palliative and will not cure the shock entirely. Thus, therapeutic approaches, such as possible cardiac surgery preceded by emergency coronary arteriography, should carefully be considered if indicated (see Chapters 24 and 25).

PROGNOSIS

Prognosis of the patient with cardiogenic shock depends largely upon various factors, including the extent of heart muscle damage, involvement of various coronary arteries, the presence or absence and degree of other major complications, the response to therapy, and the patient's age. By and large, the overall prognosis of patients with cardiogenic shock remains grave in spite of modern and sophisticated management. Unfortunately, the mortality rate is still between 70 and 80 percent in cardiogenic shock.

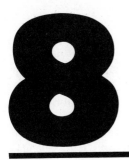

HEART SOUNDS
AND
HEART MURMURS

Sound, regardless of its cause, origin, nature, and type, is the subjective perception and interpretation of vibrations that reach the auditory apparatus in the ears and are transmitted to the brain. Of course, no heart sound is produced unless sufficient blood is circulated constantly through the heart and blood vessels.

There are four heart sounds associated with human heart function, but only the first and second are readily audible through a stethoscope. The third heart sound, however, is not uncommonly audible in healthy children and young adults (called the "physiological third heart sound"), but this sound gradually disappears as the individual gets older. The fourth heart sound is not audible in healthy individuals because of its very low intensity. Nevertheless, the heart sounds, which are not audible to human ears, can be recorded on the phonocardiogram (a graphic recording of heart sounds, using special electronic equipment; see Chapter 24). A conventional stethoscope consists of a diaphragm and a bell. The diaphragm is suitable for listening to high-pitched sound, whereas the bell is designed for listening to low-pitched sound. By careful analysis and interpretation of various heart sounds, physicians may be able to diagnose a variety of heart diseases, since a diseased heart (e.g., congenital cardiac defects, valvular heart diseases) often causes abnormal heart sounds. The genesis of various heart sounds was discussed in Chapter 2.

The term *heart murmur* is used to describe an abnormal sound that is commonly generated by blood flow through an abnormal heart valve (e.g., a narrowing or leaking valve) or by a defect in the heart (e.g., abnormal communication or a

155

hole between two heart chambers, such as atrial septal defect or ventricular septal defect; see Chapters 10 and 11). Physicians can diagnose a variety of heart diseases (e.g., rheumatic heart disease, congenital heart diseases) by recognizing various types of heart murmur. It should be pointed out, however, that the presence of heart murmur is not necessarily indicative of heart disease; many healthy subjects may have low- to mild-intensity heart murmur (better known as "functional heart murmur"). In addition, many patients with noncardiac diseases (e.g., anemia, hyperthyroidism) may have heart murmur. The genesis of heart murmurs was discussed in Chapter 2.

NORMAL VS. ABNORMAL HEART SOUNDS

Various types of heart disease may cause abnormal heart sounds. The intensity of the first or second heart sounds may be increased or decreased. In addition, the timing of the sounds may be altered depending on the nature and severity of different heart diseases.

The First Heart Sound

The onset of the left and right ventricular contractions occurs almost simultaneously. In general, left ventricular contraction precedes slightly the right ventricular contraction. As a result of this asynchrony of ventricular contractions, theoretically, splitting of the first heart sound is expected. However, in a practical sense, the first heart sound is audible as a single heart sound because the tricuspid component is usually faint, compared with the mitral component. When there is any factor (e.g., right bundle branch block) that produces delayed right ventricular contraction, the tricuspid component is heard late enough to be recognized as a sound separated from the mitral component leading to wide splitting of the first heart sound. In severe mitral stenosis (narrowing of mitral valve), the onset of the mitral valve closure is often delayed, and then the tricuspid closure sound may be unmasked. Such a tricuspid closure sound is occasionally audible because its intensity is often augmented by concomitant pulmonary hypertension (increased pressure in the pulmonary artery). By and large, the first heart sound is best heard at the apex of the heart (below the nipple).

The intensity of the first heart sound may be altered in a variety of clinical circumstances. For example, increased intensity of the first heart sound is often caused by physical exercise, epinephrine infusion, and hyperthyroidism, because the pressure rise in the ventricles is very rapid and tension develops quickly. Another good example of a loud first heart sound is observed in patients with mitral stenosis. On the other hand, the intensity of the first heart sound is often diminished in elderly people, and in those with advanced CHF, cardiogenic shock, pericardial effusion, and pulmonary emphysema. In addition, a faint first heart sound usually occurs in patients with first-degree A-V block (prolonged P-R interval; see Chapter 9). When the P-R interval (conduction time from the atria to the ventricles; see Figure 2.1) changes constantly, the intensity of the first heart sound will vary from beat to beat. The best example of this is complete A-V block, in which the atria and the ventricles beat independently (see Figure 3.6, and Chapter 9). In this circumstance, intermittent occurrence of a loud first heart sound is termed "cannon sound," and this finding is a useful criterion for diagnosing complete A-V block during physical examination. When the heart rhythm is grossly irregular (e.g., atrial fibrillation; see Chapter 9), the first as well as the second heart sounds occur irregularly, and the intensity of the heart sounds may vary from beat to beat, depending upon the length of the cardiac cycle.

The Second Heart Sound

Since the right ventricular systolic ejection time is longer than that of the left ventricle, the pulmonic second heart sound (P_2) occurs slightly later than the aortic second heart sound (A_2). This normal or physiological asynchrony of the second heart sound is exaggerated during inspiration, when venous return to the right side of the heart increases; and pulmonic second sound is further delayed so that it follows aortic closure by 0.03 to 0.06 second or more. During expiration, on the other hand, this disparity in ejection times of the right and left ventricles is minimized. Consequently, splitting of the second heart sounds becomes less pronounced or is almost absent. This phenomenon is called "physiological splitting of the second heart sounds" and is a normal finding. The second heart sounds, as a rule, are best heard at the base of the heart (just below the junction of the two clavicles —collar bones). The P_2 is less intense than the A_2 in healthy individuals; therefore, only A_2 can normally be heard at the apex. When P_2 is clearly heard at the apex, this finding usually indicates significant pulmonary hypertension and/or right ventricular enlargement.

The splitting of the second heart sounds is further exaggerated when there is a delayed activation of the right ventricle (e.g., right bundle branch block) causing late occurrence of P_2. In addition, wide splitting of the second heart sounds also occurs when there is prolonged mechanical right ventricular systolic ejection due to outflow obstruction as seen in pulmonic stenosis (narrowing of the pulmonic valve). Under this circumstance, the second heart sound may be audible as a single heart sound when the P_2 becomes very faint as a result of severe pulmonic stenosis. Wide splitting of the second heart sounds also occurs in atrial septal defect (a congenital communication or hole between two atrial chambers). In this condition, P_2 is delayed because with each beat, the right ventricle is ejecting a larger volume of blood than is the left ventricle. In addition, the wide splitting of the second heart sounds is relatively fixed in atrial septal defect. In other words, physiological splitting of the second heart sounds is no longer present in atrial septal defect. Therefore, it can be said that the relatively fixed and wide splitting of the second heart sounds is a characteristic feature of atrial septal defect.

Conversely, delayed occurrences of the A_2 may be observed so that splitting may become narrower than usual. In this circumstance, if the delay of A_2 is sufficiently pronounced, the sequence of the second heart sounds may be reversed. Thus, the P_2 precedes the A_2 in this situation. This is called "paradoxical splitting of the second heart sounds," in which inspiration results in the two components of the second heart sounds coming closer together and at times fusing; during expiration the two sounds are more widely separated. The most common causes of paradoxical splitting of the second heart sounds include left bundle branch block (delayed activation of the left ventricle due to a block in the left bundle branch system; see Figure 1.3), aortic stenosis (narrowing of the aortic valve), and patent ductus arteriosus (a form of congenital heart disease; see Chapter 10). As far as the intensity of the second heart sounds is concerned, the higher the diastolic pressure (pressure during diastolic or expansion phase) the semilunar valve (aortic or pulmonic valve) supports, the louder the second heart sounds. Most commonly, loud A_2 occurs in hypertension, and at times, the sound becomes ringing or tambourlike in quality.

The Third Heart Sound, Fourth Heart Sound, and Gallop Rhythm

As described previously, the third heart sound (often described as S_3) is commonly heard in healthy children and young adults. It is called the "physiological third heart sound" and occurs during passive rapid filling of the ventricles. The third heart sound occurs from 0.12 to 0.20 second following the A_2. It is a dull, low-pitched sound, heard best at the apex with the individual lying on the left side. The third heart sound usually waxes and wanes during respiration and is most audible at the beginning of expiration. This physiological third heart sound gradually disappears with age. When a third heart sound is heard in an older individual, it usually indicates either CHF or mitral insufficiency (leaking of the mitral valve). This third heart sound in older people is called a "ventricular or protodiastolic gallop sound" or "S_3 gallop"; it is definitely an abnormal finding. The ventricular gallop rhythm may be originating from either left ventricle or right ventricle, depending upon which ventricle is diseased. The left ventricular gallop is more consistent than the physiological third heart sound with less respiratory variation. It is heard best at the apex as the physiological third heart sound. A right ventricular gallop is heard in patients with right ventricular failure, and is best heard at the xiphoid (lower edge of breastbone) or left lower sternal border. The right ventricular gallop usually has a striking respiratory variation, becoming much louder during inspiration. When there is biventricular failure, of course, both right and left ventricular gallop rhythms may be heard. Gallop rhythm is generally expressed as "triple heart rhythm," which is comparable to a waltz tempo in dancing.

The fourth heart sound (often designated as S_4) is not audible in healthy people because of its very faint intensity. If the fourth heart sound is heard, therefore, the finding is definitely indicative of abnormal cardiac function. Audible fourth heart sound is called "pre-systolic or atrial gallop" or "S_4 gallop"; it occurs about 0.20 second after the P wave on the ECG (the P wave is due to atrial activation; see Figure 2.1). In general, atrial gallop is frequently observed in hypertensive heart disease, CAD, cardiomyopathy, and aortic stenosis. In addition, atrial gallop may also occur in patients with severe anemia, severe hyperthyroidism, and large peripheral atriovenous fistula (abnormal communication between artery and vein from various causes). Atrial gallop is best heard with the patient recumbent and the bell of the stethoscope placed lightly against the skin. The atrial gallop rhythm, like ventricular gallop rhythm, produces triple heart rhythm. When the atrial gallop and the ventricular gallop coexist, the end result is called "summation gallop," which may be audible as triple or quadruple heart rhythm. Left atrial gallop is best heard at the apex or at a point between the apex and the xiphoid, whereas right atrial gallop is heard best at the left xiphoid area. Right atrial gallop has the classical inspiratory augmentation characteristic of sounds arising from the right side of the heart.

HEART MURMURS

A heart murmur is an abnormal noise generated by the heart, and it is commonly produced by diseased heart valves or congenital heart lesions. In other words, the heart murmur is a relatively prolonged series of auditory vibrations that can be characterized and expressed according to the intensity (loudness), frequency (pitch), configuration (contour or shape), quality, duration, direction of radiation (transmission), and timing of the cardiac cycle. It should be pointed out, however, that the presence of heart murmur is not necessarily indicative of heart disease. Conversely, many cardiac patients do not have heart murmurs.

The intensity of heart murmurs is commonly graded from 1 to 6 in medical practice. A *grade 1* is so faint that it can be heard only with special effort. Thus, a grade 1 heart murmur is often unrecognized by inexperienced physicians. A *grade 2* murmur is faint but readily audible. A *grade 5* murmur is the loudest murmur and can be heard through a stethoscope placed on the chest wall. A grade 5 murmur is not audible with the stethoscope removed from the chest wall. A *grade 6* murmur is so loud that it can be heard even when the stethoscope is not touching the chest wall. *Grade 3 and 4* murmurs are intermediate in intensity. The *grade 3* murmur is prominent but not loud, whereas a *grade 4* murmur is loud. By and large, the heart murmurs of grade 3 or more in intensity are hemodynamically significant, and the presence of loud heart murmurs usually signifies a serious heart disease. When a heart murmur of any type is very loud (greater than grade 4 or 5), there is often a palpable thrill on palpation as a result of transmission of a loud murmur through the chest wall. The medical term *palpable thrill* means the feeling of fine vibration when a palm or fingers are placed above the chest wall where the heart murmur is loudest. The feeling of the palpable thrill of the heart murmur is somewhat comparable to the sensation experienced when one's palm is placed on the chest wall of a cat while it is purring.

Frequency or pitch of a heart murmur varies from high to low, but they may be intermediate. The configuration may be crescendo (progressive increment in intensity), decrescendo (progressive reduction in intensity), crescendo-decrescendo (diamond-shaped—progressive increment of intensity to a peak followed by progressive reduction in intensity), or plateau (sustained—relatively constant intensity throughout its course).

The quality of a heart murmur is often described as harsh, rough, rumbling, scratchy, buzzing, grunting, blowing, musical, squeaky, whooping, and so on. The duration of a heart murmur may be long or short, or it may be any length in between. A long heart murmur may occupy the entire length of a systolic phase or diastolic phase of the cardiac cycle. On the other hand, a short heart murmur occupies a relatively brief period of systole or diastole. Sometimes, a very long heart murmur may occupy the entire cardiac cycle—the systolic as well as diastolic phases (e.g., patent ductus arteriosus—a form of congenital heart diseases). A loud heart murmur, as a rule, radiates from its site of maximum intensity to a variety of locations depending upon the nature and severity of the underlying heart disease. The direction of transmission may provide useful information regarding the mechanism of the heart murmur and the nature of the underlying heart disease.

As far as the timing of heart murmurs is concerned, there are three major categories—systolic, diastolic, and continuous. A systolic murmur (a heart murmur during pumping phase of the ventricles) begins with or after the first heart sound and ends at or before the second heart sound. A diastolic murmur (a heart murmur during expansion phase of the ventricles) begins with or after the second heart sound and ends before the first heart sound of the subsequent heart beat. A continuous heart murmur begins in systole and continues without interruption through the time of the second heart sound into all or part of diastole. Systolic murmurs again are classified according to their time of the onset and termination as midsystolic, holosystolic (pansystolic), early systolic, or late systolic. A midsystolic murmur begins after the first heart sound and ends before the second heart sound. A holosystolic murmur begins with the first heart sound and ends with the second heart sound. In other words, holosystolic murmur occupies the entire systolic phase of the cardiac cycle. Diastolic murmurs, likewise, may also be classified according to their time of the onset as early diastolic, middiastolic, or late diastolic (presystolic). An early diastolic murmur begins with either the A_2 or P_2, depending upon its side of origin. A middiastolic murmur begins at a clear interval after the second heart sound. A late diastolic murmur (presystolic murmur) begins in the period immediately before the first heart sound.

The intensity and configuration of heart murmurs may be changed from time to time, and they may be altered according to the individual's body position. Changing heart murmurs may be due to cardiac tumors, bacterial endocarditis, and advanced CHF. In addition, the intensity is often increased during inspiration when the murmur originates from the right side of the heart.

Recognition of various heart murmurs and their characteristic features is extremely important to make the correct diagnosis of a variety of heart diseases.

Systolic Murmurs

The most common types of systolic murmurs include midsystolic and holosystolic murmurs, whereas early systolic or late systolic murmurs are much less common.

Midsystolic Murmurs (Ejection Systolic Murmurs)

Midsystolic murmurs are the most common heart murmurs in humans. These murmurs may occur in healthy individuals as well as patients with diseased heart. Midsystolic murmurs characteristically occur when blood is ejected across the semilunar (aortic or pulmonic) valves during pumping phase of the ventricles. This is the reason why the terms *midsystolic murmurs* and *ejection systolic murmurs* are used interchangeably in the medical literatures. Ejection of blood occurs when the ventricular pressures rise sufficiently to open the aortic and pulmonic valves, so that the systolic murmur begins at this time. As ejection of blood increases, the murmur increases its intensity (crescendo in shape); as the ejection reduces, the murmur also reduces its intensity (decrescendo in shape). Thus, typical midsystolic murmur shows crescendo-decrescendo shape, which is often described as a "diamond-shaped" murmur. The murmur ends before ventricular pressure drops enough to permit closure of the aortic or pulmonic valve leaflets.

There are four major causes of midsystolic murmurs. They include

1. obstruction of ventricular outflow,
2. dilation of the aortic root or pulmonary trunk,
3. an increased rate of blood flow into the great arteries, and
4. morphologic changes (e.g., valve deformity) in the semilunar valves or their lines of attachment without obstruction.

The murmur of aortic stenosis is the prototype of the left-sided midsystolic murmur, beginning after the first heart sound or with an ejection sound, rising in crescendo to a systolic peak, declining in decrescendo to the end before the time of aortic valve closure. The quality of aortic stenosis murmur is usually harsh, rough, and grunting, particularly when it is loud. The intensity varies from grades 1 to 6. By and large, the shorter and softer the murmur and the earlier the systolic peak, the greater the probability of mild aortic stenosis. In valvular aortic stenosis, the murmur is loudest in the second right intercostal space, with radiation upward, to the right, and into the neck. In supravalvular aortic stenosis, the murmur is occasionally loudest even higher, with disproportionate radiation into the right carotid artery (artery along right side of neck). In hypertrophic obstructive cardiomyopathy (asymmetric septal hypertrophy with obstruction), the murmur originates well below the valve, within the left ventricular cavity, and is typically loudest at the lower sternal edge and apex, with relatively little radiation to the base and neck. In elderly people with aortic stenosis due to calcific deposits on the surfaces of aortic valves, the murmur in the second right interspace tends to be harsh and noisy, while the murmur at the apex may be pure and musical in quality.

The midsystolic murmur of valvular pulmonic stenosis is characteristically loudest in the second left interspace next to the sternal edge, although it may be equally loud in the third interspace. The pulmonic stenosis murmur commonly radiates upward and to the left, and it may be audible in the suprasternal notch (above the collar bones) and the base of the neck, usually on the left side when the murmur is loud. The greater the stenosis of the valve, the longer the duration of right ventricular ejection and the longer the systolic murmur.

It should be emphasized that midsystolic murmurs may also be encountered during rapid ejection of blood into a normal aorta or pulmonary trunk in various noncardiac conditions including pregnancy, thyrotoxicosis (hyperthyroidism), anemia, and fever. In addition, midsystolic murmur may also occur in pure aortic regurgitation (leakage of aortic valve) as a result of rapid ejection of blood from vigorous left ventricular contraction. Furthermore, midsystolic murmur is commonly observed in patients with atrial septal defect as a result of rapid blood flow across the pulmonic valve (functional pulmonic stenosis).

Innocent or functional (normal) murmurs are typically midsystolic in timing. A common form of innocent systolic murmur in children is the vibratory murmur, which is a short, buzzing, pure, and medium-frequency murmur. This innocent systolic murmur is believed to originate from periodic vibrations of the pulmonic leaflets at their attachments. On the other hand, innocent pulmonic midsystolic murmur in children, adolescents, and young adults may be due to an exaggeration of normal ejection vibrations in the pulmonary trunk. A similar innocent midsystolic murmur may be present in patients with narrow anteroposterior chest dimensions (straight back syndrome) because of proximity of the pulmonary trunk to the chest wall. An aortic systolic murmur is the commonest form of innocent systolic murmur in elderly individuals and is considered to be due to degenerative fibrous thickening and stiffening of the base of the aortic cusps without obstruction. By and large, innocent systolic murmurs are seldom more than grade 3 in intensity.

Holosystolic (Pansystolic) Murmurs

The term *holosystolic murmur* or *pansystolic murmur* is used when the murmur occupies the entire systolic phase of the cardiac cycle. These holosystolic murmurs are generated when there is blood flow from a heart chamber or a large blood vessel whose pressure throughout the systolic phase is greater than the pressure in the other adjacent heart chamber or blood vessel. Therefore, holosystolic murmurs are commonly due to mitral or tricuspid regurgitation (leakage of the mitral or tricuspid valve) and to ventricular septal defect.

The term *regurgitation* means that the direction of blood (or any type of liquid) flow is reversed so that it flows backward to the location from which it originated. For example, the term *mitral regurgitation* is used when the blood is flowing backward to the left atrium from the left ventricle, because the mitral valve has an inability to close during the systolic phase of the ventricle as a result of a diseased mitral valve. As described previously, the mitral valve has to close completely during systole so that blood is ejected to the aorta from the left ventricle by pumping action in a normal heart to supply blood circulation to the entire body (see Chapter 2). Tricuspid regurgitation is the same phenomenon that occurs in the right cardiac chambers.

In ventricular septal defect, the left ventricular pressure is constantly higher than the right ventricular pressure so that characteristically the murmur occupies the entire systolic phase—holosystolic murmur. The murmur of the ventricular septal defect is usually loudest at the third or fourth intercostal space along the left sternal border.

It is very important to emphasize that the presence of holosystolic murmur is unequivocally indicative of serious heart disease and that immediate medical attention is necessary. In other words, holosystolic murmurs are *never* innocent murmurs and are *never* found in healthy individuals. By and large, holosystolic murmurs are loud, and the intensity is at least grade 3 or 4 (often greater than grade 4 or 5).

Early Systolic Murmurs

Early systolic murmurs may occur in all conditions that cause holosystolic murmurs, including ventricular septal defect and mitral or tricuspid regurgitation. These early systolic murmurs begin with the first heart sound with a decrescendo in quality and end well before the second heart sound, at or before the middle of the systole. In large ventricular septal defect with pulmonary hypertension, shunting (blood flow through an abnormal communication in the ventricular septum) at the end of systole may be minimal or completely absent, leading to the occurrence of an early systolic murmur.

Severe mitral regurgitation of acute onset may cause an early systolic murmur or a holosystolic murmur. An early systolic murmur also may occur in patients with mitral regurgitation secondary to papillary muscle dysfunction (dysfunction of the structures supporting the mitral valve—a relatively common complication of heart attack). In addition, an early systolic murmur is a common finding of tricuspid regurgitation with normal right ventricular systolic pressure. A good example of this is tricuspid regurgitation resulting from infective endocarditis in patients with drug addiction (see Chapter 13). Remember that tricuspid regurgitation with elevated right ventricular systolic pressure usually produces a loud holosystolic murmur. As a rule, an early systolic murmur is often soft and pure, with medium to low frequency.

Late Systolic Murmurs

Mitral valve prolapse syndrome (deformity of mitral valve and its adjacent structures—a form of congenital heart disease; see Chapter 10) typically produces systolic click(s) and late systolic murmurs. The late systolic murmur begins with or just follows the click(s) and is usually crescendo in quality up to the aortic component of the second heart sound. Mitral regurgitation occurs under this circumstance when the prolapse of mitral valve is sufficient to disrupt leaflet apposition (closure of mitral valve). Mitral valve prolapse syndrom is discussed fully in Chapter 10.

Diastolic Murmurs

Heart murmurs that occur during the diastolic (expansion) phase of the ventricles are termed "diastolic murmurs." By and large, diastolic murmurs are much less common than systolic murmurs, and the intensity of diastolic murmurs is usually much less than that of systolic murmurs. Diastolic murmurs are generally classified according to their timing—early, middiastolic, and late diastolic (or presystolic). As a rule, diastolic murmurs are not observed in healthy individuals. Thus, the presence of diastolic murmurs of any type necessitates immediate medical evaluation by a competent cardiologist.

Early Diastolic Murmurs

Heart murmur of aortic regurgitation is a typical example of an early diastolic murmur. This murmur begins at the time of the aortic valve closure, as soon as the left ventricular pressure falls below the pressure of the aortic root. The shape of this early diastolic murmur is, as a rule, decrescendo, because there is a progressive reduction in the volume and rate of regurgitation during the course of diastole. Since the quality of the early diastolic murmur is very similar to the breathing sound, it may not be recognized readily, especially when the murmur is not loud. Thus, a faint diastolic murmur of aortic regurgitation must be specifically sought by applying very firm pressure with the diaphragm of the stethoscope at the second or third intercostal space along the left sternal border while the patient sits, leans forward, and holds the breath in full expiration. Aortic regurgitation is most commonly due to rheumatic heart disease (see Chapter 11), but it may result from other causes, such as syphilis (see Chapter 14).

The early diastolic murmur of pulmonary regurgitation begins with the P_2, and the shape of the murmur is, likewise, decrescendo. Since the early diastolic murmur in pulmonary regurgitation due to pulmonary hypertension was first described by Graham Steell in 1888, the murmur is often designated as the "Graham Steell murmur." In a practical sense, however, it is very difficult or almost impossible to distinguish between the early diastolic murmur of aortic regurgitation and pulmonary regurgitation from the auscultatory finding alone. Therefore, it is necessary to evaluate the heart murmur in conjunction with all other available information, including clinical, X-ray, ECG, and other laboratory findings.

Middiastolic Murmurs

A typical example of middiastolic murmur occurs in mitral stenosis (narrowing of the mitral valve), and it characteristically follows the opening snap (discussed later). The middiastolic murmur of mitral stenosis can occur whether the heart rhythm is normal (sinus rhythm) or grossly irregular (atrial fibrillation; see Chapter 9). The middiastolic murmur in mitral stenosis is often designated the "diastolic rumble" because of its rumbling quality. This murmur is best heard when the bell of the stethoscope is placed at the site of the left ventricular impulse and the patient is turned toward the left side. Mitral stenosis is nearly always due to rheumatic heart disease, and mitral stenosis is the most common valve lesion in rheumatic heart disease (see Chapter 11). A middiastolic murmur comparable to mitral stenosis murmur also occurs in tricuspid stenosis (narrowing of the tricuspid valve), and this murmur typically becomes louder during inspiration. The greater intensity of the murmur during inspiration in this circumstance is due to the fact that inspiration results in a larger venous return and a parallel increment in the gradient and flow rate across the tricuspid valve.

Middiastolic murmurs may be generated across the mitral valve as a result of increased flow without mitral stenosis. For instance, ventricular septal defect or patent ductus arteriosus and mitral regurgitation can cause middiastolic murmurs because of increased flow across the mitral valve. For the same reason, atrial septal defect or tricuspid regurgitation often produces middiastolic murmur because of increased flow across the tricuspid valve. This type of "relative" mitral or tricuspid stenosis murmur is typically short and medium-pitched.

Less common causes of mitral or tricuspid stenosis murmurs include large thrombi (large blood clots) or tumor (e.g., myxoma) in the left or right atria. Under these circumstances, narrowing of the mitral or tricuspid valves can occur by obstruction of the valve orifice by the thrombi or tumor (see Chapter 14).

Middiastolic murmur that is very similar in quality to the mitral stenosis murmur may represent the "Austin Flint murmur." The Austin Flint murmur is considered to be due to forward flow across the mitral valve, which is closing rapidly because of left ventricular filling from the aortic regurgitation. Thus, aortic regurgitation may produce two types of diastolic murmurs—the typical early diastolic murmur of aortic regurgitation itself and the middiastolic Austin Flint murmur.

Late Diastolic or Presystolic Murmurs

Late diastolic or presystolic murmurs begin during the period of ventricular filling that follows atrial contraction (contraction of upper chambers). As the name designates, these murmurs occur just before the systolic (pumping) phase of the ventricles. Clinically, late diastolic murmurs most commonly occur in patients with mitral stenosis just like middiastolic murmurs. Of course, presystolic murmurs are produced only during normal (sinus) rhythm under this circumstance. Remember that atrial contraction during normal sinus rhythm causes a P wave (small and round deflection) on the ECG (see Figure 2.1 and Chapter 24), and the atrial contraction is necessary to produce a presystolic murmur. Of course, a presystolic murmur may also occur in tricuspid stenosis. In mitral stenosis, the increased left atrial pressure exerted against the narrowed orifice of the mitral valve produces a low-pitched rumbling middiastolic murmur that becomes louder during the presystolic phase as additional blood flow is generated by atrial contraction. In some cases with mitral stenosis, the middiastolic murmur may be faint or not audible so that only the presystolic murmur can be heard clearly.

One of the characteristic features of tricuspid stenosis is the increased intensity of middiastolic or presystolic murmur during inspiration. As described previously, the volume of the right atrium increases during inspiration as a result of the increased systemic venous return. Consequently, the right atrium contracts with greater intensity, and this leads to a larger gradient, a more rapid velocity of blood flow, and an increase in intensity of the murmur in tricuspid stenosis.

Like middiastolic murmurs, a tumor or a large thrombus in the left or right atrium may cause presystolic murmurs that may closely resemble murmurs of mitral or tricuspid stenosis. A unique feature of murmurs produced by a cardiac tumor (or large thrombus) is the changing intensity of murmurs according to the position of the patient (see Chapter 14).

Continuous Murmurs

The term *continuous murmurs* is applied to heart murmurs that begin in systole and continue without interruption through the time of the second heart sound into all or part of diastole. Continuous murmurs occur usually because blood flow from a higher-pressure area to a lower-pressure area continues without interruption from systole into diastole of the ventricles. Therefore, a heart murmur that extends into the diastolic phase without interruption at the second heart sound is also called "continuous" even if the murmur ends before the first heart sound of the subsequent beat. Continuous murmur is a hallmark of patent ductus arteriosus, one of the most common congenital heart diseases (see Chapter 10). In addition, continuous murmurs may also occur in a variety of other clinical conditions, including pulmonary hypertension, congenital or acquired systemic atriovenous fistula (an abnormal communication between the arterial and venous systems), anomalous origin of the left coronary artery from the pulmonary artery (a form of congenital heart disease), and communications from the sinus of Valsalva to the right side of the heart. The innocent "venous hum," first described by Potain in 1867, is an example of a continuous murmur resulting from altered blood flow patterns in veins.

There are various abnormal extra heart sounds that may be heard in patients with a variety of heart diseases. Some extra heart sounds, such as an opening snap or gallop rhythm, are extremely important to recognize in the diagnosis and management of cardiac patients, whereas some other extra heart sounds (e.g., artificial valve sounds or extra cardiac sounds produced by artificial cardiac pacemakers) may not be significant clinically.

Opening Snap

It is important to note that the opening of a normal mitral valve produces no audible sound. On the other hand, a diseased mitral valve, usually caused by rheumatic mitral stenosis (see Chapter 11), causes a definite audible extra heart sound in early diastole, about 0.04 to 0.12 second following the A_2. This extra heart sound is termed "opening snap" because it has a snapping quality. The opening snap in mitral stenosis is best heard along the lower left sternal border and apex, and it is a very important physical sign. This is particularly true when other physical signs (such as a loud first heart sound, an accentuated P_2, and the diastolic rumbling murmur) are present to confirm the diagnosis of mitral stenosis. The opening snap due to mitral stenosis is observed later than the usual (physiologic) splitting of the second heart sound but earlier than the physiologic third heart sound. The opening snap occurs in well over 90 percent of patients with mitral stenosis, and it is present either in normal (sinus) rhythm or in atrial fibrillation. The opening snap often persists even after commissurotomy (surgical repair for mitral stenosis), although the intensity may be reduced after surgery.

     The opening snap also occurs as a result of tricuspic stenosis comparable to the opening snap in mitral stenosis. The general features of the opening snap due to tricuspid stenosis are very similar to those of the opening snap in mitral stenosis, but it is best heard closer to the midline along the lower left sternal border. Occasionally, the opening snap of tricuspid stenosis is best heard along the lower right sternal border. In a practical sense, tricuspid stenosis nearly always coexists with mitral stenosis. Thus, the recognition of the opening snap of tricuspid stenosis is often difficult, especially when the opening snap is concealed by coexisting diastolic rumble of mitral stenosis.

Gallop Rhythm

The medical term *gallop rhythm* is used to describe abnormal extra heart sounds causing triple or sometimes quadruple sounds that are somewhat comparable to the canter of a horse. It is important for physicians to recognize the gallop rhythm

167

because it is often one of the earliest physical signs to support organic heart disease. Gallop sounds (or rhythm) have been discussed in detail earlier in this chapter.

Ejection Sounds

An ejection sound is produced at the time of ejection of blood from the left ventricle into the aorta in patients with aortic stenosis, or from the right ventricle into the pulmonary artery in patients with pulmonic (pulmonary) stenosis. Ejection sounds do not occur in healthy individuals.

The pulmonary ejection sound is best heard over the pulmonary valve area (second interspace along the left sternal border) or third left sternal border, and it is often misinterpreted as the first heart sound. However, it should be remembered that the first heart sound is, as a rule, not well heard at the pulmonary valve area. Conversely, the pulmonary ejection sound is very faint or not heard at all at the apex of the heart. The pulmonary ejection sound is commonly observed in mild to moderate pulmonary stenosis, but it may not be obvious or not be heard at all in advanced pulmonary stenosis. At times, the pulmonary ejection sound is encountered in patients with pulmonary hypertension due to a variety of underlying heart diseases (e.g., ventricular septal defect, patent ductus arterosus, atrial septal defect; see Chapter 10). The intensity of the second heart sound is increased in pulmonary hypertension.

The aortic ejection sound is heard in patients with aortic stenosis, most commonly congenital in origin. It may also occur in patients with aortic regurgitation, coarctation of the aorta (narrowing of a segment of the aorta, a form of congenital heart disease), and aneurysm of the ascending aorta. In contrast to pulmonary ejection sounds, aortic ejection sounds are usually well audible at the apex of the heart.

Systolic Clicks

The systolic click is an extra heart sound that occurs in the systolic phase of the ventricle; it has a "clicking" quality. This is why the term *systolic click* is used. The systolic click usually has a single component, although, at times, two or more multiple clicks may be observed in the same patient. The timing of the systolic click is usually constant, but it may be slightly variable. Although the systolic click was considered an extracardiac sound some years ago, it is now believed to be cardiac in origin. It is generally agreed that the systolic click is related to a prolapse during systole of the mitral valve leaflets (most commonly, posterior leaflet). In other words, the presence of a systolic click(s) usually indicates mitral valve prolapse syndrome (see Chapter 10).

Systolic clicks may occur in early systole, midsystole, or late systole, but most commonly they are midsystolic in timing. The systolic click is usually best heard when the patient is recumbent and in the left lateral position. Systolic clicks may or may not be associated with late systolic or pansystolic murmur at the cardiac apex. The intensity of the systolic click is often accentuated by mild physical exercise (e.g., running for a few minutes).

Artificial Valve Sounds

Artificial heart valves are most commonly inserted in the aortic and mitral valve areas; less commonly the tricuspid valve may be replaced. The caged ball and disc valve types are the most popular artificial heart valves employed today, and they produce characteristic opening and closing sounds. Of course, these artificial valves produce considerably different sounds depending upon the types of prosthetic valve. Some artificial valve sounds are louder than the normal heart sounds and have a different quality, whereas others have sounds similar to normal heart sounds. When double heart valves are replaced, each valve has an opening sound as well as a closing sound. Since most artificial valves produce their unique sounds, identification is not difficult if a physician has the opportunity to hear the various types of artificial heart valve sounds. Therefore, it is essential for every physician to become familiar with the characteristic features of various artificial heart valve sounds.

When the artificial heart valve does not function properly, various abnormal sounds may occur. For instance, abnormal valve sounds may be a series of rattles or clicks that may closely resemble the rolling of dice or ball traversing a roulette wheel. In some cases, artificial valve sounds may be multiple rather than single and may occur in systole and/or diastole. When these abnormal sounds are observed, the possibility of blood clot formation or some other complications of the artificial heart valves should be considered. It should be emphasized that a change in the time of occurrence or intensity of artificial heart valve sounds may be the first clue to malfunction. When artificial heart valve sounds disappear completely, disruption of sutures of a prosthetic valve should be considered. When a prosthetic valve, such as a discoid type of mitral valve, gets stuck in its open position, the heart murmur of mitral regurgitation may reappear following valve replacement.

Artificial Pacemaker Sounds

By and large, no extra heart sounds are produced following implantation of artificial cardiac pacemakers in most cases. However, occasionally, an artificial pacemaker may produce a sound in the presystolic phase that is actually related to skeletal muscle contraction rather than being of cardiac origin. At times, it is possible to see precordial muscle contraction coincident with the sound, and the patient may be aware of it, rarely feeling some discomfort. In this circumstance, repositioning the pacemaker electrode or reducing pacemaker energy output usually eliminates the problem. The artificial pacemaker may cause unusual musical sounds such as a whoop or honk. These pacemaker sounds are often loud and occur in late systole. Again, repositioning the pacemaker electrode usually eliminates the abnormal sounds. When a patient with a permanent artificial pacemaker develops pericardial friction rub (discussed shortly), penetration of the heart muscle or rupture of the heart should be strongly considered, and immeidate medical attention is mandatory.

Pericardial Friction Rubs

Pericardial friction rubs are hallmarks of pericarditis (inflammation of the pericardial sac) with or without pericardial effusion (fluid accumulation around the heart; see Chapter 13). These pericardial friction rubs are very high-pitched sounds, scratchy in quality, and they seem close to the ears. They are usually best heard with the patient leaning forward after blowing air out completely. In most cases, the friction rubs have two components that occur at the time of atrial systole and ventricular systole, although a third component may be heard during the diastole of rapid ventricular filling leading to triple component rubs. Typically, pericardial friction rubs possess scratchy sounds with a "to-and-fro" quality rather than a continuous sound. The friction rubs may occur only intermittently or may be continuous depending upon the underlying disorder.

Pericardial Knock

The pericardial knock is a unique feature of constrictive pericarditis (thickening and hardening of the pericardial sac as a result of long-standing pericarditis; see Chapter 13). The pericardial knock occurs early in diastole, generally 0.10 to 0.12 second following the second heart sound, and is produced in the rapid-filling phase of the ventricular diastole. The term *pericardial knock* is used because the extra sound is somewhat comparable to the sound of a knock on a door. The knocking sound is produced when the blood is rapidly flowing against the hardened and constricted pericardial wall, preventing the usual expansion of the ventricles during the systolic phase. The pericardial knock occurs slightly later than the opening snap of mitral stenosis but earlier than the normal physiologic third heart sound. It may be single and sharp, but at times it may exhibit considerable variations in intensity as well as in the number of components. The pericardial knock may persist even after surgical repair for constrictive pericarditis, or it may disappear completely following surgery.

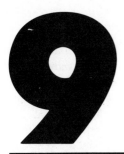

HEART RHYTHM
ABNORMALITIES

In the normal heart, the cardiac impulse originating from the primary pacemaker (the sinus node) passes the sinoatrial junctional tissue and spreads throughout the atria radially, like the wave formed in a pond after a stone is thrown into it. The P wave (a small, round wave) is recorded on the ECG during atrial activation (see Figure 2.1). The average time required for atrial depolarization (activation) in the normal heart varies from 0.08 to 0.10 second. The activation process spreads through the atrial muscle and passes down the A-V nodal tissue. Then, the cardiac impulse continuously spreads down along the A-V bundle (His bundle), both bundle branches, and, finally, the terminal Purkinje fibers to activate the ventricles (see Figures 1.3 and 2.1). The time interval required from the beginning of atrial depolarization to the beginning of ventricular depolarization is represented by the P-R interval (A-V conduction time) on the ECG (Figure 2.1); its average value in normal adults varies from 0.12 to 0.20 second. The ventricular depolarization (activation) produces the QRS complex on the ECG, and its average duration is between 0.06 and 0.10 second in normal adults (see Figure 2.1). The QRS complex is the largest deflection on the ECG (see Figure 2.1). Following ventricular depolarization, the ventricles are repolarized, and this process produces another deflection (somewhat triangular shaped), which is termed a "T wave" (see Figure 2.1). At this time, one cardiac cycle is ended, and the same electrical events continue as long as there is no disturbance in cardiac impulse formation and conduction. Thus, one cardiac cycle contains P wave (atrial depolarization), QRS complex (ventricular depolarization), and T wave (ventricular repolarization; see Figure 2.1). Following the T wave, there is another low-amplitude wave, called a "U wave" (see Figure 2.1); its exact genesis is not clearly understood.

When this electrical system is not working properly, the heart rhythm becomes abnormal. In broad terms, any abnormality of heart rhythm is called a "cardiac arrhythmia" or "cardiac dysrhythmia." (The author prefers the former term.) Although there are various types of cardiac arrhythmias, they are generally classified into two major categories: (1) disturbances of cardiac impulse formation and (2) disturbances of conduction. In many cases, however, cardiac arrhythmias may be manifested in disturbances of both impulse formation and conduction, especially in advanced cardiac patients.

It is important to emphasize that the presence of cardiac arrhythmias is not necessarily indicative of heart disease. For example, sensitive individuals may develop various cardiac arrhythmias as a result of excessive use of coffee, tea, cola drinks, and cigarette smoking, as well as anxiety in the absence of any known disease. In addition, certain noncardiac diseases often cause cardiac arrhythmias. The best example is thyrotoxicosis (hyperthyroidism), which frequently causes paroxysmal atrial fibrillation (chaotic, rapid, and irregular rhythm arising from the atria). As can be expected, some arrhythmias are relatively benign, whereas others may be so serious that sudden death may occur. Thus, it is very important to distinguish between benign and serious cardiac arrhythmias. It is also known that some less serious arrhythmias may lead to life-threatening arrhythmias. Therefore, preventive measures are likewise very important to avoid serious arrhythmias and possible sudden death, particularly in patients with acute MI.

The heart rhythm originating from the primary pacemaker (the sinus node) is called "sinus rhythm" (Figure 9.1). The term *ectopic beats* or *rhythm* is used to describe any heartbeat or rhythm originating from any location in the heart other

FIGURE 9.1. Normal electrocardiogram.

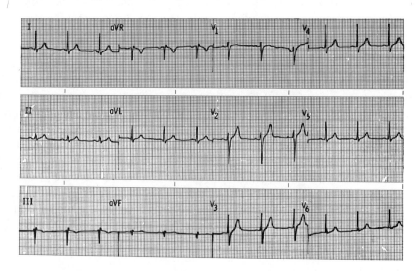

than the usual primary pacemaker (sinus node). The ectopic beats or rhythm may arise from the atria, A-V node, conduction tissue, or ventricles. When the ectopic beats occur consecutively (usually six or more beats), the term *ectopic rhythm* is applied. Any ectopic beat may occur as a single, isolated beat in the presence of underlying normal (sinus) rhythm. The most common cardiac arrhythmia in humans is probably extrasystoles (premature contractions) from various origins (atria, A-V junction, or ventricles).

The term *heart block* is used when the conduction of the cardiac impulse takes place with slower than usual speed. Thus, *heart block* has the same meaning as *conduction disturbance*. The heart block is somewhat comparable to the electrical wire system of a house that fails to supply adequate electricity because of malfunction (e.g., misconnected or broken wire). The heart block may occur in any portion of the heart, including the sinoatrial junction, atria, A-V junction, His bundle, right and left bundle branches, and ventricles (see Figure 1.3). The most common form of heart block involves the A-V junction, and it is called "atrioventricular (A-V) block." The heart block may be minimal and produce only slight delay in conduction, but it may be so advanced that no conduction is possible. When there is no conduction at all in this circumstance, the term *complete heart block* is used. Complete heart block often involves the A-V conduction so that complete A-V block is the end result. Although some physicians often use the terms *heart block* and *A-V block* interchangeably, A-V block is actually one of the most common forms of heart block.

Clinically, cardiac arrhythmias may be suspected when any of the following occurs singly or in combination.

1. Feelings of palpitations, skipped beats, or any peculiar sensation in the chest
2. Slow pulse or heart rate (slower than 40 to 50 beats/min.)
3. Irregular pulse or heart rhythm
4. Rapid pulse or heart rate (faster than 140 to 160 beats/min.)
5. Feelings of dizziness, near-syncope, syncope, angina, or shortness of breath with or without any obvious abnormality in pulse or heart rate

Almost every known type of cardiac arrhythmia may be associated with recent heart attack, and various other heart diseases can cause a variety of cardiac arrhythmias. One of the most common causes of various cardiac arrhythmias is digitalis intoxication (digitalis poisoning; see Chapter 17). Digitalis is an essential drug in treating heart failure and various tachyarrhythmias, but if the patient develops digitalis intoxication, the drug is no longer beneficial. By and large, MI and digitalis intoxication are two major causes in producing almost every known type of cardiac arrhythmia. It is important to emphasize that various cardiac arrhythmias may precipitate other serious complications, such as CHF or cardiogenic shock, and vice versa. This is the reason why clinically significant cardiac arrhythmias should be recognized early and why proper treatment must be provided immediately.

As far as the therapeutic approach is concerned, the first and most important step is to identify the possible underlying cause of the cardiac arrhythmia. If the underlying cause (e.g., excessive use of coffee, cigarette smoking) is found, it should be eliminated if possible. When the underlying cause is not certain or when it cannot be eliminated readily, clinically significant arrhythmias have to be treated medically. There are various therapeutic methods available for a variety of cardiac arrhythmias, but medications, direct-current (DC) shock, and artificial pacemakers are the most commonly employed in modern medicine (see Chapters 16, 17, and 18). For urgent situations, DC shock is the treatment of choice for rapid rhythm. On the other hand, very slow heart rhythm is best treated with an artificial pacemaker. Antiarrhythmic drugs are used either for prevention or direct suppression of various cardiac arrhythmias, depending upon the type and nature of the heart rhythm (see Chapter 17). Occasionally, a surgical approach (e.g., CABS, ventricular aneurysmectomy) is necessary for drug-resistant and refractory cardiac arrhythmias in selected cases (see Chapter 25). The therapeutic result is greatly influenced by various factors, including the type and nature of a given arrhythmia, the presence or absence and severity of the underlying heart disease, the presence or absence and severity of other cardiac complications (e.g., CHF), the presence or absence of other coexisting disorders (e.g., diabetes mellitus, chronic obstructive pulmonary disease), the patient's age, and the response to treatment.

Disturbance of Sinus Impulse Formation and Conduction

Arbitrarily, the term *normal sinus rhythm* is used when the heart rate is between 60 and 100 beats/min., providing that the cardiac impulses arise from the sinus node (see Figure 9.1). When the sinus rhythm is slower than 60 beats/min., the term *sinus bradycardia* is used (*brady* means "slow"). Conversely, the term *sinus tachycardia* is applicable when the sinus rhythm has a rate faster than 100 beats/ min. (*tachy* means "rapid"). All healthy people exhibit fluctuations of sinus rate according to their daily activity. For instance, the sinus rate speeds up during physical exercise and becomes slow in the resting state, particularly at night during sleep. These changes are perfectly normal. The usual rate of sinus tachycardia ranges from 101 to 160 beats/min., but the rate may become faster than 180 or even 200 beats/min. during vigorous physical exercise, especially in young, healthy individuals. The usual rate of sinus bradycardia is between 45 and 59 beats/min. Many healthy athletes have very slow (even slower than 40 beats/min.) sinus bradycardia without any problem.

In addition to the usual variations of sinus rate in healthy people, sinus tachycardia is commonly associated with a variety of disorders, including fever, anemia, shock, thyrotoxicosis, and various cardiac as well as pulmonary diseases (such as pulmonary embolism). Furthermore, various medications also cause transient sinus tachycardia. Therefore, persisting sinus tachycardia should be evaluated by a physician. Sinus tachycardia is often triggered by emotional excitement, ingestion of coffee or tea, and cigarette smoking. When the sinus rate is persistently and markedly slow (slower than 40 beats/min.) without any explanation, a physician should be consulted. This is particularly true when there is any associated symptom such as dizziness, near-syncope, syncope, anginal pain, or shortness of breath.

When the sinus node is unable to produce adequate cardiac impulses as a result of dysfunction (often due to degenerative-sclerotic change in the sinus node), the term *sick sinus syndrome (SSS)* is used. SSS is, in a sense, comparable to generator failure in an automobile. The initial stage is manifested by progressive slowing of the sinus rate, but eventually the sinus node may not produce any cardiac impulse. The term *sinus arrest* or *sinus pause* is used when the sinus node fails to produce any cardiac impulse, leading to the absence of a P wave on the ECG. Sinus arrest is one of the common findings of advanced SSS. In this circumstance, intermittent or persistent atrial fibrillation (AF) frequently occurs to take over the cardiac activity, and the heart rate is usually very slow (see Figure 3.7). For SSS, implantation of a permanent artificial pacemaker is the treatment of choice (see Chapter 16 and Figure 3.7). It should be pointed out that various drugs (e.g., digitalis) frequently cause sinus bradycardia (see Chapter 17). Drug-induced sinus bradycardia is by no means SSS.

The term *sinus arrhythmia* is used when the sinus cycle varies from beat to beat. A cyclic increase in sinus rate with inspiration and a cyclic slowing with expiration is called "respiratory sinus arrhythmia," which is the rule rather than an exception in healthy children and young adults. Respiratory sinus arrhythmia is considered to be reflex changes from vagal nerve influence on the sinus pacemaker, and it usually disappears upon holding one's breath or acceleration of the heart rate by any cause. However, sinus arrhythmia unrelated to the respiratory cycle (nonrespiratory sinus arrhythmia) in older individuals is frequently associated with a variety of heart diseases.

Atrial Arrhythmias

A varity of atrial arrhythmias may be observed in healthy people as well as in patients with a diseased heart. An ectopic focus anywhere in the atria (either right or left atrium) may be capable of producing an isolated atrial premature contraction and also various atrial tachyarrhythmias, including atrial fibrillation (AF), atrial flutter, and atrial tachycardia (Figure 9.2). Thus, it can be said that the production of these atrial tachyarrhythmias is usually initiated by an isolated atrial premature contraction. Atrial premature contraction is diagnosed by recognizing an ectopic P wave that appears earlier than the P-P cycle of the basic sinus rhythm, and the premature P wave is followed by a normal QRS complex on the ECG (Figure 9.2). Remember that the P wave is due to atrial depolarization whereas the QRS complex is due to ventricular depolarization. Atrial tachycardia is nothing

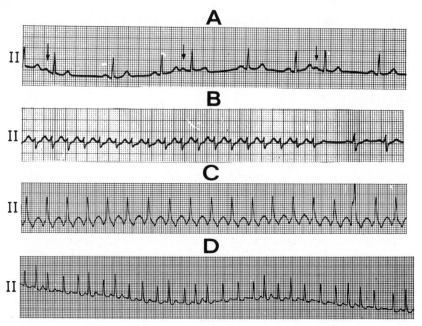

FIGURE 9.2. Atrial arrhythmias. A: Atrial premature contractions (indicated by arrows). B: Atrial tachycardia. C: Atrial flutter. D: Atrial fibrillation.

but consecutively occurring atrial premature contractions, and it produces a rapid and regular tachycardia (usual rate: 160 to 250 beats/min.) with normal QRS complex (see Figure 9.2). Each QRS complex is preceded by a P wave.

AF (Figure 9.2) produces a grossly irregular rhythm, and no discernible P wave is present because fine and chaotic AF waves replace P waves. Uncomplicated (pure) AF usually has a very rapid rate (120 to 250 beats/min.). It should be remembered that AF is the most common ectopic heart rhythm in humans. In other words, AF is the next most common rhythm to normal sinus rhythm. Atrial flutter characteristically produces flutter waves with sawtooth appearance, and every other flutter wave is conducted to the ventricles in most cases (see Figure 9.2). The usual atrial rate in atrial flutter is between 250 and 350 beats/min.

The term *aberrant ventricular conduction* is used when the configuration of the QRS complex in these atrial arrhythmias is bizarre (different from a normal beat). The aberrant ventricular conduction occurs when the atrial impulse is conducted to the ventricles during their partial refractory period. In other words, aberrant ventricular conduction occurs because the atrial impulse is conducted while the ventricles are *not* fully recovered for full responsiveness.

Clinically, atrial tachyarrhythmias may occur in healthy people from excessive use of coffee, tea, or cola drinks, from cigarette smoking, or from severe anxiety; but more commonly, they occur in patients with heart disease. In addition, thyrotoxicosis is often associated with AF. The term *paroxysmal* is often used because these atrial tachyarrhythmias start suddenly and also stop suddenly. One of the unique cardiac conditions is "Wolff-Parkinson-White syndrome," which is frequently associated with very rapid heart action (discussed shortly in this chapter). Digitalis intoxication also may cause atrial tachyarrhythmias, particularly atrial tachycardia.

The most important therapeutic approach is to eliminate the direct cause of the arrhythmia if possible. Otherwise, there are many available methods, including various medications and DC shock; less commonly, an artificial pacemaker; and, rarely, a surgical approach. Among various antiarrhythmic agents, digitalis, quinidine, and propranolol (Inderal) are most commonly used (see Table 6.2 and Chapter 17). For very urgent situations or in cases of drug-resistant tachyarrhythmias, immediate application of DC shock is the treatment of choice, particularly when the heart rate is very rapid (see Chapter 18). In addition, atrial tachycardia may be terminated by carotid sinus stimulation (massage of the side of the neck—either left or right, but one side at a time).

A-V Junctional Arrhythmias

The A-V junction (A-V node and the surrounding tissue) also may produce various arrhythmias in a way similar to the production of atrial arrhythmias. A-V junctional arrhythmias include A-V junctional premature contractions, A-V junctional tachycardia, and A-V junctional escape rhythm (see Figure 9.3). A-V junctional tachycardia is often initiated by an isolated A-V junctional premature contraction. A-V junctional tachycardia is of two types—paroxysmal and nonparoxysmal. Paroxysmal A-V junctional tachycardia starts suddenly and also terminates suddenly, as the name indicates, whereas nonparoxysmal A-V junctional tachycardia does not possess such characteristics. In addition, the paroxysmal form has a rapid rate (160 to 250 beats/min.) as in paroxysmal atrial tachycardia, but the nonparoxysmal form has a relatively slow rate (70 to 130 beats/min.; see Figure 9.3). The clinical significance of paroxysmal A-V junctional tachycardia is similar to that of paroxysmal atrial tachycardia. On the other hand, nonparoxysmal A-V junctional tachycardia is predominantly due to two clinical conditions—digitalis intoxication and diaphragmatic MI (a heart attack involving the lower portion of the left ventricle). The A-V junction may produce a slow heart rhythm—called "A-V junctional escape rhythm." The usual rate of A-V junctional escape rhythm ranges from 40 to 60 beats/min. A pure form of A-V junctional escape rhythm may occur (see Figure 9.3), but it is a common heart rhythm secondary to complete A-V block. In A-V junctional arrhythmias, a retrograde (inverted) P wave may precede or follow each QRS complex, but the P wave is often not discernible because of its superimposition to the QRS complex. In addition, P waves are often not present because of the preexisting, underlying AF. In this case, AF and A-V junctional tachycardia or escape rhythm coexist, leading to complete A-V dissociation. The term *A-V dissociation* is used when the atrial and ventricular activities are independent.

The therapeutic approach to A-V junctional arrhythmias is similar to the

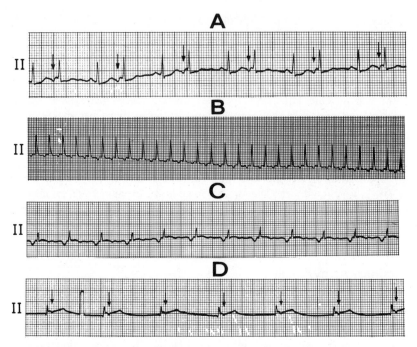

FIGURE 9.3. A-V junctional arrhythmias. A: A-V junctional premature contractions (indicated by arrows). B: Paroxysmal A-V junctional tachycardia. C: Nonparoxysmal A-V junctional tachycardia. D: A-V junctional escape rhythm (note retrograde P waves indicated by arrows).

approach to atrial arrhythmias. An artificial pacemaker may be indicated when the heart rate is very slow and especially when the patient suffers significant symptoms (such as dizziness, syncope, angina) directly from the slow rhythm itself.

Ventricular Arrhythmias

Ventricular arrhythmias (abnormal heart rhythms originating from the pumping chambers) are the most serious arrhythmias, and they are often a precursor to sudden death. Ventricular arrhythmias may include ventricular premature contractions (VPCs), ventricular tachycardia, ventricular flutter, ventricular fibrillation (VF), ventricular escape rhythm, and ventricular standstill. VPCs often lead to ventricular tachycardia and VF (Figures 3.5 and 9.4), and sudden death may be the end result unless treated immediately. This is particularly true in recent heart attack. Recognition of a VPC is relatively easy because of its bizarre and broad QRS comples (Figure 3.5). Ventricular tachycardia is actually consecutively (usually six or more) occurring VPCs. Very rapid ventricular tachycardia (160 to 250 beats/min.) starts suddenly and terminates suddenly. Therefore, the term *paroxysmal ventricular tachycardia* (Figure 9.4) is used, and it is a life-threatening ar-

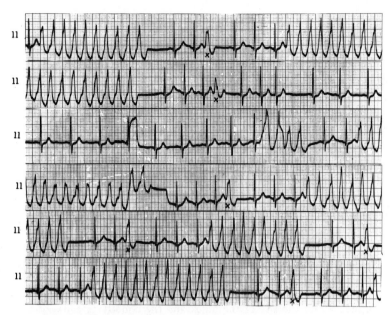

FIGURE 9.4. Paroxysmal ventricular tachycardia with frequent VPCs (marked X). All rhythm strips of lead II are continuous.

rhythmia that should be terminated promptly. On the other hand, a slow ventricular tachycardia (commonly called "nonparoxysmal ventricular tachycardia" or "accelerated idioventricular rhythm") is relatively benign, and it is clinically insignificant in most cases (rate: 70 to 130 beats/min.).

Ventricular escape rhythm (idioventricular rhythm) is the slowest heart rhythm encountered in the human heart (rate: 25 to 35 beats/min.) and is commonly the end result of complete A-V block (see Figure 3.6). The term *Adams-Stokes syndrome* is used to describe unconscious episodes associated with complete A-V block. An artificial pacemaker is indicated in this circumstance (Figure 3.6). For urgent clinical situations from paroxysmal ventricular tachycardia or VF, immediate application of DC shock is the treatment of choice. When the situation is *not* urgent, however, intravenous injection of lidocaine (Xylocaine) is preferred for paroxysmal ventricular tachycardia (see Table 6.2). For long-term therapy or a preventive measure, procainamide (Pronestyl) and quinidine are the most commonly used antiarrhythmic agents (see Table 6.2). Remember that VF has to be terminated within four minutes by DC shock. Otherwise, the patient will die. Even if cardiac function is restored by electric shock, brain function may *not* be restored when treatment is delayed (see Chapter 3). In addition, all necessary CPR measures have to be applied for cardiac arrest (see Chapter 15). It should be pointed out that the most common heart rhythm causing cardiac arrest is VF (see Figure 3.5), and ventricular standstill soon follows when cardiac function further deteriorates. VF is totally ineffective, irregular, and chaotic ventricular rhythm (see Figure 3.5), and ventricular standstill means no cardiac activity at all. VF is the usual mode of sudden death in patients with recent heart attack.

A-V Block

A-V block is the most common form of heart block, and it means that the conduction is slower than normal from the atria to the ventricles. When conduction becomes extremely slow, then of course no conduction occurs from the atria to the ventricles. In other words, A-V block occurs when the refractory period of the conduction is prolonged. For example, the cardiac impulses are conducted to the ventricles more slowly than normal or are conducted only occasionally when the A-V conduction system is *partially refractory*. On the other hand, no cardiac impulses are conducted to the ventricles at all when the conduction system is *absolutely refractory*.

A-V block may be due to a block at different locations in the A-V conduction system. Namely, a block may be in the A-V node itself (called "A-V nodal block"), in the His bundle (called "intra-His block"), or below the His bundle (called "infra-His block"; see Figure 1.3). The clinical significance of A-V block is greatly influenced by the site of the block and the underlying cause of the block. A-V block is classified into three major categories according to the degree of the block. The term *first-degree A-V block* is used when the A-V conduction is slightly prolonged. In this case, the P-R interval (A-V conduction time) is prolonged (more than 0.20 second), but every atrial impulse is conducted to the ventricle (see Figure 9.5). *Second-degree A-V block* is used to describe intermittent or occasional conductions of the cardiac impulses from the atria to the ventricles. Thus, second-degree A-V block is a more advanced form than first-degree A-V block. Second-degree A-V block is again divided into two types—Mobitz type I and type II A-V block. The Mobitz type I (another term for it is *Wenckebach A-V block*) A-V block is characterized by a progressive lengthening of the P-R intervals until a blocked P wave occurs (see Figure 9.5). On the other hand, the Mobitz type II A-V block does not possess the characteristic features of the Wenckebach A-V block, and the P-R intervals of all conducted beats are constant (see Figure 9.5). The terms *Mobitz* and *Wenckebach* are used to describe second-degree A-V block because classification of A-V block was defined independently by these two physicians for the first time.

Clinically, the Mobitz type I (Wenckebach) A-V block is commonly associated with acute diaphragmatic MI or digitalis intoxication, and A-V block is usually transient in nature. Thus, no active treatment is required for the Wenckeback A-V block. Conversely, the Mobitz type II A-V block is usually caused by permanent damage·in the conduction system due to acute anterior MI (heart attack involving an anterior wall of the left ventricle) or a sclerotic-degenerative change. Therefore, a permanent artificial pacemaker implantation is indicated for every patient with a Mobitz type II A-V block. It should be noted that the Mobitz type I

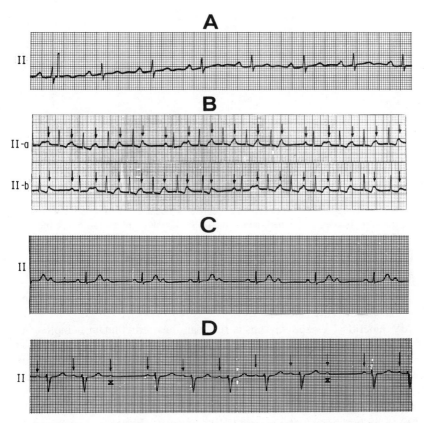

FIGURE 9.5. Incomplete (partial) A-V blocks. A: First degree A-V block. B: Wenckebach A-V block (arrows indicate sinus P waves). Leads II-a and b are continuous. C: 2:1 A-V block (note that every other P wave is not followed by QRS complexes). D: Mobitz type II A-V block (arrows indicate P waves, and blocked P waves are marked X). Note constant P-R intervals in all conducted beats.

(Wenckebach) A-V block represents A-V nodal block (block in the A-V node) whereas the Mobitz type II A-V block represents infranodal block (block below the A-V node).

Complete (or third-degree) A-V block means that no conduction occurs between the atria and the ventricles, so atrial and ventricular activities are independent throughout the cardiac cycle (see Figure 9.6). Complete A-V block may be due to a block in the A-V node (A-V nodal block), or it may be due to a block below the A-V node (infranodal block). Complete A-V nodal block is commonly due to digitalis intoxication or acute diaphragmatic MI, and the block is usually reversible. On the other hand, complete infranodal block is irreversible because it is usually caused by permanent damage in the conduction system due to anterior MI or a sclerotic-degenerative change. In general, complete infranodal block is due

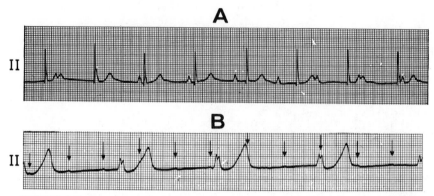

A

II

B

II

FIGURE 9.6. Complete A-V blocks. A: Complete A-V nodal block (note normal QRS complexes with relatively fast ventricular rate). B: Complete infranodal block (note bizarre QRS complexes with very slow ventricular rate). Arrows indicate P waves that are independent of QRS complexes.

to a block involving both right and left bundle branch systems (see Figure 1.3). In other words, complete infranodal block usually represents complete bilateral bundle branch block (discussed shortly).

A-V junctional escape rhythm is the main heart rhythm in complete A-V nodal block, while ventricular escape rhythm is the main heart rhythm in complete infranodal block (Figure 9.6). As described previously, A-V junctional escape rhythm is a relatively stable heart rhythm with a reasonably good heart rate (45 to 60 beats/min.) and normal QRS complexes (see Figure 9.6). Conversely, ventricular escape (idioventricular) rhythm is a very unstable heart rhythm with a very slow rate (20 to 35 beats/min.) and bizarre QRS complexes (Figure 9.6). A permanent artificial pacemaker implantation is mandatory for all patients with complete infranodal A-V block with ventricular escape rhythm (see Figure 3.6). On the other hand, a permanent artificial pacemaker is only occasionally indicated for complete A-V nodal block with A-V junctional escape rhythm.

Wolff-Parkinson-White Syndrome

Wolff-Parkinson-White (WPW) syndrome is a unique cardiac condition that is frequently associated with very rapid heart actions. WPW syndrome is a form of congenital cardiac anomaly, and one or more accessory conduction pathways are present in the heart between the atria and the ventricles. The accessory pathway is responsible for producing a unique ECG finding (short P-R interval with broad QRS complex due to initial slurring of the QRS complex—see Figure 9.7) as well as various rapid heart actions. The rapid heart action is considered to be due to a reentry cycle (circus movement) via an accessory pathway and the normal A-V conduction system.

The most common rapid heart action associated with WPW syndrome is a regular and rapid tachycardia (rate: 140 to 250 beats/min.) with normal QRS

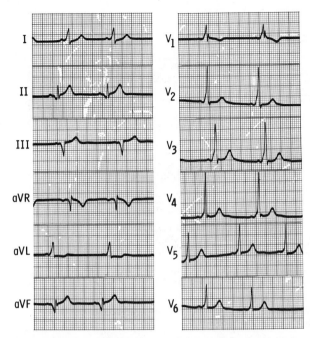

FIGURE 9.7. Wolff-Parkinson-White syndrome in a twenty-four-year-old man.

complexes (termed "reciprocating tachycardia"; see Figure 9.8). The drug of choice in this circumstance is propranolol (Inderal), and the second choice is digitalis (see Table 6.2). A less common rapid heart action in WPW syndrome is AF or flutter with a very rapid ventricular rate (160 to 300 beats/min.) and very bizarre QRS complexes as a result of anomalous A-V conduction (see Figure 9.8). The drug of choice is intravenous lidocaine (Xylocaine) for urgent situations, and procainamide (Pronestyl) or quinidine is very effective as a preventive measure in this circumstance. If rapid heart action occurs frequently in individuals with WPW syndrome, they must take one or more appropriate antiarrhythmic agents (see Table 6.2) indefinitely. When the clinical situation is extremely urgent (e.g., causing serious symptoms like near-syncope or syncope from rapid heart action), immediate application of DC shock is the treatment of choice (see Chapter 18).

Bundle Branch Blocks

The bundle branch system consists of a right bundle branch and a left bundle branch, and the left bundle branch is further divided into left anterior and posterior divisions (see Figure 1.3). Each branch of the bundle branch system is called a "fascicle." Thus, a human heart consists of three fascicles—right bundle branch, and left anterior (superior) and posterior (inferior) divisions of the left bundle branch system (see Figure 1.3).

A

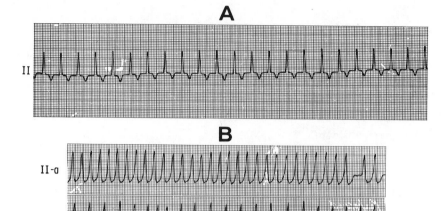

II

B

II-a

II-b

FIGURE 9.8. Tachyarrhythmias associated with Wolff-Parkinson-White syndrome. A: Reciprocating tachycardia (note regular heart cycle with normal QRS complexes). B: Atrial fibrillation with bizarre QRS complexes because of conduction via an accessory (anomalous) pathway. Leads II-a and b are continuous.

The right or left bundle branch system may be blocked either temporarily or permanently (see Figure 1.3). Under these circumstances, the terms *right bundle branch block (RBBB)* and *left bundle branch block (LBBB)* are used, respectively. RBBB and LBBB are forms of heart block, and an isolated RBBB or LBBB alone is insignificant clinically. However, when both the right and left bundle branch systems are blocked together, the end result is a bilateral bundle branch block, causing complete A-V (infranodal) block with ventricular escape rhythm (see Figure 9.6), a very serious problem, as described previously.

RBBB causes a delayed activation of the right ventricle, whereas LBBB produces a delayed left ventricular activation (see Figure 9.9). Many elderly people gradually develop LBBB or RBBB, even in the absence of apparent heart disease. Likewise, many people with no heart disease may develop a block in one of the divisions of the left bundle branch system—called "hemiblocks." Remember that the left bundle branch system consists of two divisions—left anterior and posterior fascicles (see Figure 1.3). The blocks in the divisions are called "left anterior hemiblock" and "left posterior hemiblock," respectively (the term *hemi* means "half"). No treatment is indicated under these circumstances. On the other hand, many physicians use a temporary artificial pacemaker as a prophylactic measure when someone develops LBBB or RBBB suddenly, as a result of acute MI, with the hope that the possible occurrence of complete A-V block (as a result of bilateral bundle branch block) can be managed immediately. This is particularly true when RBBB with left anterior or posterior hemiblock occurs suddenly as the result of a heart attack. A combination of RBBB and a hemiblock is called "bifascicular block,"

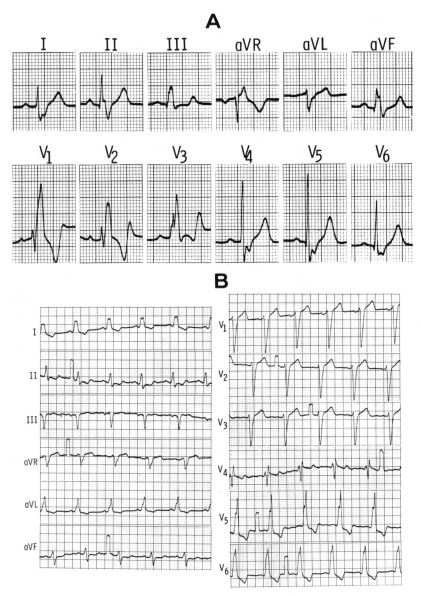

FIGURE 9.9. Bundle branch blocks. A: Right bundle branch block. B: Left bundle branch block.

which is a form of incomplete bilateral bundle branch block (the term *bifascicular* means "two fascicles"). When three fascicles are all blocked, of course, the end result is "trifascicular block" which is actually complete bilateral bundle branch block causing complete A-V block (the term *trifascicular* means "three fascicles").

185

Remember that some individuals with heart attack progressively but rapidly develop RBBB or LBBB, soon followed by complete bilateral bundle branch block, causing complete A-V block within a few hours or days. In these cases, prophylactic artificial pacing is extremely valuable and is often a life-saving measure.

Treatment and Prevention

It is not necessary to treat every individual with any type of cardiac arrhythmia. The two most important factors that indicate the need for treatment are the presence of heart disease and significant symptoms (e.g., dizziness, near-syncope, syncope, shortness of breath, angina). In other words, asymptomatic arrhythmias in individuals with no evidence of heart disease do not likely require active treatment. Elimination of the direct cause (e.g., excessive use of coffee, tea, or cola drinks or cigarette smoking) is often sufficient. Only an occasional occurrence of extrasystoles requires no treatment. When any arrhythmia is considered to be due to digitalis intoxication, discontinuation of digitalis alone is sufficient to stop the arrhythmia (see Chapter 17).

When any arrhythmia is associated with serious heart diseases, particularly recent heart attacks, active treatment is most likely indicated (see Figure 3.5). For extremely urgent or life-threatening tachyarrhythmias (Figures 3.5 and 9.4), immediate application of DC shock is the treatment of choice. For less urgent ventricular tachycardia (see Figure 9.4), however, lidocaine (Xylocaine) is the treatment of choice. Digitalis is the drug of choice for paroxysmal AF or flutter (Figure 9.2). Treatment for various rapid heart actions in the WPW syndrome has been discussed earlier. Remember that many patients with recurrent arrhythmias require one or more antiarrhythmic agents for months, years, or even indefinitely for the prophylactic purpose.

For SSS and for established complete A-V block (usually infranodal block) or Mobitz type II A-V block, a permanent artificial pacemaker is indicated in most cases. In addition, a prophylactic temporary artificial pacemaker is recommended for *new* onset of LBBB or RBBB, particularly bifasicular block associated with acute MI. Of course, all necessary CPR measures must be provided when a patient develops cardiac arrest (see Chapter 15). In selected cases with refractory arrhythmias, surgical treatment (e.g., ventricular aneurysmectomy, CABS, ligation of an accessory pathway in WPW syndrome) may be indicated (see Chapter 25).

10

CONGENITAL
HEART DISEASES

Congenital heart disease is a form of cardiovascular disease that is present at birth, resulting from a developmental abnormality. In spite of the congenital cardiac anomaly, clinical symptoms may not appear until later in childhood or even in adult life in some forms of the defect. Conversely, some forms of congenital heart defect may be so severe that they may be incompatible even with fetal life (life in the uterus before birth) and are often responsible for miscarriages. Of course, some mild forms of congenital cardiac lesions may be totally asymptomatic.

The incidence of congenital heart disease is reported to be eight to ten per 1,000 live births, and congenital lesions account for approximately 2 percent of all types of heart disease in adults. The incidence of congenital cardiac anomaly is somewhat higher, approximately twenty-seven per 1,000 stillbirths. From the group of about 25,000 newborn who are disabled annually from various forms of congenital heart disease, approximately 7,000 babies die each year in America alone. Although there is a controversy regarding a specific classification of mitral valve prolapse syndrome (discussed shortly), most physicians believe that the syndrome is a form of congenital heart disease. Therefore, the incidence of congenital heart disease will be even higher when this syndrome is included. In fact, mitral valve prolapse syndrome is probably the most common form of congenital heart disease today.

If mitral valve prolapse syndrome is not included, ventricular septal defect (abnormal communication through the wall between two pumping chambers) is the most common congenital cardiac malformation, and is encountered in approximately 30 percent of all patients with congenital heart disease. Atrial septal defect (abnormal communication between the wall of two atria) is probably the next most common congenital heart defect. Other common congenital heart diseases include patent ductus arteriosus, coarctation of the aorta, tetralogy of Fallot, pulmonic or aortic stenosis, and transposition of the great vessels. Certain congenital cardiac lesions are more common in one sex than the other. For example, patent ductus arteriosus and atrial septal defect are more common in females, whereas aortic stenosis, coarctation of the aorta, and transposition of the great vessels are more common in males.

In most cases (up to 95 percent) with congenital heart disease, the exact cause is unknown, but in some, possible etiologic factors can be identified. Some women on long-term anticonvulsive medications (e.g., trimethadione and paramethadione) and those exposed to teratogenic substances have been reported associated with giving birth to a higher than average percentage of babies with congenital heart disease. A few babies with malformed limbs due to thalidomide medication given their mothers when pregnant have congenital cardiac anomaly. In addition, significant numbers of babies have congenital heart disease when their mothers suffered from infection with rubella (German measles) during the first trimester (the first three months) of pregnancy. It has been shown that the hypoxia (inadequate oxygen supply to tissues) of high altitude after birth and the respiratory distress syndrome of premature babies may be responsible for the production of patent ductus arteriosus in some cases. Genetic factors seem related to the occurrence of certain cases with congenital heart disease. Chromosomal abnormalities such as Down's syndrome (e.g., mongolism) and Turner's syndrome are also responsible for some types of congenital cardiac defect. Medical studies indicate that the incidence of congenital heart disease increases when a baby is born to an older woman (above thirty-five or forty years of age). Congenital noncardiac anomalies often coexist with congenital heart diseases (up to 20 percent in some reports). Dextrocardia (reversed anatomic positions of all cardiac chambers, valves, and other structures) may be associated with situs inversus (reversed anatomic positions of all intestines).

There are very few symptoms of a congenital heart disease unless it is the defect that causes cyanosis (bluish-purplish color of the skin and mucous membrane) or CHF. Thus, one should look beyond the symptoms and signs the patient exhibits. This lack of recognizable symptoms is due not only to the growing child but also to the fact that for the individual born with a congenital cardiac defect, it is difficult or even impossible to know what is really normal. The way such individuals feel is normal for them on an individual basis. In many cases, it is not until after surgical repair has improved the clinical situation that a child or parents realize, in retrospect, that the child had definitely been less physically active or unusually thin before the operation.

CHF is most commonly observed in the first weeks or months of life. Common symptoms include rapid and even labored breathing, fatigue on feeding, and slow weight gain. In advanced cases of CHF, there is often edema that may be present in the legs and ankles when the individual is ambulatory, but with young infants who cannot sit, the edema is usually generalized. Cyanosis is relatively easy to recognize. Bluish-purplish coloration is often shown under the nails, mucous membranes, and skin, and cyanosis is frequently associated with clubbing of fingers and toes (enlargement of the tips of fingers and toes). Cyanosis and clubbing are the result of an insufficient supply of oxygen because of the congenital cardiac defect. Many patients with various congenital heart defects show cardiomegaly and a variety of heart murmurs or abnormal heart sounds, depending on the nature and type of defect (see Chapter 8). It can be said that the presence of a loud (grade 3 or more in intensity) heart murmur at birth usually indicates a form of congenital heart disease. Thus, it is very important to have periodic medical checkups as soon as a baby is born in order to detect any congenital cardiac defect early, so that appropriate treatment and possibly surgical repair can be provided. Vital signs (BP, pulse, respiration, and temperature), particularly BP and pulse, are often abnormal in certain types of congenital cardiac defects. In addition to careful medical examination and detailed history taking, there are many diagnostic tests available for the confirmation of a specific type of congenital heart disease. A specific heart chamber enlargement, an abnormal communication between chambers or the large blood vessels, an abnormal heart valve, and any other abnormality of cardiac anatomy can be determined by various tests (see Chapter 24).

Since the exact cause is unknown in most cases, it is difficult to prevent the occurrence of congenital heart disease. Nevertheless, some cases are preventable. The elimination of maternal rubella through immunization with a rubella vaccine reduces the incidence of congenital heart disease (the average annual incidence of congenital cardiac lesions is reduced by less than 2 percent). Better genetic understanding permits counseling of families, and intrauterine detection of some of the conditions can lead to interruption of pregnancy. Of course, a harmful environment should be avoided, as should medications that may cause congenital cardiac anomaly. Frequent and careful medical checkups are necessary, particularly for older women during pregnancy.

Treatment greatly varies depending upon the type, nature, and severity of the congenital heart disease. Any patient with a significant congenital heart lesion causing a heart murmur runs a slight risk of bacterial endocarditis (see Chapter 13). Therefore, the prophylactic antibiotics (e.g., penicillin) should be given for three days, beginning immediately before dental procedures, oral surgery, or similar operative procedures and continuing for three full days. For genitourinary tract surgery or vaginal delivery, an antibiotic for gram-negative infection should be added.

The outlook for good health and normal activity is excellent for those with physiologically insignificant congenital heart lesions and for those whose anomalies have been surgically repaired with good success. Surgical results are excellent (more than 90 percent success rate) with minimum mortality in most cases with uncomplicated congenital lesions, and medical treatment as well as surgical techniques continuously improve today. CHF and various cardiac arrhythmias, of course, must be treated with digitalis, diuretics, various antiarrhythmic agents, and so forth, regardless of the underlying congenital lesion. It is also important to know that some congenital lesions (e.g., a small ventricular septal defect) may disappear spontaneously as a child grows. Therefore, it can be said that not every congenital heart lesion is serious. Mirror-image dextrocardia (reversed position of the entire heart) without another coexisting congenital cardiac malformation functions perfectly normally.

VENTRICULAR SEPTAL DEFECT

Ventricular septal defect is the most common congenital heart disease if mitral valve prolapse syndrome is not included. The hallmark of a ventricular septal defect is a holosystolic (pansystolic) murmur at the lower left sternal border, overlying the ventricular septum (see Chapter 8). On palpation, palpable thrills (see Chapter 8) are almost always present when the holosystolic murmur is loud (grade 4 or more). A small ventricular septal defect is often asymptomatic, and spontaneous closure of the defect is said to occur in as many as 30 to 50 percent of cases. When the heart size and heart sounds are normal and the only abnormal finding is a holosystolic murmur at the lower left sternal border, the diagnosis of a small ventricular septal defect with no hemodynamic significance is almost certain.

In this congenital lesion, a persistent opening in the upper portion of the ventricular septum due to failure of fusion with the aortic septum permits blood to pass from the left ventricle to the right ventricle (left-to-right shunt). The blood flow through the defect is from the left ventricle to the right ventricle because of higher pressure in the left ventricle. In one-fourth to one-third of the cases, the shunt (abnormal blood flow through the defect) is not large enough to overload the heart. With large shunts, however, both left and right ventricular overload may occur. In advanced cases with large defects, the shunt may become small or even reversed (a right-to-left shunt instead of a left-to-right shunt), especially when there is significant pulmonary hypertension. With large shunts, the right or left ventricle (or both), the left atrium, and the pulmonary arteries are enlarged, and pulmonary vascularity is increased. These findings are readily recognized on chest X-ray films. Enlargement of various cardiac chambers is also shown on the ECG and through other noninvasive studies (e.g., echocardiogram). A definitive diagnosis is made by cardiac catheterization (see Chapter 24).

Infants with large ventricular septal defects usually develop CHF, which causes various symptoms and signs. Of course, large defects may cause death from CHF in early infancy. A small ventricular septal defect without any symptoms requires no immediate treatment. Thus, surgery should be deferred until late childhood unless the disability is severe, with a variety of symptoms, or unless there is significant hemodynamic abnormality (e.g., pulmonary hypertension).

Remember that spontaneous closure of the ventricular septal defect is not uncommon, especially when the lesion is small.

The ideal case for surgical repair with cardiac bypass techniques is one with a large left-to-right shunt, associated with left ventricular hypertrophy (enlarged left pumping chamber) and only moderate pulmonary hypertension. The surgical mortality risk increases to 50 percent when pulmonary hypertension is severe (pulmonary arterial pressures above 85 mmHg) and the left-to-right shunt is small. Surgical treatment is contraindicated when the shunt is reversed. Patients with a small ventricular septal defect without any other abnormality are expected to have a normal life expectancy other than suffering the threat of bacterial endocarditis (bacterial infection of the heart). When the shunts are large, CHF usually develops early in life, and survival beyond age forty is rather unusual in this circumstance.

ATRIAL SEPTAL DEFECT

Atrial septal defect is the second most common congenital heart disease, and it is much more common in females. The most common form of atrial septal defect is persistence of the ostium secundum in the midseptum; a less common form is the ostium primum defect (a defect in the low portion of the septum involving the endocardial cushion). In ostium primum defect, mitral or tricuspid valve abnormalities may coexist. When these valve lesions coexist with atrial septal defect (ostium primum type), of course, cardiac function deteriorates further, and the outcome is more serious.

Most patients with a mild form of ostium secundum defects are asymptomatic. When there are large shunts, however, exertional dyspnea or other manifestations of heart failure are observed. Prominent right ventricular pulsations are readily recognizable by a simple inspection, and they are also easily palpable. On auscultation, an ejection systolic murmur (see Chapter 8) with moderate intensity is usually present in the second and third interspaces on the left sternal border as a result of increased blood flow across the pulmonic valve (called "relative pulmonic stenosis"). Likewise, soft middiastolic rumbling murmur (see Chapter 8) is often present at the xiphoid area (lower edge of the breastbone) because of increased blood flow across the tricuspid valve (called "relative tricuspid stenosis"). Characteristically, these heart murmurs originating in the right-sided heart increase their intensity during inspiration (see Chapter 8). Palpable thrills are rather uncommon in atrial septal defect. One of the unique and diagnostic features of atrial septal defect is relatively fixed but widely splitting second heart sounds (see Chapter 8).

Chest X-ray findings may be normal in a small atrial septal defect without significant hemodynamic abnormality. On the other hand, advanced cases often show a variety of abnormal X-ray findings, including large pulmonary arteries with vigorous pulsations, increased pulmonary vascularity, an enlarged right atrium as well as right ventricle, and a small aortic knob.

ECG provides valuable information in the diagnosis of atrial septal defect. That is, in more than 95 percent of cases with atrial septal defect (both secundum and primum types), incomplete or complete RBBB (see Chapter 24) is present. Therefore, the diagnosis of atrial septal defect is extremely unlikely when RBBB is not present. In addition, left anterior hemiblock (superior and leftward deviation of the electrical forces during ventricular activation as a result of a block in the anterior division of the left bundle branch system) often coexists with RBBB in ostium primum defect. Right atrial enlargement (called "P-congenitale") as well as right ventricular hypertrophy may be present (see Chapter 24). First-degree A-V block (prolonged P-R interval) is relatively common, and various atrial arrhythmias may occur (see Chapter 9). WPW syndrome often coexists with atrial septal defect. Recent medical studies indicate that SSS (Figure 3.7) not uncommonly develops eight to ten years following surgical repair for atrial septal defect. In this circumstance, a permanent artificial cardiac pacemaker is indicated.

Cardiac catheterization with angiocardiography (see Chapter 24) confirms the degree and the exact site of atrial septal defect with various hemodynamic abnormalities and coexisting cardiac lesions such as mitral regurgitation. Hemodynamic evidence of CHF also can be ascertained. In general, CHF is usually associated with the late development of AF in older patients. It is not uncommon to discover atrial septal defect in late adult life (even after age sixty or seventy) when the individual develops far-advanced CHF. Echocardiogram also enables one to diagnose atrial septal defect in most cases.

By and large, surgery is not indicated for small atrial septal defects. However, surgical closure should be performed in atrial septal defects with a large left-to-right shunt (more than two to three times systemic flow) associated with slight or no increased pulmonary arterial resistance. Surgical repair is rather hazardous in patients with pulmonary hypertension associated with reversed shunt because of the risk of acute right heart failure. In ostium primum defects, in addition to surgical repair of the defect, surgical suture of the valve clefts (especially those of the mitral valve) is recommended if significant mitral regurgitation coexists.

As far as the prognosis is concerned, patients with small defects without coexisting anomalies or complications may live a normal life. On the other hand, large shunts often cause disability by age forty, and this is particularly so in ostium primum defect. Major complications include CHF, pulmonary hypertension, and various cardiac arrhythmias, particularly AF. The surgical mortality is low (less than 1 percent) in patients under age forty-five who do not have CHF and who have pulmonary artery pressures below 60 mmHg. The surgical mortality increases up to 6 to 10 percent in patients older than age forty associated with CHF and/or significant pulmonary hypertension (above 60 mmHg). Remember that some patients develop SSS approximately ten years following successful surgical repair for atrial septal defect.

Patent ductus arteriosus occurs more frequently in females, in the offspring of women whose pregnancies were complicated by rubella during the first trimester, in premature infants, and in children born at high altitudes. Although patent ductus arteriosus usually occurs as an isolated defect, it may coexist with other congenital malformations, particularly coarctation of the aorta, ventricular septal defect, pulmonic stenosis, and aortic stenosis. A continuous "machinery" murmur that occupies the systolic phase as well as the diastolic phase of the cardiac cycle is a hallmark of patent ductus arteriosus (see Chapter 8). Paradoxical splitting of the second heart sounds (see Chapter 8) may occur when there is significant left ventricular hypertrophy.

Patent ductus arteriosus is a form of arteriovenous fistula (an abnormal communication between the arterial and venous systems), and blood flows from the aorta through the ductus into the pulmonary artery continuously in systolic as well as diastolic perods of the cardiac cycle, leading to an increase in the work loads of the left ventricle. Patent ductus arteriosus is thought to occur because the embryonic ductus arteriosus fails to close normally and persists as a shunt connecting the left pulmonary artery and aorta, usually near the origin of the left subclavian artery. In some cases, pulmonary hypertension develops, and consequently the shunt may become bidirectional or even reversed.

As far as clinical manifestations are concerned, there are usually no appreciable symptoms until CHF is produced. Heart size may be normal or slightly enlarged, with a forceful apex beat. Pulse pressure (difference between systolic and diastolic pressures—see Chapters 2 and 5) is characteristically wide, and diastolic pressure is very low. On the chest X-ray film, the heart may be normal in size and contour, but there may be left ventricular hypertrophy as well as left atrial enlargement. The pulmonary artery, aorta, and left atrium are often prominent. ECG may be entirely normal, but it may show, again, left ventricular hypertrophy. Final confirmation of the diagnosis is usually made by cardiac catheterization (see Chapter 24).

As far as management is concerned, the presence of a patent ductus arteriosus is generally considered a sufficient indication for surgical correction unless there is a clear contraindication. Although there are somewhat different opinions among surgeons, the optimal age for surgery is considered to be one to two years. Patients with CHF or considerable retardation in growth as infants should undergo surgical correction promptly; results even in the first few months of life are reported to be excellent in most cases. When there has been bacterial endocarditis, the patient should be given appropriate antibiotics and the operation performed approximately six weeks later. Contraindication of surgery is severe pulmonary vascular disease associated with marked pulmonary hypertension and reversal of shunt. The surgical mortality is negligible in uncomplicated cases.

Obviously, large shunts result in a high mortality rate from CHF early in life. Smaller shunts are said to be compatible with long survival, but CHF is the most common and serious complication. In addition, the chance of suffering bacterial endocarditis is, of course, greater as long as the surgical correction is not performed. Prophylactic antibiotics are recommended when dental procedures are scheduled for every patient before surgical correction of the ductus. When the surgical correction is performed early in life, most patients may be able to live a normal life span without any problem, providing no serious complication was present before or after the operation.

COARCTATION OF THE AORTA

Coarctation of the aorta is characterized by a narrowing or constriction of the lumen of the aorta that may involve any location along its length. The narrowing of the aorta is most commonly localized just distal to the origin of the left sub-clavian artery near the insertion of the ligamentum arteriosum. Coarctation of the aorta occurs in about 7 percent of patients with congenital heart diseases and is twice as common in males as in females. This congenital lesion is most commonly encountered in patients with Turner's syndrome (a form of chromosomal abnormality).

It is important to emphasize that coarctation of the aorta is one of the common forms of secondary hypertension (see Chapter 5), and hypertension is cured through the surgical correction of the lesion in most cases. Coarctation of the aorta may occur as an isolated congenital lesion, but it often coexists with other congenital cardiac malformations, including bicuspid aortic valve, aortic stenosis, patent ductus arteriosus, ventricular septal defect, and mitral insufficiency. Thus, clinical manifestations are greatly influenced by the location and extent of the narrowing as well as the presence or absence and severity of coexisting congenital cardiac lesions. Many children and young adults with an isolated coarctation of the aorta may be completely symptom free. Although headache, epistaxis (nose bleeding), cold lower extremities, and claudication on exertion (leg pain with physical exercise) may be experienced by some patients, coarctation of the aorta is often suspected on the basis of a heart murmur or hypertension in the arms on a routine physical checkup. Although the exact reason for hypertension in patients with coarctation of the aorta is uncertain, mechanical factors are considered to play the primary role rather than those of renal origin. When there is diffuse narrowing of the aorta located proximal to the ductus arteriosus, right ventricular hypertrophy develops, and pulmonary hypertension and CHF are common in early life.

The characteristic features include markedly reduced (even completely absent in some cases) or delayed pulsations in the femoral arteries (arteries in the groin) and a low or even unobtainable BP in the legs, with hypertension in the arms. In older children and adults, enlarged and pulsatile collateral vessels (reserved blood vessels) may be palpable in the intercostal spaces (between ribs) anteriorly, in the axillae, or in the back (in the interscapular area). In some patients, the arms and thorax may be more developed than the legs because of better blood circulation in the upper portion of the body, with inadequate blood supply to the legs. On auscultation, a midsystolic murmur is best heard over the anterior part of the chest (often at the second or third intercostal space) and the upper portion of the back. The murmur is continuous in some cases when the narrowing of the lumen is severe enough to cause a high-velocity jet across the lesion of the aorta throughout the cardiac cycle (see Chapter 8).

As far as laboratory tests are concerned, ECG often reveals left ventricular hypertrophy of varying degree depending upon the severity of hypertension proximal to the narrowing and the patient's age. In mild cases, however, ECG may be entirely normal. Chest X-ray may disclose a dilated left subclavian artery high on the left mediastinal border and a dilated ascending aorta. It may be said that indentation of the aorta at the site of coarctation and prestenotic and poststenotic dilatation along the left paramediastinal shadow are almost diagnostic of coarctation of the aorta. In addition, notching of the ribs resulting from dilated collateral blood vessels on the chest X-ray film is a unique feature of this condition. The rib notching becomes more pronounced with age and is readily recognizable between the ages of six and twelve years. The precise degree, length, and site of the coarctation of the aorta can be ascertained by cardiac catheterization and aortography (see Chapter 24). In addition, coexisting congenital malformations, of course, can be identified by catheterization.

As far as treatment is concerned, all patients with uncomplicated coarctation of the aorta must have surgical correction. The surgical treatment consists of resection of the narrowed segment of the aorta and end-to-end anastomosis (suturing both ends). The surgical result is excellent in most cases. When the narrowed segment of the aorta is very long, however, it may be necessary to use a tubular graft or patch in the surgical repair. The ideal time for the surgical repair in asymptomatic patients is considered to be between the ages of four and eight. It should be noted that some patients may develop paradoxical hypertension of short duration in the immediate postoperative period. In addition, some other patients may develop the late onset of hypertension following successful surgical correction. Thus, periodic medical checkups are essential even following surgery for all patients with coarctation of the aorta, and appropriate antihypertensive treatment should be provided as needed (see Chapter 5). The major and serious complication associated with coarctation of the aorta result from severe hypertension. They may include CHF, rupture of the aorta, infective endocarditis, and cerebral (brain) aneurysms or hemorrhage.

The term *pulmonic (pulmonary) stenosis* is used to describe the narrowing of the right ventricular outflow tract. The narrowing may be localized to the supravalvular (above the valve), valvular (pulmonic valve itself), or subvalvular (below the valve), but valvular pulmonic stenosis is the most common form of isolated right ventricular outflow tract narrowing or obstruction. At times, multiple sites may show narrowing in different degrees. At any rate, the most important influence over clinical manifestations and their course is the degree of narrowing in the pulmonic valve area rather than the specific site of stenosis. Pulmonic stenosis is said to be mild when the gradient (pressure difference) between the right ventricle and the pulmonary artery across the narrowing is less than 50 mmHg. Pulmonic stenosis is considered moderate when the gradient is between 50 and 80 mmHg, whereas a gradient of more than 80 mmHg is labeled as severe pulmonic stenosis.

By and large, most patients with mild pulmonic stenosis are symptom free and demonstrate little or no progression in the severity of the narrowing as they get older. On the other hand, in patients with moderate to severe pulmonic stenosis, the degree of narrowing tends to get worse with time. Clinical manifestations and symptoms vary significantly according to the degree of narrowing. In extreme cases, for example, infants with pulmonic atresia (complete obstruction of the pulmonic valve) often die from hypoxia. Older patients with moderate to severe narrowing frequently experience fatigue, dyspnea, right ventricular failure, and syncope, because an increment of pulmonary blood flow is prevented by the narrowed pulmonic valve, especially with physical exercise. In fact, sudden death may occur with vigorous physical exercise when pulmonic stenosis is severe.

Various physical findings in pulmonic stenosis have been described in Chapter 8. The presence of the right parasternal lift and a harsh, ejection-type systolic murmur with palpable thrills at the second or third interspaces along the left sternal border supports the clinical diagnosis of pulmonic stenosis.

As far as laboratory tests are concerned, the ECG is usually normal in mild pulmonic stenosis. On the other hand, evidence of right ventricular hypertrophy is readily recognized on the ECG when pulmonic stenosis is moderate to severe. In addition, P waves are usually tall and peaked in leads II, III, aVF, and V_{1-3}, indicating right atrial enlargement (called "P-congenitale"). The chest X-ray often reveals a heart of normal size with normal vascularity of the lungs in mild to moderate pulmonic stenosis. In severe pulmonic stenosis, of course, right atrial as well as right ventricular enlargement is demonstrated on the chest X-ray film. In the presence of significant pulmonic valvular stenosis, poststenotic dilatation of the main and left pulmonary arteries may be shown on the chest X-ray. In addition, pulmonic vascularity is often reduced in severe pulmonic stenosis. The exact site and degree of the narrowing of the pulmonic valve are confirmed by cardiac catheterization and angiocardiography (see Chapter 24). In addition, any coexisting congenital cardiac malformation can be documented by these invasive diagnostic tests.

As far as treatment is concerned, moderate to severe degrees of pulmonic valvular and subvalvular stenosis should be corrected surgically. The surgical mortality rate is low, and excellent results are expected in most cases. However, multiple sites of narrowing of the peripheral pulmonary arteries are usually not operable. In patients with pure pulmonic stenosis, the incidence of infective endocarditis is approximately 1 percent per year. Patients with mild pulmonic stenosis may have a normal life expectancy unless infective endocarditis occurs.

AORTIC STENOSIS

Congenital malformations causing narrowing of the left ventricular outflow tract include valvular aortic stenosis (narrowing of the aortic valve itself), the discrete form of subaortic stenosis (narrowing of the area below the aortic valve), supravalvular aortic stenosis (narrowing of the ascending aorta above the aortic valve), and idiopathic hypertrophic subaortic stenosis. The discussion primarily concentrates on valvular aortic stenosis because of its common occurrence. Valvular aortic stenosis is observed in about 4 percent of patients with congenital heart diseases and occurs three to four times more often in males than in females. Congenital bicuspid aortic valve may become stenotic with time or be the site of infective endocarditis. At this time, the lesion may be recognized in adult life and may be difficult to distinguish from aortic stenosis of rheumatic origin. Remember that aortic stenosis is also one of the most common valvular lesions resulting from rheumatic fever (see Chapter 11). Congenital aortic stenosis may coexist with other congenital cardiac malformations, including patent ductus arteriosus and coarctation of the aorta.

A congenitally deformed and rigid aortic valve frequently leads to thickening of the valve cusps and, in later life, to the production of calcification that is readily recognized on the chest X-ray film. When narrowing of the aortic valve is severe, concentric hypertrophy of the left ventricular wall and dilatation of the ascending aorta will be produced. The narrowing of the aortic valve is considered critical when a peak systolic pressure gradient between the left ventricular outflow tract and the aorta across the aortic valve is beyond 70 mmHg in association with a normal cardiac output, or with an effective aortic valve orifice less than 0.6 cm^2 per square meter of body surface. By and large, cardiac output in the resting state is within normal limits but often does not increase normally during physical exercise.

As far as clinical manifestations are concerned, most children with aortic stenosis are completely symptom free and grow normally. Therefore, in most asymptomatic children, aortic stenosis is detected by recognizing a typical ejection-type systolic murmur in the aortic area during a routine physical checkup. On the other hand, children with moderately severe narrowing often complain of easy fatigability and dyspnea on exertion. When aortic stenosis is severe, exertional syncope may occur, because the left ventricle is unable to increase cardiac output and maintain sufficient blood circulation to the brain during physical exercise. For the same reason, patients with severe aortic stenosis frequently suffer from anginal pain because myocardial oxygen requirements, particularly during physical activity, exceed the oxygen supply to the left ventricle. As a rule, symptomatic patients have significant aortic stenosis, but a lack of the symptoms by no means excludes the possibility of serious narrowing of the aortic valve. Patients are strongly advised not to engage in any rigorous physical activity when aortic stenosis is diagnosed or suspected, because sudden death is always a possibility. Although the precise mechanism that causes sudden death is not clearly understood in this circumstance, ventricular arrhythmias, particularly VF (see Chapter 9) associated with acute myocardial ischemia (a sudden lack of adequate blood supply to the heart muscle), are considered responsible.

Various physical findings of aortic stenosis were discussed in Chapter 8. The systolic murmur of aortic stenosis is typically ejection-type (diamond-shaped), loud and harsh in quality, and best heard at the base of the heart (at the second intercostal space along the left or right sternal border). The murmur often radiates to the neck and to the cardiac apex.

With regard to laboratory tests, ECG shows left ventricular hypertrophy in moderate to severe aortic stenosis, but mild aortic stenosis often discloses a normal ECG. It should be noted, however, that a normal ECG does not exclude moderate to severe aortic stenosis in some cases. On the chest X-ray film, the overall heart size is often normal or only slightly enlarged. In moderate to severe aortic stenosis, left atrial enlargement as well as concentric left ventricular hypertrophy are usually evident. In addition, poststenotic dilatation of the ascending aorta is also frequently present. The exact site and degree of the narrowing of the aortic valve can be confirmed by cardiac catheterization, and coexisting congenital cardiac malformations will also be identified. It should be stressed that heart catheterization must be performed every five to ten years in patients with mild to moderate aortic stenosis, because the narrowing not uncommonly gets worse.

As a preventive measure against infective endocarditis, prophylactic antibiotic therapy is indicated. In patients with CHF as a result of diminished cardiac reserve, digitalis and diuretics are indicated, and sodium intake should be restricted while surgical correction is awaited. Vigorous physical activity or any form of competitive sports should be avoided by patients with moderate to severe aortic stenosis, even if the individual is symptom free, because sudden death is always a possibility. It is important to remember that the decision regarding indication versus nonindication of surgical correction primarily depends on the severity of the narrowing of the aortic valve rather than on the symptoms experienced by the patient. Surgical correction is highly recommended for all patients with critical stenosis of the aortic valve regardless of the presence or absence of symptoms. In addition, surgery is also indicated even in milder aortic stenosis when significant symptoms (e.g., syncope, anginal pain, CHF) are present.

TETRALOGY OF FALLOT

Tetralogy of Fallot consists of four components:

1. Ventricular septal defect
2. Narrowing of the right ventricular outflow tract or pulmonic stenosis
3. Overriding of the aortic orifice above the ventricular septal defect
4. Right ventricular hypertrophy

Among these, ventricular septal defect and pulmonic stenosis are the major lesions. The incidence of tetralogy of Fallot is estimated to be about 10 percent of all types of congenital cardiac diseases; it is the most common congenital heart malformation producing cyanosis in children after the age of one year. In this disorder, ventricular septal defect is usually as large as the size of the aortic valve orifice. In 25 percent of cases, a right-sided aortic knob, arch, and descending aorta are observed.

The hemodynamic abnormalities and clinical manifestations are greatly influenced by the relationship between the resistance to blood flow from the ventricles into the aorta and into the pulmonary vessels. Thus, the degree of narrowing of the right ventricular outflow tract is the major determining factor. In other words, severe cyanosis and polycythemia (increased numbers of red blood cells), associated with various clinical manifestations of systemic anoxia or hypoxia (insufficient or no oxygen supply to the tissues), occur when the right ventricular outflow narrowing is severe because the pulmonary blood flow is markedly diminished and a large volume of unsaturated systemic venous blood (blood with insufficient oxygen content) is shunted from the right to the left ventricle across the ventricular septal defect. Most children with these malformations are cyanotic from birth or before one year of age. Tetralogy of Fallot is the most common cause of cyanotic congenital heart disease in adults, although survival to adult life is uncommon without surgical correction. Common clinical manifestations include dyspnea on exertion, retarded growth and development, clubbing of extremities (enlargement of tips of fingers and toes), and polycythemia. Infants with tetralogy of Fallot characteristically assume a squatting posture when they rest following physical exertion. Frequent episodes of marked anoxia and cyanosis constitute a major threat to the survival of these children.

On inspection, underdevelopment and cyanosis of varying degrees associated with clubbing fingers and toes are obvious and particularly pronounced after the first year of life. A right ventricular impulse and systolic thrill are often palpable along the left sternal border, but generalized cardiomegaly is usually not present. On auscultation, the second heart sound is single, and the P_2 is seldom heard. An ejection-type systolic murmur is usually present at the base of the heart as a result of blood flow across the narrowed right ventricular outflow tract or pulmonic valve (see Chapter 8).

As far as laboratory tests are concerned, the ECG usually reveals right ventricular hypertrophy and, less commonly, right atrial enlargement. It is also not uncommon to observe RBBB (Figure 9.9). Chest X-ray film discloses a normal-sized but boot-shaped heart (often called "coeur en sabot") with prominence of the right ventricle and a concavity in the region of the pulmonary conus. One of the characteristic features is markedly diminished pulmonary vascular markings, so that the lung fields are abnormally clear. Cardiac catheterization with selective angiocardiography will confirm the diagnosis and assess precisely the degree and site of these combined congenital cardiac malformations (see Chapter 24).

As far as management is concerned, total surgical correction is ultimately advisable for almost all patients with tetralogy of Fallot. When dealing with infants who exhibit severe cyanosis and serious clinical symptoms, however, the risk of primary surgical correction is very high unless it is performed in a medical institution prepared properly for intracardiac surgery and a palliative operation designed to increase pulmonary blood flow may be recommended. In this circumstance, total surgical correction can be performed later, in older childhood or during adolescence, when the surgical risk is expected to be lower. Before surgery, the paroxysmal cyanotic episodes may be treated with oxygen (effectiveness is usually prompt when the child is placed in the knee-chest position) and morphine. Common complications include iron-deficiency anemia, infective endocarditis, paradoxic embolism, polycythemia, coagulation defects, and cerebral infarction or abscess. These complications, of course, must be prevented, or minimized and treated if they occur.

MITRAL VALVE PROLAPSE SYNDROME (BARLOW'S SYNDROME)

Although a controversy exists among physicians, mitral valve prolapse syndrome (Barlow's syndrome) is considered a form of congenital heart disease. Some physicians feel that the syndrome is a form of valvular heart disease, because mitral regurgitation is often one of its common manifestations. On the other hand, the syndrome is considered a form of cardiomyopathy (heart muscle disease; see Chapter 12) by others, because myxomatous degeneration of the mitral valve is the usual finding.

Prolapse of the mitral valve occurs when one or both of the leaflets protrude abnormally into the left atrium during the systolic phase of the ventricles. The syndrome was described about two decades ago by Barlow, and the characteristic features include the nonejection click (or clicks) with or without the mitral regurgitation murmur often associated with atypical chest pain and palpitations. Mitral valve prolapse syndrome is often unrecognized on casual medical examination, but 10 to 15 percent of the population is found, through the availability of echocardiography, to have this syndrome. It has been shown that female cases predominate over male cases with a two-to-one ratio. Myxomatous degeneration of the mitral valve is considered responsible for producing this syndrome, although the fundamental underlying cause is unknown. There seems to be no relationship to coronary or valvular heart disease. However, it has been shown that atrial septal defect often coexists with mitral valve prolapse syndrome. Some familial incidence of this syndrome has been reported.

As far as clinical manifestations are concerned, there are two major symptoms, including atypical chest pain and various complaints (e.g., palpitations, skipped heartbeats) due to a variety of cardiac arrhythmias. The chest pain is often sharp and localized to the left chest, and it is not necessarily related to physical activity but may be relieved by rest or NG. In older individuals, the chest pain superficially mimics coronary pain. In fact, in many cases of this syndrome, the diagnosis of angina pectoris is often made erroneously. A variety of cardiac arrhythmias may be observed, but VPCs and atrial tachycardia are probably most commonly observed. Slow heart rhythms (e.g., complete A-V block) may occasionally occur. Sudden death from a variety of abnormal heart rhythms has been reported (very rare).

The characteristic physical findings in this syndrome were discussed in Chapter 8. Abnormal heart rhythms can be detected during physical examination, and the signs of left ventricular hypertrophy and CHF may be present in advanced cases.

As far as laboratory tests are concerned, echocardiography is the most valuable diagnostic test in confirming mitral valve prolapse syndrome (see Chapter 24). One or both mitral valve leaflets may be observed moving in a posterior direction during systole. Thus, the diagnostic feature is a posterior excursion of the mitral valve leaflets during the systolic phase of the ventricles. ECG findings are not diagnostic, and nonspecific abnormality of S-T segment and T waves is common. Various cardiac arrhythmias, especially VPCs, are frequently observed. In advanced cases, left ventricular hypertrophy may be diagnosed. Cardiac catheterization and angiocardiography confirm the diagnosis, but these invasive tests are unnecessary because the diagnosis can be made accurately in almost all cases (nearly 100 percent) by echocardiography and clinical background.

As far as management is concerned, prophylactic antibiotics should be given for all dental or other surgical procedures, especially in patients with significant heart murmur. Antibiotics should be administered the day before, the day of, and two days after the surgical procedure. For the treatment of chest pain or cardiac arrhythmias, propranolol (Inderal) is the drug of choice (10 to 30 mg, three to four times daily by mouth; see Table 6.2). For AF, digitalis is the drug of choice. Mitral valve replacement may be necessary in patients with significant mitral regurgitation associated with increasing symptoms and increasing heart size. On rare occasions, artificial pacemaker implantation is indicated for a very slow heart rhythm (e.g., complete A-V block). In completely asymptomatic individuals, no treatment (other than prophylactic antibiotics for dental procedures) is indicated, even when the diagnosis is unequivocally established. The average life span of individuals with this syndrome differs very little from that of normal people. Factors that may lead to the reduction of life expectancy include progressive worsening of mitral re-gurgitation, bacterial endocarditis, and serious cardiac arrhythmias. Sudden death is always a possibility, although it is extremely rare.

MISCELLANEOUS CONDITIONS

Mirror-image dextrocardia is a congenital cardiac disease in which the anatomic positions of the heart are completely reversed, so that the heart is situated on the right rather than the left side of the chest. Aside from abnormal positions, the function of the heart is entirely normal unless there is a coexisting congenital cardiac malformation. Dextrocardia is not uncommonly associated with situs inversus (reversed position of the digestive system—e.g., liver on the left side of the abdomen instead of the right side, as in normal people).

Cardiac arrhythmias may be congenital in origin. For instance, complete A-V block may occur at birth. In congenital complete A-V block, exercise tolerance is often normal during childhood, but eventually a permanent artificial pacemaker is indicated as the individual gets older, because of a slow and inadequate heart rhythm. Congenital complete A-V block not uncommonly coexists with other congenital heart diseases. WPW syndrome is considered a form of congenital heart disease (see Chapter 9), and it may be associated with other congenital heart diseases, such as atrial septal defect, mitral valve prolapse syndrome, idiopathic hypertrophic subaortic stenosis, and Ebstein's anomaly (downward displacement of the tricuspid valve).

11

RHEUMATIC FEVER AND RHEUMATIC HEART DISEASE

Many children may recover completely from rheumatic fever without any permanent damage to the heart valves, whereas others may eventually develop various heart valve lesions months or even years later after recovering from an acute attack of rheumatic fever. It can be said that rheumatic fever is the most common cause of valvular heart diseases, and among them, mitral stenosis is the most common valvular lesion from rheumatic fever. The first part of this chapter deals with rheumatic fever and the last, with rheumatic heart disease (RHD).

RHEUMATIC FEVER

By definition, rheumatic fever is an inflammatory disease that develops as a delayed response to pharyngeal infection with group A streptococcus (a kind of bacteria). The disease process primarily involves the heart, joints, central nervous system, skin, and subcutaneous tissues. In the typical acute form, clinical manifestations are characterized by migratory polyarthritis (changing locations of arthritis involving multiple joints simultaneously); fever; carditis (inflammation of the heart), often associated with Sydenham's chorea (defined later); subcutaneous nodules; and erythema marginatum (pinkish rash).

203

Of greatest clinical significance is the involvement of the heart, leading to RHD as a chronic condition due to scarring and deformity of the heart valves, particularly the mitral and aortic valves. It has been shown that the mitral valve is involved in 75 to 80 percent of cases, the aortic valve in 30 percent, and the tricuspid and pulmonic valves in less than 5 percent. Among these lesions, mitral stenosis is the most common occurrence. It can be said that mitral stenosis nearly always represents a manifestation of RHD. Various valve lesions may develop months or years after the initial attack of rheumatic fever. Fortunately, many children may recover from rheumatic fever completely, without any sequelae, when proper treatment is provided. It should be emphasized that no single symptom, sign, or laboratory test is diagnostic of rheumatic fever; rather, various combinations of them may be diagnostic.

Although rheumatic fever may involve any age group, it is rather uncommon in infancy and in children younger than four and in adults after fifty. It most commonly affects children aged five to fifteen years. The overall incidence of RHD is in third rank behind coronary and hypertensive heart disease. Thus, rheumatic fever is the most common precursor of heart disease among individuals under the age of forty. The incidence of rheumatic fever is reported to increase to as high as 5 to 50 percent following streptococcal infection in individuals who have suffered from rheumatic fever in the past. In addition, the incidence of recurrent attacks of rheumatic fever following streptococcal infection is reported to be considerably higher in patients with known RHD than in those who have recovered from previous attacks of rheumatic fever completely without cardiac damage. Rheumatic fever is still a worldwide disease, particularly in underdeveloped countries where conditions are such that overcrowding and less-than-desirable housing situations are unavoidable. For the same reason, it is common to observe several children suffering from rheumatic fever in a single family, and often there is a family history of rheumatic fever. Fortunately, the mortality rate of acute rheumatic fever has been declining steadily in the past thirty years, but still it is the major cause of death and disability in children and adolescents.

Clinical Manifestations and Diagnosis

For the diagnosis of rheumatic fever, modified Jones's criteria are commonly utilized in the medical literature. Major and minor Jones's criteria are as follows:

Major criteria include (1) carditis; (2) polyarthritis; (3) chorea; (4) erythema marginatum, and (5) subcutaneous nodules.

Minor criteria include (1) fever; (2) arthralgia; (3) prolongation of the P-R interval (delayed A-V conduction time) on the ECG; (4) increased sedimentation rate or positive C-reactive protein, and (5) previous history of rheumatic fever or any evidence of RHD.

By and large, the diagnosis of rheumatic fever is established with a reasonable certainty when two or more major criteria are present. The most reliable findings among them include carditis and migratory polyarthritis. In addition, various other factors indicating evidence of preceding streptococcal infection also support the diagnosis. They include a history of recent scarlet fever, positive throat culture for group A streptococcus, and increased antistreptolysin O (ASO) titer or other streptococcal antibodies.

Major Criteria

Carditis   Carditis is the most common and the most reliable manifestation. Therefore, the diagnosis of acute rheumatic fever is extremely doubtful in the absence of carditis. The inflammatory process of rheumatic fever usually involves the entire heart diffusely, including myocardium (heart muscle) as well as pericardium (pericardial sac). The heart murmurs of mitral or aortic regurgitation (see Chapter 8) are often the first sign of acute rheumatic carditis, and mitral regurgitation occurs more frequently. Various signs and symptoms of acute pericarditis and of CHF often occur in advanced cases. Of course, permanent valvular damage may be produced subsequently, and death may result from intractable CHF under this circumstance. It should be noted, however, that rheumatic carditis may vary from a low-grade and very mild inflammatory process to a life-threatening and fatal clinical course. In mild cases of carditis, there may be no significant or apparent symptoms referable to the cardiac illness.

In most cases of acute rheumatic carditis, there is usually tachycardia disproportionate to the degree of fever, and gallop rhythm is often present. First degree A-V block often occurs, and at times second-degree Wenckebach A-V block may appear (see Chapter 9). In addition, nonspecific abnormality of the S-T segment and T wave is also relatively common. It can be said that acute rheumatic carditis should be strongly suspected when any child develops first-degree A-V block unless proven otherwise. Acute pericarditis often produces a friction rub (see Chapter 8) and precordial pain, often associated with diffuse S-T segment elevation in many leads on the ECG.

By and large, acute rheumatic carditis is diagnosed with reasonable certainty when one or more of the following can be found: (1) the appearance of new heart murmurs or changing character of the murmurs; (2) enlargement of the heart documented by chest X-ray or fluoroscopy; (3) signs and symptoms of acute CHF; (4) evidence of acute pericarditis or pericardial effusion; and (5) first-degree or Wenckebach A-V block.

The diagnosis of acute rheumatic carditis is further confirmed under these circumstances when any of the following is definitely established: (1) a history of rheumatic fever; (2) valvular lesion(s) clearly rheumatic in origin, and (3) evidence of streptococcal infection of the upper respiratory tract within the preceding four weeks.

Polyarthritis   The term *polyarthritis* means that two or more joints are involved, and it should be associated with at least two minor Jones's criteria to establish the diagnosis. The arthritis of acute rheumatic fever is characteristically a migratory polyarthritis of gradual or acute onset associated with signs and symptoms of acute febrile illness. The large joints of the extremities are most frequently involved, but arthritis may affect the hands and feet and even the spine in some children.

The polyarthritis manifested by hot, red, swollen, and tender joints changes the location to other joints sequentially as the inflammatory process of the involved joints subsides. In some cases, joint effusions may occur, but acute inflammatory process in the joints subsides within one to five weeks without residual deformity in most cases. A definitive diagnosis requires one of the additional Jones's major criteria, particularly carditis. It should be remembered that polyarthritis and carditis are the most common and reliable diagnostic clinical manifestations of acute rheumatic fever. As a rule, there is a high titer of antistreptolysin O (ASO) or some other streptococcal antibody.

Chorea   Chorea (Sydenham's chorea or Saint Vitus's dance) is a disorder of the central nervous system characterized by purposeless, irregular, jerky movements of the extremities, trunk, and facial muscles often associated with muscular weakness and emotional instability. Chorea is actually a delayed clinical finding of rheumatic fever, because all other clinical findings may or may not exist at the time chorea occurs. Arthritis usually subsides before chorea occurs. It has been shown that chorea may occur after a long latent period (up to several months) following the preceding streptococcal infection and at a time when other manifestations of acute rheumatic fever have subsided.

For unknown reasons, girls seem to be more frequently involved with chorea, and adults are only rarely affected. Patients may be extremely nervous and may have difficulty in writing or drawing. These children tend to stumble or fall and drop things, and they frequently make facial grimaces. In advanced cases, it becomes difficult or impossible to walk, talk, or sit up. Chorea usually gets worse with emotional excitement, effort, or fatigue, but subsides during sleep. Speech disturbance in varying degrees is very common. Chorea usually lasts several weeks, but it may last even months.

Erythema Marginatum   Erythema marginatum is a round, pinkish rash that often assumes the shape of rings or crescents with clear centers. The rash varies markedly in size, but occurs primarily on the trunk and proximal part of the extremities. It never occurs on the face, however. The erythematous areas may be slightly raised and confluent. Erythema marginatum is often transient and migratory, and the rash may be brought out by applying heat. It is nonpurulent; it is not indurated and it branches on pressure. The rash is frequently associated with skin nodules.

Subcutaneous Nodules   Subcutaneous nodules are usually small (2 cm or less in diameter), pea-sized, firm, and painless swellings over bony prominences such as the elbows, the dorsal surfaces of the hands and feet, the margins of the patellae (knee caps), the scalp, the scapulae, and the vertebral spines (backbones). The skin moves freely over the nodules. They may be few or many, and they may persist for days or weeks. The skin nodules are often recurrent, but they are relatively uncommon except in children. Many children may not recognize the skin nodules unless they occur at multiple locations.

Minor Criteria

Various manifestations considered to be Jones's minor criteria are valuable in supporting the diagnosis of rheumatic fever only when more specific features (e.g., carditis, polyarthritis) are present. These minor criteria play only a supportive role in the diagnosis of rheumatic fever when there are two or more major Jones's criteria coexisting, because these minor criteria may also be due to many other disorders.

In addition to the aforementioned minor criteria, rheumatic fever is often associated with other manifestations, including general malaise, anorexia, weight loss, abdominal pain, and epistaxis. The abdominal pain may result from liver engorgement, sterile rheumatic peritonitis (inflammation of a sac in the abdominal cavity), or rheumatic arteritis (inflammation of an artery). At times, the abdominal pain may be extended from the inflammation of the pleura (pleurisy) or pericardium (pericarditis). On rare occasions, the abdominal pain is so intense that unnecessary abdominal surgery may be performed for possible diagnosis of appendicitis or cholecystitis (inflammation of the gallbladder).

Laboratory Tests

Although no laboratory test is specific for the diagnosis of rheumatic fever, various abnormal test results are valuable in supporting the diagnosis when clinical manifestations are compatible. In addition, careful evaluation of the results of laboratory tests is also very useful when clinical features of rheumatic fever are not apparent.

Antistreptolysin O (ASO) Test

Streptococcal antibody titers are usually elevated in the early stages of acute rheumatic fever. However, these antibody levels may be low or declining when detection of the acute streptococcal infection has been delayed for more than two months, or when the presenting manifestation is only chorea. In addition, these antibody titers may be low in patients who suffer only from carditis. Other than these clinical circumstances, the diagnosis of acute rheumatic fever is very unlikely in the absence of a significant elevation of streptococcal antibody titers.

The ASO test is the most commonly used and reliable streptococcal antibody test. By and large, the ASO titers above 250 Todd units in adults and 333 Todd units in children older than five years are considered abnormally elevated for the diagnosis. In general, a very low ASO titer, especially a value of less than 50 Todd units on repeated tests, is strong evidence against the diagnosis. There are some other streptococcal antibody tests available, but these tests are not commonly utilized today.

Throat Culture

The term *throat culture* means an isolation of the bacteria on the materials obtained from the surface or inner layer of the throat utilizing a special culture substance. Although many patients with acute rheumatic fever may constantly show evidence of group A (beta-hemolytic) streptococcus on a throat culture, particularly at the onset of the disease, the bacteria may be difficult to isolate in a single throat culture. Similarly, the administration of penicillin or other antibiotics may also result in failure to isolate the streptococcus. Another diagnostic problem is that a significant number of normal people, especially children, may have group A streptococcus in the upper respiratory tract all the time without any evidence of rheumatic fever. Thus, throat cultures are less reliable than the evaluation of the ASO titer as supportive evidence for the diagnosis of acute rheumatic fever. Nevertheless, the throat culture is positive for group A streptococcus in about 50 percent of cases with acute rheumatic fever.

Other Laboratory Tests

Other laboratory tests, including the erythrocyte sedimentation rate (ESR), the test for C-reactive protein (CRP), blood tests for white cell counts and hemoglobin or hematocrit value, and urine tests for red blood cells and protein, provide objective but nonspecific confirmation of the inflammatory process in the body. The first-degree A-V block on the ECG is again not specific for rheumatic fever, but the finding strongly supports the diagnosis, especially in children and young adults. First-degree A-V block is observed in approximately 25 percent of cases with acute rheumatic fever. This ECG finding is nearly always encountered when the presenting manifestation of rheumatic fever is primarily carditis. Other ECG abnormalities (e.g., S-T segment and T wave changes) are also common in patients with rheumatic carditis.

Complications

The immediate and major complication of acute rheumatic fever is CHF in very sick patients. Other immediate complications may include various cardiac arrhythmias, rheumatic pneumonitis (inflammation of the lungs), pericardial effusion, and pulmonary embolism. The most serious late complication is the development of permanent heart valve damage months or years following the first attack of acute rheumatic fever. Valvular heart diseases are most commonly produced by rheumatic fever, and in some cases, rheumatic valvular lesions may be detected even in late adulthood.

Treatment

Unfortunately, no specific cure for rheumatic fever is available. However, immediate and appropriate supportive therapy with the proper use of various medications can reduce the morbidity and mortality considerably. One of the most important therapeutic approaches is prevention of initial rheumatic attacks, as well as long-term prevention of the recurrence of rheumatic fever, especially in schoolchildren and young adults.

General Measures

Bed rest is the most important aspect, and it should be continued as long as any sign or symptom of acute rheumatic fever is present. In particular, all patients with rheumatic fever need bed rest until the body temperature returns to normal without medications (e.g., salicylates) and until other signs of acute attack (e.g., rapid heart or pulse rate) have subsided. When all manifestations of acute rheumatic attack are considered to have disappeared, the patient may then be allowed up slowly, and daily activity may be increased progressively as tolerated. It usually takes several months to regain full strength unless the rheumatic fever is extremely mild. It is also important to maintain general health with good nutrition. Of course, bed rest is mandatory when there are major complications (e.g., congestive heart failure).

Medications

By and large, the drug therapy for acute rheumatic fever consists of penicillin, salicylate, and costicosteroids (adrenal hormones).

Penicillin   As soon as the diagnosis is established, a course of penicillin therapy should be initiated promptly in order to eliminate group A streptococci. Penicillin therapy is indicated even if the throat cultures for streptococci are negative on repeated examinations, because the bacteria may be present where ordinary throat-swabbing techniques cannot isolate them.

The most effective kind of penicillin therapy is a single intramuscular injection of 1.2 million units of benzathine penicillin (Bicillin). Alternatively, 600,000 units of procaine penicillin may be injected intramuscularly for ten consecutive days with the same effect. Even after completion of penicillin therapy for acute rheumatic attack, prophylactic penicillin therapy is extremely important for the prevention of recurrence, especially in schoolchildren and young adults. Unfortunately, administration of large doses of penicillin early in the acute rheumatic attack does not seem to prevent ultimate heart damage.

Salicylate   Salicylate is a very effective drug in relieving acute polyarthritis and in reducing fever. As long as there is no evidence of carditis, the use of corticosteroids is not indicated. The dosage should be increased until the drug produces either a clinical effect or signs of toxicity (e.g., tinnitus—ringing in the ears; head-ache; or hypercapnea—very rapid breathing). In general, salicylate may be started at 15 to 20 mg/kg in children and 6 to 8 g in adults, given in four to five divided doses/day. Among various salicylate preparations, ordinary aspirin is the cheapest and is also very effective. A variety of gastrointestinal problems (e.g., stomachache, indigestion, bleeding from the stomach) are often produced by salicylate. Thus, it is advisable to take aspirin after meals. Antacids should be taken with aspirin when the aforementioned problems occur. Optimal doses of aspirin should be continued as long as the signs and symptoms of acute rheumatic fever persist, providing there is no major side effect or drug toxicity.

Corticosteroids   Corticosteroids (adrenal hormones) are potent antiinflam-matory agents, but they frequently produce side effects (e.g., acne; hirsutism—abnormal hair growth on the body and face; and moonface). In addition, the clinical manifestations of acute rheumatic fever often recur following termination of therapy. For these reasons, it is preferable to start with salicylates first, without corticosteroids. Remember that corticosteroids are not indicated when there is no evidence of carditis. Corticosteroids should be administered promptly when salicylates fail to reduce fever and also when other manifestations do not respond to these agents in patients with rheumatic carditis. A commonly used corticosteroid is prednisone, which can be given orally in doses of from 60 to 120 mg in four divided doses daily. If necessary, the dosage of prednisone may be increased as the clinical circumstance persists. When the manifestations of acute rheumatic fever are considered to be brought under control by salicylates and/or corticosteroids, treatment must be continued until the sedimentation rate is reduced to near-normal or normal values, and then must be maintained for another several weeks thereafter.

Treatment of Chorea   Various sedatives and tranquilizers may be necessary for patients with chorea because salicylates and corticosteroids have little or no effect on chorea. If chorea is severe, large doses of phenobarbital may be necesary to control purposeless movements, because tranquilizers alone are often ineffec-tive. Librium and Valium are commonly used for milder cases. Complete emotional and physical rest is very important, because many patients are emotionally unstable and the manifestations of chorea are frequently exaggerated by various emotional traumas. In advanced cases, padded sideboards for the bed may be needed to avoid injury.

It is advisable to allow gradual resumption of physical activity when most abnormal movements from chorea are relatively well controlled, providing other manifestations of acute rheumatic fever are no longer present. It may take many months until all manifestations of chorea disappear. Fortunately, chorea is a self-limited disorder that is not followed by significant neurologic sequelae. Com-plete recovery is usually expected when appropriate medical treatment is provided in conjunction with good nursing care and a cooperative attitude in patients themselves.

Treatment for Complications

Treatment for CHF has been discussed in Chapter 6. When pericarditis develops as a complication of rheumatic fever, it should be treated as any acute nonpurulent pericarditis (see Chapter 13). For cardiac arrhythmias, one or more antiarrhythmic agents may be needed (see Chapter 9).

Prevention

Prevention of rheumatic fever is extremely important because there is no complete cure once an individual suffers from the disease. In addition, it is difficult or even impossible to prevent permanent damage in various heart valves in many cases when an individual has already suffered acute rheumatic fever. Therefore, prevention is a key issue. It should include (1) prevention of initial rheumatic attacks and (2) long-term preventive measures for recurrence of rheumatic fever.

Prevention of Initial Rheumatic Attacks

Initial attacks of rheumatic fever can be prevented in most cases when adequate treatment of pharyngeal infection resulting from group A streptococci is provided promptly. Thus, the spread of streptococcal infection in a given population, particularly in schoolchildren, can be prevented or significantly modified when clinical manifestations with laboratory findings of streptococcal infection are properly identified, particularly with throat cultures, and adequately treated.

By and large, pharyngitis (sore throat because of pharyngeal infection) due to streptococcal infection is adequately treated with a single intramuscular injection of 600,000 units of benzathine penicillin (Bicillin) in children younger than ten, or with 1.2 million units in older children and adults. Alternatively, 600,000 units of procaine penicillin can be injected intramuscularly for ten consecutive days. If oral penicillin is chosen (e.g., due to inconvenience of penicillin injection for some people), at least 800,000 units/day in four divided doses should be given for ten consecutive days in order to achieve therapeutic results comparable to those of a single injection of Bicillin. When an individual is allergic to penicillin, erythromycin in daily doses of 1 g for ten days may be given in place of penicillin with similar therapeutic results. Tetracycline (a kind of broad-spectrum antibiotic) is not recommended because the drug is not effective for some strains of group A streptococci. It should be emphasized that the most effective preventive approach is a single intramuscular injection of Bicillin.

Long-Term Preventive Measures

For long-term preventive measures against group A streptococci, again the best therapeutic regimen is a monthly intramuscular injection of 1.2 million units of Bicillin. Long-term prophylaxis is critically important for individuals with known

RHD, a recent episode of acute rheumatic fever, and exposure to an environment in which the prevalence of streptococcal infection is high. When a monthly intramuscular injection of Bicillin cannot be tolerated, 1 g of sulfadiazine daily in a single dose or 200,000 units of penicillin twice daily on an empty stomach may be given by mouth. Although it is difficult to determine the exact duration of the preventive treatment, many high-risk individuals may require prophylaxis indefinitely. It is generally agreed that continuous prophylactic treatment is indicated for children younger than eighteen years. In addition, a minimum period of five years is highly recommended for individuals even older than eighteen years who suffer from acute rheumatic fever with no known evidence of carditis.

Needless to say, individuals with known RHD are more susceptible to reactivation of rheumatic fever if a streptococcal infection occurs. Furthermore, all individuals who have suffered from rheumatic carditis in the past are much more likely to suffer from carditis again in a subsequent rheumatic attack. These high-risk individuals should receive the prophylactic penicillin treatment vigorously at least until the age of twenty-five. The actual necessity of prophylaxis after the age of twenty-five must be determined by a physician on an individual basis, but it may be safe to continue the preventive penicillin even until the age of fifty years for very high-risk patients with great susceptibility to streptococcal infection. In addition, even older adults should receive the prophylaxis against rheumatic fever for about five years after an acute rheumatic attack. In addition, each susceptible individual should try hard to avoid any contact with persons who suffer from upper respiratory infections, particularly those due to streptococcal infections, if possible. Whenever the possibility of rheumatic fever is raised clinically, especially in high-risk individuals, a physician should be contacted immediately for proper advice and treatment. Improvement in environmental factors, especially in housing and hygiene as well as nutrition and climate, will contribute considerably to the prevention of rheumatic fever.

Prognosis

It is difficult to predict the course and prognosis of rheumatic fever at the onset of the disease because they vary considerably from patient to patient. By and large, however, about 75 percent of acute rheumatic attacks subside within six weeks, 90 percent within twelve weeks, and less than 5 percent more than six months. As a rule, severe rheumatic carditis and/or prolonged attacks of chorea are responsible for persisting rheumatic activity. In some cases, the rheumatic fever may last as long as several years under these circumstances. Recurrence of rheumatic fever does not likely occur in the absence of a new streptococcal infection when all manifestations of acute rheumatic fever have disappeared and when more than two months have elapsed following discontinuation of treatment with salicylates and/or corticosteroids. In general, recurrence of rheumatic fever is more frequent within the first five years after initial rheumatic attack. The frequency of recurrence progressively declines thereafter, with increasing duration of freedom from rheumatic activity. The frequency of recurrences is greatly influenced by the frequency and severity of streptococcal infection, the presence or absence of RHD following a rheumatic attack, the duration of freedom from the last rheumatic attack, and the degree of faithfulness to, as well as the therapeutic result of, preventive measures.

It has been shown that the immediate mortality in rheumatic fever is about 1 to 2 percent. Of course, the prognosis is worse when there is persisting rheumatic activity with markedly enlarged heart, CHF, myocarditis, and pericarditis. Under these circumstances, 30 percent of children may die within ten years of the initial rheumatic attack. RHD may be detected in about a third of the children after the initial rheumatic attack. RHD may occur in adults later, and it is usually less severe. The mitral and aortic valves are the most commonly involved in rheumatic fever, and about 20 percent of patients who have suffered from chorea may develop RHD, even after a long latent period of apparent well-being.

RHEUMATIC HEART DISEASE (RHD)

Following one or more attacks of acute rheumatic fever, permanent deformity and damage of one or more heart valves may be produced months or, more commonly, many years later. Stenosis and/or regurgitation of one or more heart valves will be produced. The term *rheumatic heart disease* (RHD) is used to describe a variety of valvular lesions in this circumstance. The incidence of various valvular lesions has been described earlier. A history of rheumatic fever is documented in not more than 50 to 60 percent of patients with RHD. The earliest clinical evidence of RHD, regardless of the heart valve involved, is a significant heart murmur, and two or more different types of heart murmurs may be heard. When the valve lesion is not severe, the patient may have few or no symptoms. Likewise, there may be no cardiomegaly on physical examination, chest X-ray film, or ECG. Therefore, RHD may be detected accidentally during a routine physical examination by recognizing a heart murmur(s).

On the other hand, various cardiac symptoms (e.g., dyspnea on exertion, chest pain, poor exercise tolerance, syncope, or near-syncope) eventually develop in patients with advanced RHD, because heart function is significantly reduced by the diseased heart valve(s). In addition, one or more heart chambers will be enlarged, and a variety of complications (e.g., CHF, abnormal heart rhythms) will be encountered in advanced cases.

Mitral Stenosis

The mitral valve (see Figure 1.1) orifice (opening) in healthy adults ranges from 4 to 6 cm^2 in area. When this orifice has narrowed to less than half the normal opening, the pressure in the left atrium must be elevated in order to maintain normal blood flow across the mitral valve to the left ventricle, and a normal cardiac output. This narrowing of the mitral valve is termed "mitral stenosis," and it is the most common valvular lesion other than mitral valve prolapse syndrome (see Chapter 10). The increased left atrial pressure due to the narrowing of the mitral valve orifice produces a pressure difference between the left atrium and the left ventricle during the diastolic phase of the ventricles. The term *gradient* is used frequently in the medical literature to designate the pressure difference between cardiac chambers (at times, large blood vessels). The degree of the gradient indicates the severity of the narrowing of the heart valve.

It has been shown that mitral stenosis is nearly always rheumatic, and congenital mitral stenosis is extremely rare. Mitral stenosis is estimated to occur in about 40 percent of all patients with RHD, and females are involved twice as often as males. The interval between the acute rheumatic attack and the development of mitral stenosis varies considerably. It may be as short as a few months to two or three years, but may be as long as ten to twenty-five years. Valvulitis (inflammation of the heart valve) from the preceding rheumatic fever is considered the fundamental reason for producing mitral stenosis. That is, the healing process of the acute inflammation of rheumatic fever eventually leads to scar formation followed by calcification of the mitral valve. This chronic inflammatory process causes fusion of the commissures, rigidity of the valve leaflets, and thickening and matting of the chordae tendineae. Thus, mitral stenosis is produced by adhesions between the mitral leaflets and the loss of mobility of the leaflets associated with fibrosis and rigidity of the chordae tendineae and papillary muscles (structures supporting the mitral valve).

In mild mitral stenosis, the left atrial pressure and the cardiac output may be nearly or even entirely normal, so that patients are often symptom free. On the other hand, dyspnea and fatigue occur only during physical exercise in moderate mitral stenosis with a valve orifice less than 1 cm^2. In advanced mitral stenosis, the left atrial pressure is significantly elevated even at rest, leading to pulmonary venous congestion that is manifested by severe dyspnea with marked limitation of exercise tolerance. Marked pulmonary congestion in severe mitral stenosis often leads to acute pulmonary edema, which may result in sudden death unless treated promptly. Many patients fail to recognize the slowly progressing symptoms, such as easy fatigability with poor exercise tolerance, in mild mitral stenosis. In addition, dyspnea, which is commonly the first symptom of mitral stenosis, may be ignored until the patient begins to experience nocturnal dyspnea (dyspnea at night so severe that the patient wakes up) and orthopnea (the patient has to breathe in a sitting position because of intolerable dyspnea in the supine position). In some cases of advanced mitral stenosis, the patient finally presents with signs and symptoms of right ventricular failure. Even in asymptomatic and mild cases, the characteristic physical signs enable the physician to diagnose mitral stenosis without any difficulty. The diagnostic physical findings of typical mitral stenosis include a middiastolic rumbling murmur (with presystolic accentuation during sinus rhythm) at the cardiac apex, loud first heart sound with tapping quality, and opening snap at the apex (see Chapter 8).

AF develops in many patients (up to 50 to 80 percent), and, not uncommonly, mitral stenosis is diagnosed for the first time after the development of AF. Because of a very rapid heart rate (120 to 250 beats/min.) in AF in most cases, the arrhythmia often triggers off the episode of acute dyspnea and even acute pulmonary edema. AF may be abolished by digitalis so that normal sinus rhythm may be restored. Otherwise, AF may persist for months, years, or even indefinitely as a chronic form. In general, however, the heart rate can be adequately controlled with digitalis and/or propranolol even if AF persists. In advanced mitral stenosis, emboli (blood clots) may occur in various locations, and hemoptysis (coughing up blood) is not uncommon.

In typical cases, mitral stenosis can be diagnosed from a clinical background alone without any difficulty. Various laboratory tests are available, however, to assist the diagnosis, and the degree of the stenosis as well as other necessary information can be obtained. On the ECG and chest X-ray film, enlargement of the left atrium and/or the right ventricle is readily recognized. In addition, pulmonary congestion or edema can be demonstrated on the chest X-ray film. AF or any other cardiac arrhythmia will be confirmed on the ECG. The echocardiogram provides an accurate estimation of the degree of mitral stenosis. Cardiac catheterization and angiography will confirm the diagnosis and the degree of mitral stenosis in less obvious cases, and these tests enable the physician to evaluate other coexisting valve lesions and ventricular function (see Chapter 24). Coronary arteriography is recommended for older patients, particularly when surgical repair is planned, since a coexisting CAD may be repaired when indicated simultaneously with mitral valve surgery, because RHD and CAD often coexist among older individuals.

As far as management is concerned, completely asymptomatic patients with very mild mitral stenosis require no treatment, but periodic medical checkups are indicated because the narrowing of the valve may progressively get worse. The clinical course varies considerably, and some individuals with a known mitral stenosis may not develop any apparent symptoms for many years. Conversely, other patients may develop various symptoms rapidly, and clinical conditions may progressively deteriorate. When the patient with mild mitral stenosis experiences an episodic shortness of breath as a result of pulmonary congestion triggered by high salt intake or extraordinary physical activity, these precipitating factors should be avoided. If necessary, mild diuretics may be given for pulmonary congestion. Digitalis is not effective for a pure mitral stenosis, but the drug is essential in the treatment of AF. Normal sinus rhythm may be restored with digitalis. Otherwise, the heart rate will be adequately reduced with digitalis even if atrial fibrillation persists. When a restoration of sinus rhythm is highly desired, quinidine may be added or DC shock may be applied if necessary (see Chapter 18). When the heart rate in AF cannot be adequately controlled with digitalis, propranolol (Inderal) may be added.

The final decision regarding indications for surgical treatment for a given patient has to be carefully determined by a cardiologist and a cardiac surgeon. In general, there are two types of surgical approach, including mitral commissurotomy (sectioning of the rigid and thickened fibrous structures surrounding the mitral valve leading to opening up the narrowed mitral valve orifice) and replacement of the mitral valve with a prosthetic (artificial) valve. Again, the proper choice of surgical approach has to be determined by physicians and surgeons. By and large, patients with moderate to severe mitral stenosis will require the surgical approach. Mitral commissurotomy provides excellent relief of symptoms for many years for properly selected patients with moderate but pure mitral stenosis. It is important to emphasize that mitral commissurotomy should not be performed when symptoms are due to coexisting mitral regurgitation or associated aortic valve lesions. Replacement of the mitral valve with an artificial valve should be considered when mitral stenosis coexists with mitral regurgitation or when the mitral valve is extremely deformed and calcified so that mitral commissurotomy is not feasible. In addition, replacement of the mitral valve with an artificial valve is indicated when the narrowing of the mitral valve occurs again following mitral commissurotomy. As a rule, this radical surgical approach is indicated in patients with advanced mitral stenosis that is manifested by severe, intolerable, and life-threatening symptoms due to severe pulmonary congestion or edema.

In some cases, continuous medical treatment is necessary even after surgical repair. On the other hand, following a successful commissurotomy or replacement with an artificial valve, many patients can return to a fully active life. Furthermore, anticoagulant (blood-thinning drugs) therapy is indicated indefinitely for all patients following mitral valve replacement. Lifelong anticoagulant therapy is also indicated for patients with a history of thromboembolic phenomenon (episodes of blood clots anywhere in the body). In fact, some physicians recommend long-term anticoagulant therapy in all patients with mitral stenosis associated with chronic AF. It is important to reevaluate every patient with mitral stenosis periodically because of the possibility of restenosis, even after mitral commissurotomy, and possible complications (e.g., CHF, infective endocarditis).

In addition, it is very important to examine all patients periodically following the artificial valve replacement of the diseased mitral valve, because various complications may occur at any time. Serious complications include thromboembolic phenomenon, hemolytic anemia (as a result of destruction of red blood cells), and mechanical or material defects in the artificial valve itself (e.g., incomplete closure, failure of the opening, or partial or complete destruction of the artificial valve). When any mechanical problem with the artificial heart valve is detected, it should be corrected promptly. Indeed, a new artificial valve is required. The degree of blood thinning should be ideally maintained with proper amounts of anticoagulants. Excessive amounts of anticoagulants cause hemorrhage, whereas insufficient amounts may produce thromboembolic phenomena. Thus, frequent blood tests are essential in maintaining the ideal therapeutic level. When any type of tissue valve is used for replacement, anticoagulant therapy is not necessary.

Mitral Regurgitation (Insufficiency)

Remember that the mitral valve has to close completely during a systolic phase of the ventricles in order to pump blood out of the left ventricle into the aorta via the aortic valve (see Figures 1.1 and 1.2). When the mitral valve fails to close during the systolic phase, however, blood flows back into the left atrium as well as into the aorta via the aortic valve. This clinical situation is called "mitral regurgitation" (insufficiency). In lay people's terms, the condition is better known as "leaking heart valve." There are various structures surrounding the mitral valve, and damage to any of these structures (the valve leaflets, chordae tendineae, papillary muscles) may cause mitral regurgitation. In some cases, mitral regurgitation is produced by dilatation of the mitral valve ring (rather than any permanent damage) as a result of marked dilatation of the left ventricle secondary to CHF. In this circumstance, the term *functional mitral regurgitation* is used. Functional mitral regurgitation often disappears as cardiac function improves following adequate management of CHF.

In mitral valve prolapse syndrome (see Chapter 10), clinically significant mitral regurgitation occurs only occasionally. Rheumatic fever is responsible for the production of mitral regurgitation in approximately half the cases. A pure mitral regurgitation of rheumatic origin occurs more frequently in males. Remember that females are involved in mitral stenosis twice as often as males. The clinical course of rheumatic mitral insufficiency is rather chronic. In rare cases, mitral regurgitation is congenital. Mitral regurgitation of acute onset is usually due to dysfunction or rupture of the chordae tendineae and/or papillary muscles secondary to recent heart attack or infective endocarditis. At times, mitral regurgitation is produced suddenly as a consequence of trauma or as a complication of cardiac surgery. In elderly people, mitral regurgitation may be caused by massive calcification of the mitral annulus for an obscure reason.

As far as clinical manifestations are concerned, many patients with mild rheumatic mitral regurgitation may be totally asymptomatic or may have only minimal symptoms (e.g., shortness of breath only during extraordinary physical activity) for many years with no progression. In advanced cases, however, the left ventricle has to work harder to maintain adequate cardiac output by compensating the leakage of blood into the left atrium. Consequently, the left atrium as well as the left ventricle will enlarge progressively. Eventually, CHF is the end result. Fundamentally, the symptoms of mitral regurgitation result from pulmonary congestion and reduced cardiac output. Thus, patients experience shortness of breath and fatigue only during extraordinary activity in the early stage, but eventually these symptoms begin to appear even at rest in advanced cases as a result of

CHF. In addition, some patients may experience palpitations from AF or other arrhythmias. Systemic emboli (blood clots) may occur in some patients, especially in the presence of AF. Mitral regurgitation frequently predisposes to infective endocarditis (see Chapter 13). Accordingly, prophylactic antibiotic therapy is essential before dental or any surgical procedure.

The characteristic feature of mitral regurgitation is a pansystolic murmur best heard at the apex of the heart; various other findings have been described in Chapter 8. As far as laboratory tests are concerned, ECG may be entirely normal in mild cases. In advanced cases, enlargement of various heart chambers (particularly the left atrium and the left ventricle) will be shown on the ECG, chest X-ray film, and echocardiogram. Various cardiac arrhythmias will be documented on the ECG. The chest X-ray film will show pulmonary congestion and other signs of CHF in advanced cases. In addition, calcification of the mitral valve is not uncommonly observed on the chest X-ray film. The diagnosis of mitral regurgitation can be made in most cases without any difficulty on the basis of the characteristic pansystolic heart murmur at the apex, in addition to other clinical and laboratory findings. However, the severity of mitral regurgitation and possible coexisting valvular lesions will be confirmed by cardiac catheterization with left ventricular angio-cardiography (see Chapter 24).

As far as management of mitral insufficiency is concerned, completely asymptomatic patients require no treatment. No restriction of physical activities is necessary in these individuals. However, even asymptomatic individuals with proven mitral insufficiency should be examined periodically and carefully advised to use prophylactic antibiotics before dental extraction or any surgical procedures to prevent infective endocarditis. In mildly symptomatic patients (e.g., those with dyspnea and fatigue on exertion), proper medical treatment, such as reduction of salt intake, avoidance of extraordinary activities, and appropriate use of diuretics and digitalis, will be sufficient. Anticoagulant therapy is recommended in the late stages of the disease and also in patients with chronic AF or with previous episodes of thromboembolic phenomena.

A surgical approach should be considered seriously in patients with severe symptoms despite proper medical treatment. Various types of prosthetic (artificial) valves are available to replace the diseased mitral valve. The immediate risk of mitral valve replacement increases markedly when there is significant CHF. Like-wise, long-term survival of these patients is considerably reduced (about 50 percent in five years). Thus, it is advisable to replace the diseased mitral valve early in the course of mitral regurgitation. When surgery is performed significantly early, results are excellent in many cases. On the other hand, some degree of inadequate heart function may persist in some patients even after successful surgical replacement of the valve. Anticoagulant therapy is indicated indefinitely following replacement of the mitral valve with an artificial valve. Many patients with mild mitral regurgitation can lead perfectly normal lives without any restrictions, but mild or moderate mitral regurgitation may progress to severe regurgitation either slowly or sometimes very rapidly.

Aortic Stenosis

The normal size of the aortic valve orifice in healthy adults ranges from 2.6 to 3.5 cm^2. When the valve orifice is reduced to between one-third and one-fifth its normal size (about 0.5 to 0.7 cm^2), the stenosis of the aortic valve is considered critical. Aortic stenosis occurs in approximately one-fourth of all patients with chronic valvular heart disease. Aortic stenosis is much more commonly encountered in men than women (about 80 percent of patients are men). Aortic stenosis may be congenital, rheumatic, or resulting from calcification of the aortic cusps of obscure origin in elderly people. Clinically, in most cases of rheumatic aortic stenosis, mitral valvular lesion(s) nearly always coexist(s), and aortic regurgitation also often coexists. The narrowing of the left ventricular outflow tract is most commonly observed at the level of the aortic leaflets (ordinary aortic stenosis), but occasionally the narrowing may be due to constriction of the ascending aorta (called "supravalvular stenosis") or to a fibrous ring or tunnel within the left ventricle just below the aortic leaflets (called "subvalvular stenosis"). Aortic stenosis is discussed here because of its common occurrence.

When there is significant narrowing at the left ventricular outflow tract, a pressure gradient will be produced between the left ventricle and the aorta across the aortic valve during the systolic ejection period of the ventricle. The pressure gradient across the aortic valve increases in a manner proportional to the degree of aortic valve narrowing. Aortic stenosis is considered severe when the gradient across the aortic valve is 75 to 100 mmHg or more. When the gradient is 50 to 75 mmHg, aortic stenosis is considered moderate, whereas mild aortic stenosis shows the gradient at less than 50 mmHg.

It is interesting to note that a significant gradient across the aortic valve may be present for many years without producing any significant symptoms, because cardiac output may remain normal in spite of aortic stenosis. In other words, the cardiac output and stroke volume are often normal at resting state in the majority of patients with moderate to severe aortic stenosis. However, adequate cardiac output may not be maintained during exercise, and consequently the patient becomes symptomatic (e.g., with angina pectoris, exertional dyspnea, and syncope). Many patients with severe aortic stenosis may remain asymptomatic because the hypertrophied left ventricle is capable of pumping blood more forcefully as a compensatory mechanism in order to supply adequate circulation to the body in spite of the narrowed aortic valve orifice. When the aortic valve orifice is narrowed to a third its normal size, most patients begin to experience symptoms, especially during the fourth or fifth decade. By and large, there are three cardinal symptoms: exertional dyspnea, angina, and syncope. Many patients gradually cut down their physical activity because they experience progressive fatigue and shortness of breath on exertion. Exertional dyspnea is usually followed by angina as the disease progresses. Angina is produced in the late stage of aortic stenosis because oxygen requirements are increased in the hypertrophied left ventricular muscle mass, so there will be insufficient oxygen supply to the heart muscle. In addition, there is often coexisting CAD.

In advanced cases of aortic stenosis, patients eventually develop various manifestations of CHF, and syncope may also occur. The syncopal episode is thought to be due to a sudden fall in cardiac output resulting from ventricular arrhythmias, particularly VF. CHF is a cause of death in a half to two-thirds of patients. Sudden death is reported in 10 to 20 percent of patients who die primarily from aortic stenosis, especially during or immediately after exercise. Thus, any form of vigorous or competitive physical activity should be avoided by all patients with aortic stenosis, even if they are asymptomatic. The characteristic physical sign of aortic stenosis is a loud, harsh, ejection-type systolic (midsystolic) murmur best heard at the base of the heart (upper chest); the murmur is often transmitted to the neck and to the apex of the heart. Detailed descriptions of physical findings are found in Chapter 8.

In mild to moderate aortic stenosis, ECG and chest X-ray film are often normal, but when the stenosis is severe, enlargement of the left atrium and left ventricle can be readily recognized. In severe aortic stenosis, calcium is seen in the area of the aortic valve on the chest X-ray film, and prominence of the ascending aorta is often present. In advanced cases, ECG may reveal left anterior hemiblock or left bundle branch block (see Chapter 9). In severe calcific aortic stenosis, complete A-V block may occur, especially in older patients. In this circumstance, permanent artificial pacemaker implantation is indicated. Cardiac catheterization is not necessary in every case of aortic stenosis, because the diagnosis can be made with reasonable certainty in most cases from clinical findings and noninvasive tests. However, cardiac catheterization with angiocardiography must be performed when the aortic stenosis is considered severe and when the surgical approach is seriously being considered. The severity of the aortic stenosis as well as possible coexisting CAD or other valve lesion(s) can accurately be assessed by these invasive tests.

As far as management of aortic stenosis is concerned, different therapeutic approaches have to be considered depending upon various factors, including the presence or absence and the degree of significant symptoms, the degree of narrowing of the aortic valve, the pressure gradient across the aortic valve, and the patient's age. By and large, no active treatment is required for asymptomatic mild aortic stenosis (gradient less than 50 mmHg), but periodic medical checkups with yearly (every three to six months in some cases) ECG and chest X-rays should be performed to assess the progress of the narrowing of the aortic valve and to recognize early findings of CHF, cardiac arrhythmias, new symptoms, and aortic valve calcification. Every patient with aortic stenosis should be advised to take prophylactic antibiotics before any dental or other surgical procedure, because these individuals are at increased risk of developing bacterial endocarditis. Vigorous or competitive physical activity should be avoided by all patients with aortic stenosis, particularly when the narrowing is severe (gradient beyond 75 mmHg), even if they are asymptomatic. The reason for this is obvious—sudden death commonly occurs in aortic stenosis during or immediately following extraordinary physical exercise. CHF and angina should be treated in the usual manner (see Chapters 4 and 6).

Surgical approaches for aortic stenosis vary significantly depending upon the patient's age, the severity of the narrowing of the aortic valve, and the degree of symptoms. In general, a simple commissurotomy of the narrowed aortic valve to open up the stenosis under direct vision is advised for children and young adults with moderate to severe aortic stenosis (gradient above 50 mmHg) with no evidence of calcification around the valve. The mortality rate is minimal (less than 3 percent). The aortic commissurotomy is generally recommended in children and young adults with moderate to severe noncalcific aortic stenosis regardless of the presence or absence of symptoms. Unfortunately, restenosis of the aortic valve may occur following the aortic commissurotomy, and then the radical surgical treatment (aortic valve replacement) is indicated.

The surgical replacement of the narrowed aortic valve with the prosthetic (artificial) valve or the tissue valve is definitely indicated in all adult patients with symptomatic and/or severe (gradient above 75 mmHg) aortic stenosis. In general, valve replacement is indicated when calcification is readily visible (on chest X-ray film) in adult patients (calcific aortic stenosis). If possible, valve replacement should be performed before significant CHF develops because of high surgical mortality (15 to 25 percent). In addition, many physicians recommend the surgical replacement of the aortic valve even in asymptomatic moderate aortic stenosis (gradient 50 to 75 mmHg).

It has been shown that considerable improvement with good surgical results is observed in approximately 85 percent of the surviving patients. Early surgical mortality is about 5 percent, whereas late mortality is reported to be 10 to 20 percent. The follow-up study indicates that the eight-year survival rate after surgical replacement of the valve in aortic stenosis is about 65 percent. On the other hand, many patients with mild aortic stenosis may remain asymptomatic for many years because the severity of the narrowing may progress very slowly. Even after successful surgical replacement of the narrowed aortic valve, sudden death may occur, especially during the first few months. Therefore, one or more antiarrhythmic agents (see Table 6.2) should be given for months, years, or even indefinitely when a patient shows significant ventricular arrhythmias. On rare occasions, permanent artificial pacemaker implantation is indicated for complete A-V block.

When there is a coexisting mitral valve lesion, of course, the mitral valve must also be replaced. Likewise, CABS should be performed simultaneously when aortic stenosis is associated with significant CAD. The same postoperative medical care is necessary, as described previously in this chapter (see "Mitral Stenosis").

Aortic Regurgitation (Insufficiency)

In the normal heart, the aortic valve must close completely during a diastolic phase of the ventricles so that blood flows normally from the left atrium to the left ventricle. When the aortic valve fails to close completely in this circumstance, the blood ejected from the left ventricle to the aorta during a systolic phase on a previous cardiac cycle will return to the left ventricle from the aorta. This clinical condition is termed "aortic regurgitation" or "aortic insufficiency"—meaning a leakage of the aortic valve. The amount of blood that returns from the aorta to the left ventricle depends upon the degree of incomplete closure of the aortic valve. In aortic regurgitation, the total blood stroke volume ejected by the left ventricle during a systolic phase is increased, because the total amount of ejected blood will be a combination of the blood volume received from the left atrium as usual and the blood volume regurgitated back from the aorta during a diastolic phase on a previous cardiac cycle.

It has been shown that about three-fourths of all patients with aortic regurgitation are males. However, the incidence of combined aortic regurgitation and mitral valve lesion is higher in females. Rheumatic fever is the most common cause of aortic regurgitation (about 80 percent), and it may be congenital in origin. Infective endocarditis may affect the aortic valve previously involved with rheumatic fever or deformed congenitally (at birth). Trauma to the heart may cause acute aortic regurgitation. Not uncommonly, aortic regurgitation is produced by syphilis, and rheumatoid disease may cause it as well. In addition, aortic insufficiency may be caused by severe hypertension, Marfan's syndrome (discussed shortly), dissecting aneurysm (a tear and dissection of the inner layer of the aorta, which may be followed by the rupture of the aorta, leading to death), and idiopathic dilatation of the aorta (enlargement of the aorta by an unknown cause).

Marfan's syndrome is a generalized hereditary disorder of the connective tissue, and the syndrome commonly involves the skeletal system, the eyes, and the cardiovascular system. Common manifestations of Marfan's syndrome include a tall and slender body structure because of very long arms and legs, hyperextensibility of the bone joints, dislocated lens of the eyes, myopia, detached retinas, aortic regurgitation, and possible dissecting aneurysm of the aorta. Treatment is primarily toward the involvement of the cardiovascular system, and surgical replacement of the aortic valve is indicated in some cases.

As far as clinical findings are concerned, it usually takes about six to eight years until hemodynamically significant aortic regurgitation develops following rheumatic attack. Many patients remain asymptomatic for another ten to twenty years in spite of moderate or even severe aortic regurgitation. As a compensatory mechanism, the left ventricle has to pump out the usual stroke volume of the blood received from the left atrium, plus the additional blood regurgitated from the aorta into the left ventricle in order to supply adequate circulation to the body. Consequently, the stroke volume of the blood ejected by the left ventricle may be more than two times greater than normal. Thus, the left ventricle progressively enlarges in order to maintain adequate circulation until the left ventricle is no longer capable of pumping sufficient blood for the body's demands. At this stage, the patient develops CHF. Many patients experience pounding heartbeats, palpitations, and even head pounding for several to many years until exertional dyspnea occurs. Exertional dyspnea is often followed by orthopnea, nocturnal dyspnea, and excessive sweating. Chest pain may occur, and various manifestations of CHF will be observed in advanced cases. CHF is the most common cause of death, and 10 to 15 percent of patients with aortic regurgitation die suddenly. Sudden death is common in the acute form of aortic regurgitation, such as in dissecting aneurysm, cardiac trauma, and infective endocarditis.

On inspection, it is often possible to recognize the jarring of the entire body and the bobbing motion of the head corresponding to each systolic cycle of the heart in advanced aortic insufficiency. In addition, the sudden distension and collapse of the large arteries can readily be noted. The characteristic feature of aortic regurgitation is a wide pulse pressure (a difference between the systolic and diastolic BP) as a result of an elevated systolic BP and a reduced diastolic BP. Other common physical findings include capillary pulsations ("Quincke's pulse"), "pistol-shot" sound over the femoral (groin) arteries, to-and-fro murmurs (Duroziez's sign) upon light compression with a stethoscope over the femoral artery, and "water-hammer pulse" (rapidly rising pulse that collapses abruptly during late systolic and diastolic phase—"Corrigan's pulse"). In a typical case, capillary pulsations characteristically exhibit an alternating paling and flushing of the skin under the nail when pressure is applied to the tip of the nails (Quincke's pulse). The most important diagnostic physical finding is the typical early diastolic murmur, decrescendo in shape and high-pitched and blowing in quality. Various physical findings have been described in Chapter 8.

Enlargement of the left ventricle will be shown on the ECG, chest X-ray film, and echocardiogram. Dilatation of the ascending aorta is observed in syphilitic aortic regurgitation. The echocardiogram is valuable to assess left ventricular function and to diagnose a coexisting mitral valve lesion. Cardiac catheterization and angiocardiography are not necessary to establish the diagnosis of aortic regurgitation. However, these invasive diagnostic tests are indicated when the surgical approach is planned. These tests are essential in diagnosing coexisting valve lesion(s) and/or CAD.

As far as management is concerned, the patient with mild or even moderate aortic regurgitation without any symptoms should be allowed to carry out a normal life. However, these individuals should have periodic medical checkups with annual ECGs and chest X-ray films. In addition, they should be instructed to take prophylactic antibiotics before dental or surgical procedures. CHF should be treated in the usual manner. NG and long-acting nitrates may be given for chest pain. A full course of penicillin therapy is definitely indicated for patients with aortic regurgitation due to syphilis.

Surgical replacement of the aortic valve with a prosthetic (artificial) valve or tissue valve should seriously be considered when significant symptoms occur as a result of CHF, especially when medical treatment is ineffective. Even in asymptomatic patients, surgical valve replacement is highly recommended when aortic regurgitation is proven to be severe (pulse pressure greater than 100 mmHg, severe left ventricular hypertrophy on the ECG and chest X-ray film, and so forth). In patients with acute and severe aortic regurgitation, surgical replacement of the aortic valve is urgently indicated, and it may be a life-saving measure. When there are coexisting valve lesion(s) and/or CAD, these lesion(s) should be surgically repaired simultaneously. Anticoagulant therapy is indicated indefinitely following surgical replacement with an artificial valve. The prognosis after surgery largely depends on the degree and length of the previous ventricular damage; the presence or absence and degree of coexisting cardiac diseases, particularly CAD; and other major complications. A late annual mortality following surgery is reported to be about 5 percent in patients with a markedly enlarged heart and prolonged impairment of left ventricular function. The surgical risks of aortic valve replacement seem greatly dependent on the stage of aortic regurgitation.

12

HEART MUSCLE DISEASES

The medical term *cardiomyopathy* (primary myocardial disease) is used when the disease process involves, predominantly or entirely, the heart muscle (*cardio* means "heart"; *myo* means "muscle"; *pathy* means "disease"). Thus, the clinical manifestations of cardiomyopathy result from dysfunction of the myocardium rather than from any abnormality in the heart valve or coronary artery. Cardiomyopathy may be totally due to an unknown cause, and the term *idiopathic cardiomyopathy* is used in this circumstance (*idiopathic* means "unknown cause"). In some other cases, on the other hand, a causative agent or disease process may be identified. For example, excessive use of alcohol (alcoholic cardiomyopathy), certain parasite infections (e.g., Chagas's heart disease), or vitamin deficiency (e.g., beriberi heart disease) may cause cardiomyopathy. In addition, cardiomyopathy may be secondary to systemic (generalized) diseases, such as amyloidosis (the widespread tissue deposition of an amorphous, hyalinelike substance of unknown cause, producing cardiomyopathy and involvement of other organs) and various connective tissue diseases (e.g., lupus erythematosus—a generalized disease with unknown cause involving heart, kidneys, skin, bone joints, and many other organs).

Regardless of the causative factor in cardiomyopathy, the clinical manifestations and the outcome are very similar. In addition, the clinical manifestations may mimic other heart diseases (e.g., CAD). The early manifestations include weakness, easy fatigability, and exertional dyspnea as a result of reduced cardiac output. Cardiomegaly is usually detected on physical examination, ECG, and chest

X-ray film when the patient already experiences the aforementioned symptoms. Sooner or later, the patient develops CHF. By and large, many patients exhibit the signs and symptoms of combined left and right ventricular failure (see Chapter 6) in the advanced stage. In addition, many people develop a variety of cardiac arrhythmias and systemic or pulmonary emboli, and sudden death is not uncommon in advanced cases.

It has been shown that cardiomyopathy may account for approximately 15 percent or more of the patients with heart disease in underdeveloped countries. In America, however, less than 1 percent of cardiac deaths are estimated to be due to cardiomyopathy. In fact, Chagas's heart disease (cardiomyopathy caused by the protozoan *Trypanosoma cruzi*) is the most common form of heart disease in South and Central America. According to some medical studies, evidence of parasite (*Trypanosoma cruzi*) infection in the heart in 95 percent or more of the population in some parts of Central and South America can be identified.

In a practical sense, cardiomyopathy should be suspected when a patient shows unexplainable cardiomegaly and/or CHF in the absence of any evidence indicating known heart disease (e.g., CAD). Likewise, the diagnosis of cardiomyopathy is always a possibility when there are unexplainable cardiac arrhythmias or other ECG abnormalities in the absence of any known heart disease or heart murmur. The treatment of cardiomyopathy is primarily toward the clinical manifestations, including CHF, abnormal heart rhythms, thromboembolic phenomena, and so forth. Cardiac transplantation has been performed in some medical centers for patients with advanced cardiomyopathy, but the result is still far from ideal (see Chapter 26).

CAUSES AND CLASSIFICATION

The most common method of classifying cardiomyopathy is according to its causative agents or underlying systemic disorders. Cardiomyopathy is generally classified into two major categories:

Cardiomyopathy as the primary myocardial involvement includes:

1. Idiopathic cardiomyopathy
2. Familial cardiomyopathy (cardiomyopathy occurring in the same family)
3. Peripartum or postpartum cardiomyopathy (cardiomyopathy during the last months of pregnancy or within five months after delivery)
4. Alcoholic cardiomyopathy
5. Beriberi heart disease (cardiomyopathy due to vitamin B_1 deficiency)
6. Idiopathic hypertrophic subaortic stenosis (IHSS)—narrowing of the left ventricular outflow tract due to hypertrophy primarily involving the ventricular septum
7. Chagas's heart disease
8. Cardiomyopathy due to drugs (e.g., Adriamycin)

9. Cardiomyopathy due to radiation
10. Endocardial fibroelastosis (commonly found in infants, unknown cause)
11. Endomyocardial fibrosis (cardiomyopathy seen in the tropics, especially in Africa, involving children and young adults)

Cardiomyopathy secondary to systemic diseases includes:

1. Amyloidosis
2. Sarcoidosis (chronic disease with unknown cause involving, most commonly, the lungs and affecting many other organs, such as skin, bones, joints, salivary glands, and heart)
3. Connective tissue diseases, such as lupus erythematosus, polyarteritis, scleroderma, and dermatomyositis (diseases involving diffusely many organs with unknown cause)
4. Neuromuscular diseases such as muscular dystrophy and myotonic dystrophy (diseases involving diffusely many organs as a result of neuromuscular disorder with unknown cause)
5. Neoplastic diseases (various forms of cancer)

Idiopathic Cardiomyopathy

The term *idiopathic cardiomyopathy* should be used only when no known cause for heart disease is found.

Chagas's Heart Disease

Certain forms of cardiomyopathy are difficult to define as a cardiomyopathy because many features are somewhat compatible with myocarditis. For instance, Chagas's heart disease (trypanosomiasis) is produced by the protozoan *Trypanosoma cruzi*, which is harbored by hematophagous insects; this cardiomyopathy is predominantly found in Central and South America. Chagas's heart disease is the most common heart disease in Central and South America, but it is very rare in the United States. Less than 1 percent of infected individuals may develop an acute form, and about 30 percent develop a chronic form about twenty years after the initial infection. About 20 percent of individuals with chronic Chagas's heart disease die from CHF within two years after the diagnosis is first established. The diagnosis is confirmed by demonstrating the parasite in the patient's blood culture, or complement fixation test. There is no specific treatment.

Beriberi Heart Disease

Beriberi is probably the most common cause of heart disease resulting from nutritional deficiency in the world. Beriberi heart disease produces high-output CHF, and common manifestations include a hyperkinetic circulation with bounding and pistol-shot pulses, venous engorgement, flushing of the skin with peripheral vasodilatation, and syncope or shock. CHF predominantly involves the right ventricle or both ventricles. Beriberi is commonly produced by the low intake of vitamin B_1 (thiamine) and a carbohydrate-rich diet. Thus, a polished rice diet is the usual cause of beriberi in many Asian countries. In Western countries, beriberi is observed primarily among chronic alcoholics. Thus, alcoholic cardiomyopathy may be due partially or totally to vitamin B_1 deficiency. Beriberi heart disease often improves after thiamine therapy.

Alcoholic Cardiomyopathy

Alcoholic cardiomyopathy is a clinical entity that is characterized by cardiomegaly and CHF in individuals with chronic alcoholism, providing there is no known cause for heart disease. Although various nutritional (particularly vitamin B_1) deficiencies are common in alcoholics, some individuals often fail to show any apparent deficiency of the essential nutrients. In general, chronic alcoholism is defined as the daily consumption of 8 oz. of whiskey, 1 qt. of wine, or 2 qt. of beer for at least five years. Of course, many patients also have other evidence of chronic alcoholism, such as liver cirrhosis. Alcoholic cardiomyopathy is often manifested by palpitations, fatigue, and exertional dyspnea, and these symptoms are soon followed by various manifestations of CHF. Thromboembolic phenomena are common. When significant symptoms are observed, three-year mortality is reported to be more than 40 percent. The treatment of alcoholic cardiomyopathy is primarily supportive and symptomatic (e.g., for CHF), and prolonged bed rest does not seem to be significantly beneficial. Alcoholic consumption should be avoided.

Cobalt-Beer Cardiomyopathy

A unique form of alcoholic cardiomyopathy is a "cobalt-beer cardiomyopathy" that was discovered in 1965 in Quebec City, Canada, for the first time among heavy beer drinkers. Cobalt-beer cardiomyopathy was manifested by severe biventricular failure associated with low cardiac output, cyanosis, cardiomegaly, pericardial effusion, and cardiogenic shock. The mortality rate was reported to be 40 to 45 percent. The toxicity of cobalt chloride contained in the beer was the cause. Similar cases of cobalt-beer cardiomyopathy have been reported in Minneapolis and Omaha and elsewhere throughout the world thereafter. Fortunately, no further occurrence of cobalt-beer cardiomyopathy has been reported, since beer manufacturers no longer use cobalt in beer.

Peripartum (Postpartum) Cardiomyopathy

When a woman develops cardiomegaly and CHF for the first time during the last month of pregnancy or during the first five months after delivery, peripartum (postpartum) cardiomyopathy should be suspected, providing there is no known cause for heart disease. Peripartum cardiomyopathy is most common among multiparous black females over age thirty. It is associated with poor nutrition, inadequate prenatal care, a previous history of hypertension, toxemia of pregnancy, and multiple births. An enlarged left ventricle usually becomes apparent within the first three months after delivery.

Clinical manifestations are very similar to those of idiopathic cardiomyopathy. Although the heart size may return to normal within six months in as many as 50 percent of patients, chronic CHF with persisting cardiomegaly is not uncommon. In addition, pulmonary or systemic emboli and various cardiac arrhythmias, especially VPCs, are frequently associated with this cardiomyopathy. When chronic CHF and significant cardiomegaly persist, of course, the prognosis is very poor, and sudden death is often unavoidable. The treatment is essentially the same as for patients with idiopathic cardiomyopathy and is purely supportive and symptomatic. In addition, the nutritional state should be improved, and further pregnancies should be avoided.

Idiopathic Hypertrophic Subaortic Stenosis (IHSS)

IHSS is a form of cardiomyopathy that is manifested by marked left ventricular hypertrophy, particularly the ventricular septum, producing a narrowing of the left ventricular outflow tract of varying degrees. The fundamental cause of IHSS is unknown, but it frequently involves close relatives (e.g., parents, siblings, and children) in the same family. Thus, it can be said that IHSS is a form of idiopathic cardiomyopathy and also familial cardiomyopathy. The common clinical findings include dyspnea on exertion, chest pain, dizzy spells, near-syncope or syncope, and CHF. An ejection-type (midsystolic) systolic murmur is commonly heard at the base of the heart (upper chest). In addition, a pansystolic murmur is not uncommonly present at the apex, because mitral regurgitation is frequently produced by displacement of the mitral valve secondary to a markedly hypertrophied left ventricular myocardium, particularly the septum. Echocardiography usually confirms the diagnosis. The clinical course varies considerably, but sudden death is not uncommon, especially during or immediately following vigorous physical activity. Digitalis is often hazardous to patients with IHSS because the left ventricular outflow obstruction is further aggravated by more forceful contractions of the left ventricle produced by the drug. Remember that the contractile force of the heart muscle is enhanced by digitalis. Beta-adrenergic blocking agents (e.g., propranolol) are beneficial in relieving chest pain and other symptoms, including near-syncope or syncope. Surgical excision or incision of the hypertrophied ventricular septum may be indicated for severely symptomatic patients with IHSS when medical treatment is ineffective.

Amyloidosis

Cardiac amyloidosis is a disease entity that commonly involves older individuals. Its cause is unknown, and it is rare in people under the age of forty. This disorder is characterized by widespread tissue deposition of an amorphous hyalinelike substance, and CHF is the most common cause of death. Amyloidosis may occur without a coexisting disease (called "primary amyloidosis"), or it may coexist with a chronic inflammatory disease (called "secondary amyloidosis"). In addition, patients with multiple myeloma (a form of malignant tumor involving bones) may show an incidence of amyloidosis as high as 15 percent. The common manifestations include fatigue, weight loss, edema, dyspnea, dizziness, near-syncope or syncope, and orthostatis hypotension (reduction of BP upon standing). On physical examination, many patients exhibit enlargement of various organs, including heart, spleen, liver, and tongue. The clinical diagnosis of amyloidosis is confirmed by tissue biopsy obtained from the rectum, kidney, or liver in over 80 to 90 percent. Treatment is primarily supportive and symptomatic.

Drug-Induced Cardiomyopathy

Although various drugs may cause toxic effects on cardiac function in varying degrees, cardiomyopathy is probably most commonly induced by Adriamycin (a drug used in the treatment of cancer) toxicity. Adriamycin often produces a variety of abnormal heart rhythms, particularly VPCs. In addition, some patients (about 10 percent) may develop progressive and severe biventricular heart failure, and death often follows within three weeks after the onset of symptoms. Cardiotoxicity seems to be dose related.

Radiation Cardiomyopathy

When 4,000 rads or more radiation therapy is given, clinically apparent cardiac damage is observed in about 5 percent of patients. The incidence of radiation cardiomyopathy may be as high as 50 percent when 6,000 rads or more radiation treatment is applied. Of course, radiation therapy is indicated for patients with many forms of malignant diseases. Cardiac damage due to radiation is most commonly manifested by a form of acute pericarditis, chronic pericardial effusion, or chronic constrictive pericarditis (see Chapter 13). Myocardial fibrosis may coexist with pericarditis, and various cardiac arrhythmias are not uncommon.

CLINICAL MANIFESTATIONS

Clinical manifestations of cardiomyopathy, regardless of type, etiologic agents, or underlying disorders, seem to be almost the same. The earliest cardiac findings include weakness, fatigue, and dyspnea on exertion as a result of a low cardiac output. At this stage, most patients show an evidence of cardiomegaly on physical examination, ECG, and chest X-ray film. The diagnosis of cardiomyopathy must be made only when all known common heart diseases (e.g., CAD) are excluded.

DIAGNOSIS

There is no specific test to establish the diagnosis of cardiomyopathy, especially the idiopathic variety. On the other hand, certain types of cardiomyopathy (e.g., Chagas's heart disease) require a specific test to establish the diagnosis. Echocardiography is extremely valuable in diagnosing IHSS in almost every case. Cardiac catheterization and angiocardiography are necessary in some patients with cardiomyopathy, primarily to exclude any other heart diseases (e.g., CAD) and to identify coexisting heart diseases.

A clinical history, with social as well as cultural backgrounds, is very important in establishing the diagnosis of beriberi heart disease, alcoholic cardiomyopathy, peripartum heart disease, radiation cardiomyopathy, and drug-induced cardiomyopathy. Cardiomyopathy should be strongly considered when a person develops cardiomegaly and CHF in the absence of apparent known heart disease.

MANAGEMENT AND PROGNOSIS

No specific treatment is available because the cause of the heart disease is unknown in most cases of cardiomyopathy. Thus, management is primarily supportive and symptomatic. When the causative agents or underlying disorders (e.g., vitamin B_1 deficiency) are known, of course, these factors should be treated or eliminated. Anticoagulant therapy (blood-thinning drugs) is recommended for all patients with cardiomyopathy, especially in the idiopathic variety and in patients with previous thromboembolic phenomena. CHF and cardiac arrhythmias should be treated in the usual manner (see Chapters 6 and 17). Beta-adrenergic blocking agents are very useful for patients with IHSS. An artificial cardiac pacemaker is indicated for very slow heart rhythm (e.g., complete A-V block), which may occur in almost all forms of cardiomyopathy. Surgical excision of the hypertrophied septum may be required for patients with IHSS when medical treatment is ineffective and symptoms (e.g., chest pain, syncope) are serious. In general, the outcome of cardiomyopathy is poor. Sudden death is usually the end result of serious cardiac arrhythmias, severe CHF, or thromboembolic phenomena in the lungs, brain, or elsewhere. Heart transplantation has been carried out in some medical centers with good technical success, but the long-term survival rate is still very poor.

13

INFLAMMATION
OR INFECTION
OF THE HEART

Inflammation or infection in the heart includes myocarditis, pericarditis, and endo-carditis. Although foreign organisms (e.g., viruses, bacteria) are a common cause, these disease processes may be due to chemical or physical agents, drugs, radiation, traumas, and neoplasms. At times, the exact underlying cause may not be obvious. Myocarditis is an infection or inflammation of the myocardium (heart muscle), whereas pericarditis is an infection or inflammation of the pericardium (a sac surrounding the heart). In many clinical circumstances, an infectious or inflam-matory process involves both the myocardium and the pericardium; the term *pancarditis* is used in this circumstance (*pan* means "entire"). Endocarditis is often called "infective endocarditis" or "bacterial endocarditis," which represents a microbial (bacterial) infection of the heart valve(s) or of the endocardium (inner layer of the heart chambers) in proximity to congenital cardiac defects or valvular lesions. The clinical course may be very mild and self-limited, or it may be so serious that sudden death may occur. The most common cause of myocarditis in the United States is various viruses. Although the most common form of acute pericarditis is said to be idiopathic (unknown cause), again various viruses are considered responsible. In addition, acute pericarditis is frequently caused by surgical injury (called "postpericardiotomy syndrome" or "postcardiotomy syn-drome") and acute MI (called "post-MI syndrome" or "Dressler's syndrome"). In these cases, an autoimmune mechanism (unusual or hypersensitive reaction to injured or damaged tissue) is considered responsible. Endocarditis is commonly caused by staphylococcus, pneumococcus, and streptococcus.

Although myocarditis means any infectious or inflammatory process involving the myocardium, it often coexists with pericarditis. In addition, myocarditis is not always distinguishable from cardiomyopathy, because a boundary between these two entities is not clear in many circumstances. Likewise, heart muscle damage caused by radiation is often considered a form of myocarditis, but it may be classified under cardiomyopathy. Furthermore, so-called idiopathic cardiomyopathy is thought to be initiated by chronic myocarditis in some cases.

Causes

Viral infection is probably the most common cause of myocarditis, particularly in the United States. Prior to the development of myocarditis, there is often a history of upper respiratory febrile illness (like flu). Group B Coxsackie viruses most often produce myocarditis; less commonly, it is due to group A Coxsackie viruses, echo viruses, and viruses of measles, mumps, and poliomyelitis. It has been shown that idiopathic pericarditis, which often coexists with myocarditis, is frequently produced by group B Coxsackie virus. Viral myocarditis commonly affects newborn infants, and a fatal outcome frequently results from rapidly progressing CHF. Myocarditis may also be caused by or associated with influenza (flu), rabies, chicken pox, German measles, and infectious mononucleosis.

Myocarditis may be due to bacterial infection in rare cases, and it usually occurs as a complication of bacterial endocarditis. Streptococci and staphylococci are the most commonly responsible organisms. Myocarditis may also occur as a complication of diphtheria and frequently leads to death. Fiedler's myocarditis, a rare entity with an unknown cause, frequently produces severe CHF, leading to a fatal outcome in most cases. Viral etiology has been considered a possible cause for this fatal myocarditis. Similarly, idiopathic giant-cell myocarditis (unknown cause), a newly recognized clinical condition, also frequently results in a fatal outcome. In very rare cases, myocarditis may be produced by rickettsial or fungal infection.

Clinical Manifestations and Diagnosis

A mild form of myocarditis, especially viral in origin, is often unrecognized by the patient and may be considered a common cold or flu. Most individuals recover completely without any complication or sequelae. On the other hand, some patients with acute myocarditis may suffer from chronic myocarditis for weeks, months, or even years. In clinically significant acute myocarditis, there may be various manifestations, including fever, weakness, anorexia, general malaise, palpitations, chest pain, shortness of breath, and edema. In advanced cases of myocarditis, various clinical findings of CHF are observed. When there is coexisting acute pericarditis, a pericardial friction rub (see Chapter 8) may be present. The tachycardia is often disproportionate to the degree of fever in many cases of acute myocarditis.

A pansystolic mumur of relative mitral or tricuspid regurgitation may be audible as a result of dilatation of the mitral or tricuspic valve ring secondary to severe CHF. A variety of ECG abnormalities and cardiac arrhythmias are observed, and S-T segment and T wave changes are the most common findings. By and large, the diagnosis of acute myocarditis is strongly suspected when any previously healthy individual develops cardiomegaly and/or CHF associated with fever and various ECG abnormalities in the absence of any known heart disease. Sudden death is not uncommon in acute myocarditis, especially in newborn infants or elderly individuals, resulting from rapidly progressing CHF and/or serious cardiac arrhythmias. Poliomyelitis is often associated with myocarditis. Various clinical manifestations of underlying viral diseases (e.g., measles, German measles, poliomyelitis) are expected when acute myocarditis is a complication of a generalized viral infection.

The causative virus or bacteria should be identified if possible. The virus may be isolated from the nasopharynx, feces (stool), or other body fluids, and changes in specific viral antibody titers are often valuable to support the clinical diagnosis of acute myocarditis of viral origin. In bacterial myocarditis as a complication of bacterial endocarditis, the causative bacteria (e.g., streptococcus, staphylococcus) must be identified by blood culture in order to select the proper antibiotics. Various abnormal heart rhythms may be encountered, but VPCs are most common. Complete A-V block may occur, especially in myocarditis due to diphtheria. Cardiomegaly will be shown on the chest X-ray film and ECG, and various findings of CHF are expected in advanced cases. Elevation of various enzymes (e.g., SGOT, LDH, CPK) in the blood will be observed when there is sufficient damage to the heart muscle.

Management and Prognosis

Management of viral myocarditis is primarily supportive and symptomatic. Bed rest is essential for every case with clinically significant myocarditis regardless of the underlying cause. Bed rest should be continued until fever disappears, the quality of heart sounds improves, signs and symptoms of CHF markedly reduce, and the ECG findings improve or stabilize. Resumption of physical activities should be gradual, extending over a period of weeks to months. CHF and cardiac arrhythmias should be treated in the usual manner (see Chapters 6 and 17). In rare cases of myocarditis, especially when it is due to diphtheria, an artificial cardiac pacemaker is indicated for complete A-V block. For bacterial myocarditis, appropriate antibiotic therapy is mandatory.

By and large, most patients with acute viral myocarditis recover completely, and the prognosis is good. However, in newborn infants and in elderly people, death often occurs as a result of severe CHF and/or serious cardiac arrhythmias. In some patients, acute myocarditis may progressively lead to chronic myocarditis, which may closely simulate cardiomyopathy. The prognosis is more serious in bacterial myocarditis. In nearly 50 percent of the cases, various ECG abnormalities may persist for weeks or months, even when clinical evidence of myocarditis has completely subsided.

PERICARDITIS

By and large, pericarditis is manifested by three major clinical categories, including acute pericarditis, pericardial effusion, and constrictive pericarditis. The disease process may start with acute pericarditis, and it may progress to pericardial effusion followed by constrictive pericarditis. In other cases, the disease of the pericardium may appear as pericardial effusion or constrictive pericarditis without apparent preceding acute pericarditis. Clinical features have changed recently in several ways. For instance, the incidence of bacterial pericarditis has been reduced markedly because of the availability of effective antibiotics. On the other hand, the incidence of postcardiotomy syndrome has increased considerably in the past decade because various cardiac operations, especially CABS, are performed very frequently, particularly in the United States. Another example is the growing recognition of postmyocardial infarction syndrome in recent years. In addition, the most common cause of constrictive pericarditis today is acute idiopathic pericarditis, although the major cause used to be tuberculosis. The reason for this is that tuberculosis has been eliminated in most parts of the world because of an improvement in living standards and a ready availability of antituberculous drugs.

Acute Pericarditis

It is a well-known fact that the early manifestation of pericardial disease is most commonly acute pericarditis. Acute pericarditis may be due to a variety of underlying causes, but idiopathic pericarditis is probably the most common form today. Acute pericarditis may be cured completely, but it may progress to pericardial effusion, subacute or chronic pericarditis, and constrictive pericarditis. Acute pericarditis may also recur in some cases.

Idiopathic Pericarditis

Idiopathic pericarditis is probably the most common form of acute pericarditis in adults. Pericarditis is often self-limited, but very serious clinical outcome, including severe pericardial effusion, cardiac tamponade (defined later), and constrictive pericarditis, may be observed. Although the exact cause is said to be unknown, it is often difficult to distinguish it from viral acute pericarditis in many aspects. On the other hand, some form of hypersensitive reaction has been considered a possible cause.

Idiopathic pericarditis most commonly affects older children, adolescents, and young adults. Pericarditis is frequently preceded by an upper respiratory infection (like common cold or flu) for a few days or several weeks before fever and chest pain occur. The febrile course with varying degrees of chest pain generally lasts from one to several weeks. In some cases, pericardial effusion may occur early, and it may be the earliest sign of idiopathic pericarditis. Many patients may feel weak for weeks or even several months after recovering from the febrile course and chest pain. A mild leukocytosis (increased number of white blood cells) is often present, and the ECG shows a typical finding of acute pericarditis (S-T segment elevation in many leads diffusely; see Figure 13.1). In the majority of cases with idiopathic pericarditis, bed rest and analgesics are sufficient to relieve fever and chest pain in one to two weeks. Aspirin and indomethacin may be used when chest pain persists. If these measures are found to be ineffective for severe chest pain, adrenal corticosteroid hormone therapy (cortisonelike drugs) may be indicated.

Infectious Pericarditis

Infectious pericarditis means acute pericarditis caused by known infectious organisms, including virus, bacteria, tuberculosis, fungus, and others like parasites. Thus, a significant number of cases of acute pericarditis represent infectious pericarditis. Among various forms of infectious pericarditis, viral pericarditis is the most common form, and it is often difficult to distinguish it from idiopathic pericarditis. The most common virus is type-B Coxsackie virus, whereas type-A Coxsackie virus is a much less common causative agent. In occasional cases, acute

FIGURE 13.1. Pericarditis. A: Acute pericarditis (note S-T segment elevation in many leads). B: Subacute pericarditis (note T wave inversion in many leads).

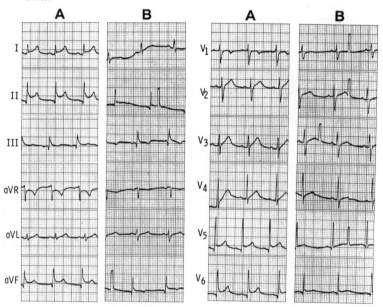

pericarditis may be caused by type-A echo virus, mumps, and infectious mononucleosis. The clinical manifestations of viral pericarditis are very similar, if not identical, to those of idiopathic pericarditis.

Bacterial pericarditis is much less common today because of the availability of many effective antibiotics. Nevertheless, pericarditis due to various bacterias still occurs, and the pericardium is often affected by direct extension of infection from foci (source of infection) in the lungs or chest cavity. Bacterial pericarditis also occurs as a complication of bacterial endocarditis or septicemia (generalized bacterial infection in the blood). Common bacterial organisms include staphylococcus, pneumococcus, streptococcus, gonococcus, meningococcus, and Hemophilus influenza. Less commonly, bacterial pericarditis may be due to Klebsiella, Pseudomonas, Proteus, and E. coli; rarely, Salmonella may cause bacterial pericarditis. It is essential to identify the causative agent so that a proper antibiotic therapy can be instituted. Significant leukocytosis is always present in bacterial pericarditis.

The incidence of tuberculous pericarditis is not too common today, especially in the United States, because of an improved living standard and the availability of many effective antituberculous drugs. Nonetheless, tuberculosis is still with us, especially in underdeveloped countries. Tuberculous pericarditis predominantly affects men, especially blacks, who show about ten times higher incidence than whites. In many cases, evidence of tuberculosis is found elsewhere (e.g., lungs) in the body. The clinical manifestations of tuberculous pericarditis are similar to those of other forms of infectious pericarditis during the acute phase, but various systemic symptoms such as weakness and low-grade fever will appear during the chronic phase. In addition, chronic tuberculous pericarditis is frequently followed by constrictive pericarditis. In fact, tuberculosis was the most common cause of constrictive pericarditis until recently. A proper antituberculous therapy is, of course, indicated when the diagnosis of tuberculous pericarditis is established or strongly suspected.

Various fungal infections (e.g., histoplasmosis, coccidioidomycosis, actinomycosis, and nocardosis) may cause pericarditis on rare occasions. Extremely rarely, pericarditis may be due to various parasites (e.g., Entamoeba histolytica).

Postmyocardial Infarction Syndrome (Dressler's Syndrome)

Post-MI syndrome is a form of acute pericarditis that usually occurs two to eleven weeks following a heart attack. Post-MI syndrome is a relatively common complication of a heart attack, and it is considered to be due to an autoimmune mechanism (a response to the injured or damaged tissue). The patient may experience recurrent chest pains weeks to months after the acute episode of a heart attack. The chest pain is usually sharp in character. It is usually precordial but may radiate to the shoulder or into the neck. The pain is often aggravated by deep respiratory movements and by lying down. On physical examination, a pericardial friction rub (see Chapter 8) is the most important diagnostic feature. There may be low-grade fever, tachycardia, and evidence of pleural effusion (fluid accumulation in the chest cavity) and/or pericardial effusion (fluid accumulation in the pericardial sac). Pulmonary rales may be heard in the chest.

There is no specific laboratory finding to diagnose, but a typical ECG finding (diffuse S-T segment elevation) supports the clinical findings of the syndrome. Of course, the preexisting MI is evident on the ECG. Chest X-ray film may disclose pulmonary infiltrates or pleural effusion. A globular-shaped heart may be observed only if there is a massive pericardial effusion. Diagnosis can be established in most cases without difficulty on the basis of recurrent chest pain after an appropriate interval following acute MI in conjunction with a typical ECG finding of acute pericarditis. However, it is very important to differentiate it from another acute MI, extension of acute MI, or pulmonary embolism. Various arrhythmias may be observed in this syndrome, and hemopericardium (hemorrhagic pericardial effusion) and cardiac tamponade are the most serious complications, especially when anticoagulants (blood thinners) are administered. In most cases, the syndrome is self-limited, and the prognosis is good. However, aspirin may be needed to relieve chest pain and fever in some patients. When symptoms are severe, indomethacin (Indocin) or steroids (cortisonelike drugs, such as prednisone), may be indicated in some cases. The post-MI syndrome does not seem to alter the prognosis of the underlying CAD.

Postcardiotomy Syndrome (Postpericardiotomy Syndrome)

Postcardiotomy syndrome is a form of acute pericarditis that occurs approximately two weeks to three months following cardiac trauma. Postcardiotomy syndrome most commonly follows various types of cardiac operations, particularly CABS. In addition, it may be due to penetrating (open) trauma to the chest and, less commonly, to blunt (closed) trauma and artificial cardiac pacemaker implantation. The mechanism that produces postcardiotomy syndrome is thought to be a hypersensitive response to blood in the pericardium and/or an autoimmune reaction to the injured myocardial or pericardial tissue. Infectious process has also been considered in some cases. Postcardiotomy syndrome is observed in approximately 10 to 30 percent of cases following cardiac surgery. Thus, postcardiotomy syndrome is one of the most common forms of acute pericarditis today, because CABS is the most commonly performed major operation.

As in other forms of acute pericarditis, there is chest pain that is usually intensified by deep breathing and lying down. Cough and shortness of breath may occur. In general, postcardiotomy syndrome is strongly suspected when there is unexplained prolongation of fever or reappearance of fever following any type of cardiac surgery or cardiac trauma. Pleural and/or pericardial effusions may be observed, and pericardial friction rub (see Chapter 8) is commonly heard. ECG and radiologic findings of the postcardiotomy syndrome are essentially the same as those seen in the postmyocardial infarction syndrome except for the absence of an MI pattern. The clinical course is generally benign, and the prognosis is excellent in most cases. On rare cases, cardiac tamponade may occur, but a variety of transient cardiac arrhythmias is not uncommon. In severe cases, indomethacin (Indocin) or corticosteroids may be required for a short time. Salicylates are often effective for mild symptoms.

Miscellaneous Conditions

Acute pericarditis may occur as a manifestation or complication of various connective tissue disorders such as lupus erythematosus, rheumatoid arthritis, periarteritis, and scleroderma. In children and young adults, acute pericarditis, of course, commonly occurs as a manifestation of acute rheumatic fever (see Chapter 11). Acute pericarditis may also occur as an allergic or unusual reaction to various agents including drugs (e.g., penicillin, procainamide, hydralazine). In addition, the occurrence of acute pericarditis as a complication of metabolic disorders such as uremia (kidney failure) and myxedema (hypothyroidism—reduced function of the thyroid gland) is well recognized. The exact mechanism for the production of acute pericarditis in patients with uremia is not clearly known, but hemorrhagic pericardial effusion often occurs in the terminal phase. Pericarditis in patients with myxedema is usually manifested by significant pericardial effusion, but thyroid replacement is usually effective in treating this condition. High-dose radiation therapy for various forms of malignancy not uncommonly causes acute pericarditis, which may lead to pericardial effusion and even constrictive pericarditis.

Pericardial Effusion

Pericardial effusion means the accumulation of serous or serousanguineous fluid in the pericardial space surrounding the heart. It should be remembered that there is about 25 to 35 ml of fluid in the pericardial space of the normal heart. Therefore, pericardial effusion is said to be present when the fluid accumulation is more than 35 ml. Pericardial effusion may be present either in an acute or chronic form, and it may be the first manifestation of acute pericarditis. The circulatory effects and clinical manifestations are directly related to the speed of accumulation of fluid in the pericardial space. For instance, the sudden and rapid development of a pericardial effusion of several hundred mililiters often produces severe hemodynamic consequences that may lead to marked reduction of cardiac output and even sudden death. Conversely, slow and gradual accumulation of fluid in the pericardial space may not provoke significant hemodynamic changes, and the patient is often asymptomatic despite accumulations of several liters.

The major reason for hemodynamic consequences and clinical manifestations is the accumulation of fluid in the pericardial space that is sufficient to interfere with the adequate filling of the heart chambers. In other words, the filling of the heart chambers is mechanically disturbed by the accumulation of fluid in the pericardial space around the heart. For the same reason, venous inflow to the heart is also markedly reduced so that accumulation of blood in the venous system leads to a marked jugular venous distension (engorgement of the neck veins) and liver enlargement. In chronic pericardial effusion, peripheral edema (e.g., swelling of the ankles) often occurs. When venous return to the heart is significantly reduced, cardiac output is also markedly diminished, and fatal outcomes may not be avoided.

Causes

Practically speaking, almost any type of acute pericarditis may cause pericardial effusion, but common causes may include tuberculosis, idiopathic pericarditis, viral pericarditis, and malignancy. Hemopericardium is often due to tuberculosis or malignancy, but it may also be associated with acute rheumatic fever and post-cardiotomy syndrome. In occasional cases with uremic pericarditis, hemopericardium may be observed. Hemopericardium is, of course, a serious complication of anticoagulant therapy, especially in patients with acute MI.

Clinical Manifestations

Clinical manifestations are greatly influenced by the speed of the accumulation of pericardial effusion. Very rapid accumulation of several hundred mililiters of fluid may cause marked reduction of cardiac output, which may lead to death. On the other hand, slowly accumulating pericardial effusion, even as much as several liters, may not produce significant symptoms. Clinical manifestations will vary according to the amounts of effusion and the underlying cardiac as well as non-cardiac disorders. Most patients with significant pericardial effusions frequently show shortness of breath, cyanosis, tachycardia, a rapid thready pulse, distended neck veins, liver enlargement, paradoxical pulse, peripheral edema, and faint heart sounds. The paradoxical pulse is almost a pathognomonic feature of pericardial effusion, particularly cardiac tamponade. The paradoxical pulse is defined as a greater than normal (8 to 10 mmHg) reduction of systolic BP during inspiration. When the paradoxical pulse is very pronounced, the arterial pulse during inspiration may be so weak that it may not be detectable at all.

The heart sounds are often distant, and the pericardial friction rub (see Chapter 8) is frequently audible by auscultation. Large pericardial effusion usually causes increased cardiac silhouette with a "water bottle" configuration on the chest X-ray film, and the cardiac apex is shifted to the left and laterally. When there is massive pericardial effusion, increased dullness at the base of the lung below the angle of the left scapula is often detected by careful percussion as a result of compression of the left lung (lower lobe) by the distended pericardial sac (called "Ewart's or Pin's sign"). The heart sound may change its intensity on every other beat so that weak and strong pulses may be felt alternately (called "pulsus alternans"). The pulsus alternans may or may not be associated with electrical alternans (an electrical version of pulsus alternans that is manifested by alternating ECG deflections). Pericardial effusion may be the first sign of acute pericarditis, but the former often occurs as a complication of the latter.

Cardiac Tamponade

Cardiac tamponade is the most serious life-threatening complication of pericardial effusion and acute pericarditis regardless of the causative agents or underlying disorders. Cardiac tamponade is produced by the accumulation of fluid in the pericardium in an amount sufficient to cause significant obstruction of the inflow of blood to the ventricles. Cardiac tamponade causes marked reduction of cardiac output and systemic venous congestion, and a fatal outcome is often unavoidable unless treated immediately. The speed of fluid accumulation in the pericardial space greatly influences the development of cardiac tamponade. For example, rapid accumulation of pericardial fluid as little as 250 ml may be sufficient to produce cardiac tamponade. On the other hand, it may require as much as 1,000 ml or more when the pericardial effusion develops very slowly. By and large, cardiac tamponade is most commonly produced by bleeding into the pericardial space following various types of cardiac surgery or trauma, tuberculosis, and malignancy. In addition, cardiac tamponade may also be due to idiopathic and viral pericarditis, postcardiotomy syndrome, and postradiation pericarditis. Hemopericardium is not uncommon during anticoagulant therapy.

In cardiac tamponade, various clinical findings are produced by marked reduction of BP secondary to the fall in cardiac output, and also by systemic venous congestion. When cardiac tamponade develops slowly, the clinical manifestations superficially resemble those of CHF. Common manifestations may include dyspnea, orthopnea, tachycardia, hepatomegaly, engorgement of neck veins, and enlarged cardiac silhouette (actual heart size is normal, but the entire outline of the heart is enlarged because of excessive fluid accumulation around the heart). Cardiac tamponade is often manifested by all physical findings of massive pericardial effusion as already described. Cardiac tamponade is usually fatal unless pericardial effusion is immediately removed.

Diagnosis

Echocardiography is the most effective and the most commonly utilized method to detect and estimate even small amounts of pericardial effusion with a high degree of accuracy (see Chapter 24). Chest X-ray film often discloses enlarged cardiac silhouette with a "water bottle" or "pear-shaped" configuration, and a variety of ECG abnormalities may be observed. Most commonly, a generalized low voltage of the QRS complexes is shown on the ECG. In addition, S-T segment elevation with T wave inversion is very common, especially when pericardial effusion is associated with acute or subacute pericarditis. At times, electrical alternans (changing configuration of various complexes on every other or every third beat) may be present, especially in hemopericardium. Preexisting other ECG abnormalities may also be present. Pericardial effusion can be documented by invasive diagnostic tests. Needless to say, the unequivocal proof of documentation of pericardial effusion is to obtain fluid (or bloody fluid) from the pericardial space by pericardio-

241

centesis (pericardial tap; discussed shortly). The diagnosis of pericardial effusion can be made, however, from the clinical background alone in many cases.

Management and Prognosis

When there is a massive pericardial effusion, pericardiocentesis (pericardial tap) is generally indicated. In the treatment of tamponade, rapid aspiration of pericardial fluid (or bloody fluid) by pericardiocentesis is only a life-saving measure. Clinically, pericardial tap is urgently needed when the patient demonstrates serious manifestations, including marked weakness, palor, dyspnea, hypotension with narrow pulse pressure (see Chapter 5), rapid and thready pulse, unclear mental status, and other signs of cardiogenic shock.

Pericardiocentesis can be performed by an experienced physician by inserting a medium-sized needle into the pericardial space. Various locations can be chosen for the pericardial tap. The needle can be inserted high in the epigastrium (upper portion of the abdomen) in the angle formed between the left border of the xiphoid process (breastbone) and the lower left rib cage. The needle is advanced slowly upward at an angle of about 30°, pointed toward the midline. The pericardium is reached usually at 3 to 4 cm from the skin surface. Another method is to insert a needle at the left fifth or sixth intercostal space about 1 cm within the area of cardiac dullness or 1 to 2 cm inside the left heart border outlined on the chest X-ray film (about 7 to 8 cm outside the left sternal border). The needle is advanced slowly inward and slightly upward. When the pericardial fluid is obtained by the pericardial tap, it should carefully be examined for the number and type of cells and the presence of bacteria (requiring bacterial and tuberculous culture); cytologic examination (to detect malignancy) under a microscope should also be performed. The contents of sugar and protein should be examined also.

It is important to treat underlying disorders or any coexisting disease. For example, antituberculous drugs should be given for tuberculous pericardial effusion, whereas thyroid hormone is indicated when pericardial effusion is due to myxedema. Appropriate antibiotics must be given for purulent (pus-forming) pericardial effusion. For uremic pericardial effusion, it is mandatory to treat the underlying kidney failure (e.g., by kidney dialysis). When hemopericardium is the end result of a trauma to the heart and adjacent structure, appropriate surgical repair may be indicated. Open surgical drainage is required for recurrent cardiac tamponade, particularly when the effusion is purulent. When pericardial effusion accumulates again and again rapidly in spite of repetitive pericardial taps, pericardiectomy (excision of the pericardium) should be considered.

Prognosis is greatly influenced by the speed of fluid accumulation in the pericardial space, causative agents, and underlying disorders. Cardiac tamponade and rapidly accumulating pericardial effusion are often fatal unless treated immediately. Pericardial effusion secondary to malignancy, uremia, and bacteremia (bacteria in the bloodstream) carries a grave prognosis. On the other hand, the prognosis is favorable when pericardial effusion is associated with idiopathic or viral pericarditis. Untreated or long-standing pericardial effusion, particularly of tuberculous origin, may lead to constrictive pericarditis.

Constrictive Pericarditis

Constrictive pericarditis is a chronic disorder in which the pericardium is thickened (often more than 1 cm in thickness) from a firm scar formation following a long-standing inflammation or infectious process. Consequently, a rigid and thickened pericardium will encase the heart and interfere with the filling (expansion) of the ventricles. In a long-standing constrictive pericarditis, the thickened pericardium often calcifies. Although the disease process in the majority of cases is chronic and slowly progressing, subacute forms may be observed. In these cases, constriction of the pericardium may occur within days, weeks, or months rather rapidly. In some cases, constriction may become significant even when pericardial effusion and cardiac tamponade are still present.

The fundamental mechanism that produces various clinical manifestations is obstruction or constriction of either the cardiac chambers or the orifices of the great veins entering the heart. As a result, the ventricles are unable to fill (expand) adequately during the diastolic phase because of the limitations imposed by the rigid and thickened pericardium. The process of the constriction may be localized predominantly to isolated chambers of the heart or even to small, localized portions of the pericardium surrounding these heart chambers, although more commonly the constriction occurs diffusely. The process of the constriction in the pericardium may be so slow that initial symptoms may not be recognized readily either by the patient or by the physician in many cases. In advanced cases, however, there will be various clinical findings, including markedly elevated venous pressure (e.g., distended neck veins, liver engorgement), diminished heart pulsation, paradoxical pulse, and ascites (fluid accumulation in the abdominal cavity) out of proportion to the degree of ankle edema.

Causes

In a practical sense, almost any type of acute pericarditis may lead to constrictive pericarditis except for that which is rheumatic in origin. Although the major cause until two decades ago was tuberculosis, it is rather uncommon at the present time. The exact cause of constrictive pericarditis is uncertain in many cases, but unproven tuberculosis or virus infection cannot be excluded in some cases. Common causes may include viral pericarditis, idiopathic pericarditis, purulent (bacterial) infection, malignancy, trauma, radiation, uremia, and various collagen (connective tissue) diseases (e.g., lupus erythematosus).

Clinical Manifestations

Common clinical manifestations of constrictive pericarditis may include weakness, fatigue, loss of weight, and anorexia associated with distended abdomen due to ascites, distended neck veins, and ankle edema resulting from systemic venous congestion. Most patients often appear to be chronically ill, with decreased muscle mass, and dyspnea is often produced by physical activity. In addition, enlargement of the liver and at times the spleen from engorgement is frequently observed as a result of systemic venous congestion secondary to impaired filling of the ventricles caused by a rigid and thickened pericardium, and various signs of abnormal liver function (e.g., jaundice) may occur. In advanced cases, edema may be so intense that anasarca (generalized edema, including the scrotum) may be observed. One of the unique features of constrictive pericarditis is ascites out of proportion to the degree of ankle edema.

The heart size is normal in about half the cases of constrictive pericarditis, and marked cardiomegaly is very unusual unless there is a coexisting heart disease. The cardiac impulse is reduced in intensity, and the heart sounds are often muffled and distant. An accentuated third heart sound (called "pericardial knock") is common (see Chapter 8), and paradoxical pulse is observed in about a third of the cases. In addition, the pulse pressure is often reduced, and AF frequently occurs in the late stages of constrictive pericarditis.

Diagnosis

Echocardiography provides very important information by demonstrating a thickened pericardium with small to normal ventricular chambers and enlarged atrial chambers. Cardiac catheterization with angiography is also a valuable tool in diagnosing constrictive pericarditis by excluding various heart diseases. Weak to almost absent pulsations of the heart can be readily demonstrated by fluoroscopy, and calcification may be visualized in about 50 percent of the cases. On the ECG, a generalized low voltage of the QRS complexes is very common, and flat to inverted T waves are frequently observed diffusely in many leads. The S-T segment may be elevated when there is a component of acute or subacute pericarditis. In most cases, the constrictive pericarditis can be diagnosed from clinical backgrounds in conjunction with various laboratory tests, particularly echocardiographic and fluoroscopic findings.

Management and Prognosis

The definitive management for constrictive pericarditis is a pericardiectomy (resection of the pericardium). Thus, as soon as the diagnosis is established, pericardiectomy should be performed immediately. The earlier this surgery is carried out, the lower the mortality and the greater the benefit. The mortality rate is reported to be not more than 3 to 5 percent in most cases, but the surgical risks are much greater in patients with long-standing constrictive pericarditis with heavy calcifications. A low-salt diet and diuretic therapy are beneficial in treating ascites, ankle edema, or generalized edema before surgery. When constrictive pericarditis is proved or even suspected to be tuberculous in origin, antituberculous therapy should be continued before and after the operation.

Endocarditis is expressed as either "infective endocarditis" or "bacterial endocarditis," and it is defined as infection involving the endocardium (inner lining of the heart chambers). Endocarditis primarily affects damaged heart valves and less commonly involves congenital defects or prosthetic (artificial) valves. When the causative bacteria are highly virulent, a normal heart may be affected. Endocarditis may develop suddenly or slowly, depending upon the nature and strength of the causative bacteria, and the disease process is often fatal unless properly and immediately treated with appropriate antibiotics. The infection caused by microorganisms with high pathogenicity (e.g., *Staphylococcus aureus*) is usually acute, whereas the infection caused by low-virulence bacteria (e.g., *Streptococcus viridans*) is generally subacute. *Streptococcus viridans* is the most common bacterium in producing endocarditis involving congenital or rheumatic heart valve lesions, and its clinical course is usually subacute. Customarily, endocarditis is divided into two major categories: (1) the acute form and (2) the subacute form, depending upon the nature and manifestations of the clinical course and the causative bacteria.

Common clinical manifestations of endocarditis include fever, heart murmurs, anemia, hematuria (bloody urine), splenomegaly (enlarged spleen), petechiae (pinpoint- to pinhead-sized hemorrhage spots in the skin), and embolic phenomena. Most patients have continuous bacteremia (bacteria in the bloodstream), and infection can spread from the vegetations (lesions with bacterial colonies) to cause abscess (pus) formation in the heart valves, especially in patients with infected prosthetic valves. Metastatic evidence (a widespread) of bacterial infection may be observed in the brain, heart, spleen, kidneys, and elsewhere in the body. Men seem to be slightly more involved than women, and the mean ages range from the mid forties to the fifties, with 50 percent or more being fifty or older. Endocarditis is uncommon in children and young adults.

Underlying Heart Disease

As far as the underlying heart disease is concerned, RHD is the most common (40 to 60 percent of all cases). In particular, the mitral valve is most commonly affected, and aortic valve infection is also common. Endocarditis involving the right heart is less than 10 percent of the total patient population with RHD and usually affects the tricuspid valve. In approximately 10 percent of cases of endocarditis, various congenital heart defects are found. The congenital heart lesions that commonly predispose to endocarditis include patent ductus arteriosus, ventricular septal defect, tetralogy of Fallot, coarctation of the aorta, pulmonic stenosis, and bicuspid aortic valve (see Chapter 10). Endocarditis seldom occurs on atrial septal defect of the secundum type (see Chapter 10).

Endocarditis not uncommonly occurs in patients with various prosthetic heart valves and rarely following the implantation of an artificial pacemaker. In addition, atriovenous or arterioarterial fistulas (abnormal communication between an artery and a vein or between two arteries) also predispose to endocarditis. Furthermore, endocarditis has been reported in patients with mitral valve prolapse syndrome, IHSS, Marfan's syndrome, and syphilitic aortic valve disease (see Chapters 10 and 14). In 20 to 40 percent of patients with bacterial endocarditis, no evidence of apparent underlying heart disease can be demonstrated.

Causes and Classifications

By and large, endocarditis is classified into two major categories, including acute bacterial endocarditis and subacute bacterial endocarditis, depending upon the clinical course. In acute bacterial endocarditis, the most common causative bacteria is *Staphylococcus aureus,* and, less commonly, pneumococci, group-A streptococci, gonococci, and other bacteria. Acute endocarditis nearly always involves normal heart valves and produces severe destruction with rapid clinical course. Commonly, metastatic foci of infection (a wide spread of infection elsewhere) occur, and most patients die within days to weeks if untreated. In fact, many patients with acute bacterial endocarditis may die even if immediate and appropriate treatment is given.

In subacute bacterial endocarditis (often called "SBE" in the medical literature), on the other hand, the most common causative organism is streptococcus of the *viridans* group. In this circumstance, the infection usually affects the already damaged heart valves, particularly from RHD. In SBE, metastatic foci of infection occur only on rare occasions, and the therapeutic result is generally favorable. As the name of the disease indicates, the clinical course of SBE is relatively slow and mild, and it takes six or more weeks and even years to be fatal if untreated. In rare cases, *Staphylococcus aureus* may cause SBE, whereas streptococci of the *viridans* group can produce acute endocarditis involving normal heart valves.

It can be said that almost every kind of bacteria may cause endocarditis, but streptococci and staphylococci are responsible in more than 90 percent of the cases. In particular, streptococci are the causative bacteria in 60 to 80 percent and the *viridans* group is the most common streptococcus to produce the infection. Staphylococci are found to be causative bacteria in 10 to 30 percent, and *Staphylococci aureus* produce the infection most commonly. *Staphylococci epidermidis* are a less common causative bacteria. The pneumococcus is a relatively uncommon bacterium that produces bacterial endocarditis, and gonococci (bacteria that cause gonorrhea) are only a rare causative bacteria. Endocarditis due to fungi (e.g., *Candida, Histoplasma*) is not common. Rarely, endocarditis may be caused by spirochetes or rickettsiae.

As far as the invasive route of the infection is concerned, various types of bacteria may enter the bloodstream following a variety of procedures leading to bacterial endocarditis, although the portal of entry for initiating bacteremia is not always apparent. An infection in the oral cavity or from various dental procedures are the most common modes of entry, particularly in endocarditis produced by *viridans* streptococci. Sigmoidoscopy (insertion of an instrument into the rectum to visualize the inside of the large intestine) and barium enema (X-ray examination of the large intestine) may cause endocarditis. In addition, various surgical or instrumental procedures involving the genitourinary tract (e.g., resection of the prostate gland, cystoscopy) and the female reproductive system (e.g., insertion of a contraceptive intra-uterine device, abortion, delivery of a baby) frequently cause endocarditis. Occasionally, endocarditis may follow instrumentation in the gastro-intestinal tract (stomach and intestine). It is also known that endocarditis is not uncommon in drug addicts because of frequent usage of contaminated (dirty) syringes with needles. In some cases, endocarditis may be caused by bacterial invasion following pneumonia, skin infection, or surgical incision of the skin and even after vigorous tooth brushing or chewing hard candy.

Clinical Manifestations

Acute endocarditis caused by highly virulent bacteria such as *Staphylococcus aureus* usually presents high fever with various manifestations (discussed later) with abrupt onset. On the other hand, SBE caused by low-virulence bacteria such as *Streptococcus viridans* produces very slowly progressing clinical findings with low-grade fever. The early manifestations of SBE commonly include night sweats, chills, malaise, anorexia, fatigue, loss of weight, myalgias (muscle ache), arthralgia (joint pain), late afternoon temperature elevation, and worsening of chronic CHF. In many patients with bacterial endocarditis, the procedure or operation that may be responsible for causing the infection cannot be identified readily. By and large, clinical manifestations of SBE start within two to three weeks following the dental or surgical procedure. On the other hand, acute endocarditis is usually manifested by acute illness with high fever abruptly, and sudden death often follows even if an appropriate treatment is provided immediately.

In bacterial endocarditis, fever is present in nearly all patients, and temperature is often low grade (less than 39.4° C.) except in acute endocarditis. Fever may be absent in elderly patients or in individuals with severe CHF, kidney failure, or marked debility. Heart murmurs (see Chapter 8) are also nearly always present, either because of preexisting valvular or congenital heart lesions or destruction of heart valves as a result of bacterial endocarditis. When any new heart murmur develops, it is usually due to aortic regurgitation. One of the characteristic features of endocarditis is said to be the changing intensity or quality of the heart murmurs or the development of a new heart murmur. The changing intensity of heart murmurs may be due to progressive valvular damage from endocarditis itself, but it may simply be due to changes in the heart rate and/or cardiac output. Heart murmurs may be absent in patients with acute endocarditis or in drug (narcotic) addicts.

There is often splenomegaly in up to 20 to 60 percent, especially in SBE. Various skin manifestations are not uncommon. For instance, petechiae are present in 20 to 40 percent and are more common in SBE. Petechiae commonly appear in the conjunctivae, palate, buccal (mouth) mucosa, and extremities. Splinter hemorrhages (linear and dark red streaks) may be observed under the nail bed, and Roth's spots (oval hemorrhages with a clear pale center) may be noted in the retina. In addition, Osler's nodes (small tender nodules commonly occurring in the pads of fingers or toes) may be encountered in 10 to 25 percent. Clubbing of the fingers (enlarged finger tips) may also occur.

Complications

CHF is a very common complication and may occur at any time during the course of endocarditis. The prognosis is grave in this circumstance. Kidney involvement is also common in patients with endocarditis, and microscopic hematuria may be observed in up to 50 percent of the cases. Proteinuria (protein in the urine) is even more common in endocarditis. These manifestations may be due to renal emboli (blood clots in the kidneys) or glomerulonephritis (infection or inflammation in the kidneys), and severe cases may lead to renal failure. Emboli may also occur in the spleen, eyes, and lungs. Emboli in the spleen often cause pain in the left upper abdomen, radiating to the shoulder, whereas retinal emboli cause blindness. Pulmonary emboli are common in drug addicts and in patients with congenital heart lesions with left-to-right shunts. In endocarditis due to fungal infections, large emboli to the lower extremities are common, and embolectomy (a removal of blood clots) should be performed immediately in this case.

Mycotic aneurysms (bulging of the blood vessels produced by growth of the microorganisms in the vessel wall) are observed in approximately 15 percent, and they are most commonly produced by less virulent bacteria. The mycotic aneurysms most commonly occur in the brain, and they may rupture. Emboli may be observed commonly in the middle cerebral artery. Other neurologic complications may include brain abscess, encephalitis or meningitis (infection or inflammation in the brain), and brain hemorrhage. These neurologic complications may produce personality changes, stroke, and even sudden death. Anemia is a very common finding in patients with bacterial endocarditis, especially in subacute form, as a result of bone marrow depression by the infection.

Diagnosis

Needless to say, the most important diagnostic test is a blood culture, which will confirm the presence of causative bacteria in the bloodstream. Thus, blood cultures must be obtained immediately when endocarditis is suspected clinically. Blood cultures are positive in over 95 percent of the patients with acute endocarditis and in 85 to 95 percent of patients with SBE. By and large, three to five blood cultures (10 ml of blood for each culture), obtained at intervals determined by the patient's clinical circumstance, are adequate to identify the bacteremia. In patients with SBE, five blood cultures are obtained over a period of twelve to twenty-four hours, and the treatment is initiated. In acute endocarditis, however, treatment should not be delayed for more than two to four hours while obtaining blood cultures. Blood cultures may not become positive for several days in patients who have received antibiotics prior to obtaining blood cultures. In this case, antibiotic therapy may be interrupted momentarily while blood cultures are obtained when clinical circumstance permits. In addition, blood cultures may be negative in rare cases with endocarditis due to unusual microorganisms such as *Histoplasma*, *Brucella*, or anaerobic streptococci. Under these circumstances, blood cultures require special nutrient media with an extended (even up to three or four weeks) incubation period.

Anemia is almost always present, especially in SBE as a result of bone marrow depression by the infection. Sedimentation rate is usually elevated. In acute endocarditis, leukocytosis is common. Rheumatoid factor (latex agglutination titer) is elevated in about half to two-thirds of patients with SBE, whereas serum cholesterol levels are generally reduced during the prolonged illness. When there is sufficient kidney damage, blood urea nitrogen (BUN) and creatinine levels are often elevated. Echocardiogram may demonstrate vegetations (colonies of bacteria) on the infected valves and enlargement of various chambers depending upon the underlying heart disease.

The diagnosis of bacterial endocarditis is certain when a patient presents common clinical manifestations (as already discussed) associated with positive blood cultures. When repeated blood cultures are negative, a rare endocarditis due to unusual microorganisms (e.g., *Histoplasma*) should be suspected.

Treatment

The best therapeutic result is expected when an appropriate antibiotic is selected and when the treatment is initiated early in the illness. Bactericidal antibiotics (agents capable of destroying bacteria) should be used rather than bacteriostatic antibiotics (agents inhibiting the growth or multiplication of bacteria). Appropriate antibiotics should be instituted as soon as three to five blood cultures are obtained over twelve to twenty-four hours in SBE. In acute endocarditis, however, the treatment should not be delayed more than two to four hours. Proper selection of the best antibiotic depends upon the sensitivity of the causative microorganism. While awaiting the result of the blood cultures or when causative bacteria are not demonstrated on repeated blood cultures, selection of the antibiotic depends on the prediction of the most probable causative bacterium and its probable antibiotic sensitivity.

In young individuals with RHD or congenital cardiac defects, endocarditis (usually the subacute category) is most commonly due to streptococci of the *viridans* group. These streptococci are usually very sensitive to penicillin G. The usual dose of penicillin is 6 to 10 million units in intravenous injection (some physicians only use 2.4 to 6 million units) daily, and the treatment should be continued for four to six weeks. The penicillin should be given intravenously at least for the first two weeks, and for the second two to four weeks, penicillin may be given by mouth (7.2 g/day) if adequate blood levels of bactericidal titer of more than 1:8 dilution are maintained. During the first two weeks of penicillin therapy, many physicians recommend additional streptomycin in a dose of 0.5 g twice daily, because there is a synergistic action between streptomycin and penicillin.

For the treatment of acute endocarditis caused by staphylococci, a penicillinase-resistant drug should be given intravenously. Commonly used antibiotics include methicillin (16 to 20 g daily), naficillin or oxacillin (4 to 8 g daily), or cephalothin or cefazolin (10 to 14 g daily). These antibiotics should be continued for six to eight weeks. If the staphylococci are found to be sensitive to penicillin G, this antibiotic should be given in a daily dose of 16 to 20 million units for six to eight weeks. Vancomycin (4 to 8 g daily) or clindamycin phosphate (1.5 to 2.5 g daily) can be administered intravenously to patients with allergic reactions to penicillin.

Endocarditis due to enterococci is difficult to treat in general. Penicillin, 20 million units with streptomycin, 1 to 1.5 g daily, has been successful in treating enterococcal endocarditis in many cases. Alternatively, ampicillin and kanamycin or gentamicin may be used. The treatment should be continued for six weeks. In some patients with allergic reactions to penicillin, the hypersensitive (allergic) reactions may be controlled by corticosteroids (cortisonelike drugs) or antihistamines. For pneumococcal endocarditis, penicillin G, 6 to 12 million units daily, should be given intravenously. Endocarditis due to fungal infection is usually fatal. In some cases, however, replacement of the infected valve and surgical removal of the vegetations and emboli with amphotericin B therapy have been successful. Surgical treatment is indicated for many patients with A-V fistula (communication between an artery and a vein), valve ring abscess, recurrent embolization, or infected artificial heart valves. In fact, surgical removal of the damaged valves and implantation of artificial heart valves may be a life-saving measure. The valve replacement should be considered early in patients with intractable CHF usually associated with severe valvular destruction (especially aortic or mitral regurgitation) resulting from the infection.

Fever usually begins to go down within three to seven days after initiation of treatment. When the therapeutic result is not satisfactory, reevaluation of the entire clinical picture with a proper choice of the antibiotic with the best sensitivity to a given causative bacterium is essential. Recurrence of endocarditis occurs in about 10 to 20 percent, and it usually develops within four weeks after termination of treatment. Thus, follow-up blood cultures should be obtained at weekly intervals for four to six weeks after treatment is terminated. When endocarditis recurs, reinstitution of antibiotic therapy is, of course, indicated, but the sensitivity of the microorganism to the antibiotic must be reexamined carefully. By and large, relapse usually indicates inadequate or inappropriate therapy or the need for surgical treatment. Supportive and symptomatic treatment for various complications (e.g., CHF) is, of course, essential.

Preventive Measures

It is highly recommended that all patients with known valvular heart disease or prosthetic heart valves and congenital cardiac lesions receive prophylactic antibiotic therapy before, during, and after dental procedures, instrumentation or surgical procedures in the genitourinary or gastrointestinal tracts, childbirth, and abortion. Penicillin should be part of any antibiotic therapy in most cases, and an aminoglycoside should be added for gastrointestinal or genitourinary tract manipulation.

The following prophylactic measures have been recommended against streptococci of the *viridans* group for dental manipulation or other surgical procedures in the mouth, nose, and throat. The prophylactic regimen consists of a single dose of 1.2 million units of aqueous procaine penicillin G, plus 1.0 g streptomycin given by intramuscular injection within thirty minutes of the procedure, followed by penicillin V 500 mg by mouth every six hours for four doses. Alternatively, the patient may be given a loading dose of 2 g penicillin V by mouth, followed by 500 mg every six hours for twenty-four hours. When the patient is allergic to penicillin, 1.0 g of vancomycin should be given intravenously over thirty minutes, one hour before the procedure; alternatively, 1.0 g of erythromycin may be given by mouth one and a half to two hours before the procedure. Either drug must be followed with 500 mg of erythromycin by mouth every six hours for four doses. For patients with prosthetic heart valves, the combined therapy of penicillin and streptomycin is recommended.

For genitourinary and gastrointestinal tract procedures or operations, the prophylactic measure is directed against enterococci. The best prophylactic regimen consists of ampicillin plus gentamicin. Ampicillin, 1 g, plus gentamicin, 1.5 mg/kg (not exceeding 80 mg), should be administered by intramuscular or intravenous injection thirty to sixty minutes before the procedure, and both drugs should be given every eight hours for two doses thereafter. When the patient is allergic to penicillin, vancomycin should be given intravenously in a dosage of 1.0 g, together with streptomycin, 1.0 g by intramuscular injection, thirty to sixty minutes before the procedure. Both drugs should be repeated twelve hours later.

For cardiac surgery, the prophylactic measure is directed against staphylococci. Recommended preventive treatment includes 2 g of methicillin, oxacillin, nafcillin, or cephalothin intravenously every four hours starting one hour before the surgery and continuing for several days. When the patient is allergic to penicillins and cephalosporine, vancomycin in a dose of 500 mg should be given intravenously every six hours for several days. For drug addicts, endocarditis may be prevented only when individuals are adequately educated so as to foresee the danger of suffering endocarditis and even death before introducing the bacteria into their own bloodstream. It can be said, without a doubt, that endocarditis in drug addicts is one of the most serious problems in society today.

Prognosis

The prognosis depends upon various factors, including causative microorganisms, the therapeutic response to antibiotics, the presence or absence and severity of complications, underlying heart disease, and the patient's age. Poor prognosis is generally expected in various clinical circumstances, including delay in diagnosis and proper treatment, inadequate response to antibiotic therapy, development of serious complications (particularly CHF), infection in the prosthetic valve, aortic valve involvement by the infection, and old age.

In streptococcal endocarditis, the cure rate is reported to be approximately 90 percent, and death usually results from CHF, emboli phenomena, renal failure, or rupture of a mycotic aneurysm. On the other hand, the cure rate in staphylococcal endocarditis is only about 50 percent, with most death due to severe staphylococcal infection itself or to advanced CHF. In general, endocarditis due to fungi and gram-negative bacilli carries a poor prognosis. Approximately 5 to 8 percent of patients who have recovered completely from one episode of endocarditis may suffer from one or more additional episodes of endocarditis over a period of years.

14

UNCOMMON
HEART DISEASES

This chapter will deal with relatively uncommon heart diseases that are clinically important. Thus, the primary discussion will deal with tumors of the heart, traumatic heart disease, and syphilitic heart disease.

TUMORS OF THE HEART

Although tumors of the heart are relatively uncommon, they should be recognized early because they can be cured completely by surgery in most cases. In addition, cardiac tumors often produce various clinical manifestations that may closely simulate other common heart diseases, particularly RHD. Therefore, it is important to distinguish cardiac tumors from other known heart diseases. Cardiac tumors may be the primary tumors (tumors originating from the heart), but they may be metastatic or secondary tumors. Over three-fourths of all primary tumors of the heart are benign, and half of these occur inside the heart chambers (intracavitary tumors). Myxomas are the most common primary tumors, and rhabdomyomas are also relatively common. Myxomas and rhabdomyomas account for more than half of all primary benign cardiac tumors. Rare primary cardiac tumors include cardiac fibromas, lipomas, angiomas, papillomas, teratomas, leiomyomas, and xanthomas. Primary cardiac tumors in infancy and childhood are nearly always

254 Uncommon Heart Diseases

benign. Primary malignant cardiac tumors are most commonly sarcomas, which account for more than 20 percent of all primary cardiac tumors. Sarcomas are only rarely reported in infancy and childhood.

The clinical manifestations are almost identical between benign and malignant primary cardiac tumors and metastatic (secondary) cardiac tumors. Various clinical findings are predominantly influenced by the location of the cardiac tumors rather than the nature or malignancy of the tumors. In fact, there are often no characteristic symptoms unless the tumors produce a disturbance in cardiac function. Consequently, only about 5 to 10 percent of all cardiac tumors may be diagnosed from clinical background. On the other hand, certain cases of cardiac tumors may produce severe and rapidly progressing CHF, which may be associated with a variety of manifestations, including pericardial effusion (frequently bloody), pericarditis, various cardiac arrhythmias, thromboembolic pheomena in various organs, and syncope. Sudden death may occur. Malignant tumors of the heart often cause hemopericardium (bloody fluid accumulation around the heart).

Myxomas

Myxomas are the most common primary tumors of the heart, and the surgical cure is expected in most cases. Myxomas most frequently occur in the atria, and the left atrium is involved three times as often as the right atrium. They are usually pedunculated, and the stem is attached to the atrial septum in the region of the foramen ovale. The atrial myxomas may be either firm and smooth or gelatinous and polypoid. When myxomas involve the ventricles, they are generally fixed to the ventricular wall. Ventricular myxomas are very rare, and metastasis of the myxomas is extremely rare. Various symptoms and physical findings are commonly due to disturbance or even obstruction of blood flow in the cardiac chambers, but they may result from emboli released from the tumors into the pulmonary or systemic arterial beds. In many cases, systemic symptoms (e.g., generalized malaise, fatigue, fever, weight loss) are observed.

Left atrial myxomas frequently produce clinical manifestations similar to mitral valvular disease, particularly mitral stenosis. Mitral stenosis is closely simulated when the pedunculated myxoma falls into the mitral valve orifice, causing narrowing or obstruction. In some cases, the clinical findings closely resemble those of combined mitral stenosis and mitral regurgitation (see Chapter 11). This is because the myxoma produces mitral regurgitation by interfering with the function of mitral valve closure. When the myxoma produces a complete obstruction of the mitral valve, episodes of syncope are commonly observed. On the other hand, various symptoms often disappear immediately when the tumor's obstruction of the mitral valve is relieved by a change in body position. Detailed descriptions of physical findings are found in Chapter 8. The myxomas may also produce various constitutional symptoms, including fever, weakness, myalgias (muscle ache), arthralgias (joint pain), general malaise, and loss of appetite, as well as abnormal laboratory findings, such as elevated sedimentation rate, anemia, and dysfunction of the liver. The clinical picture may simulate bacterial endocarditis and cardio-myopathies. Clinical findings of right atrial myxomas closely resemble those pro-duced by tricuspid stenosis and/or regurgitation. Constitutional symptoms are very similar to those seen in left atrial myxomas. Thromboembolic phenomena may occur. Myxomas of the ventricles may cause obstruction of the ventricular out-flow tract by involving the aortic or pulmonic valves or subvalvular regions. They may also produce emboli.

The diagnosis of myxomas is readily established by echocardiography or angiocardiography, which demonstrates a space-occupying lesion in the involved cardiac chamber. Surgical removal of the myxoma usually results in a complete cure. Early surgical treatment is highly recommended because high morbidity and mortality are expected, especially because of embolization, in untreated patients. The endocardial attachment should be excised because of potential recurrence of myxomas, and a follow-up medical checkup with serial echocardiography is recom-mended after surgery.

Rhabdomyoma

Rhabdomyoma is the most common primary tumor of the heart in children. This tumor is considered a hamartoma (a tumor that originates from normal embryonal elements found in the heart), and the left ventricle is most commonly involved. Multiple nodules occur in the ventricular septum and ventricular wall. Rhabdo-myoma is a benign tumor.

Sarcomas

Sarcomas are the most common primary malignant tumors of the heart, and they involve most frequently the right atrium. Sarcomas often produce obstruction of the inflow into the right atrium from either vena cava. At times, sarcomas may obstruct the right ventricular outflow. The most common clinical findings include various cardiac arrhythmias and severe CHF. Cardiac sarcomas frequently produce metastasis to other organs.

Metastatic (Secondary) Cardiac Tumors

The term *metastatic* or *secondary tumors of the heart* is used when the primary origin of the tumors is elsewhere in the body. Metastatic cardiac tumors occur most commonly (up to 60 percent) in patients with malignant melanoma (a form of skin cancer). In addition, secondary cardiac tumors are found in 37 percent of patients with leukemia and in 25 percent of patients with Hodgkin's disease (a form of cancer involving the lymph nodes and lymphoid tissues). Metastatic tumors of the heart also not uncommonly occur in patients with bronchial carcinoma (a form of lung cancer) and breast cancer. Metastases to the heart from carcinoma of the pancreas, gastrointestinal tract, and kidney may occur only occasionally. The most common clinical manifestations include a variety of cardiac arrhythmias, particularly heart blocks and AF, and hemopericardium.

TRAUMATIC HEART DISEASE

It is unfortunate that trauma is one of the leading causes of death in our society, and cardiac injury is the major cause of death. There has been an increasing incidence of trauma to the heart in recent years, primarily because of the increasing frequency of traffic accidents and social violence. Of course, various forms of injury to the human body, including the heart, may not be avoided during war. Cardiac injury also occurs during various surgical procedures and instrumentations around or in the heart. Traumatic injury to the heart may not be noticed immediately when other organs are more severely damaged, such as occurs in automobile accidents. Therefore, it is very important to consider the possibility of cardiac injury when dealing with any patient with trauma involving various parts of the body. At times, cardiac injury may be diagnosed several hours, days, weeks, or even months after it takes place. The term *traumatic heart disease* is used when the heart is injured in any way, either from a blunt or open trauma.

Blunt (Nonpenetrating) Trauma to the Heart

The most common cause of blunt trauma to the heart is the impact of the chest against an automobile steering wheel in a traffic accident. It is common to observe a variety of serious injuries to the heart even though no wound is visible in the chest. Myocardial contusion is the most common consequence, but any structure of the heart may be damaged. Not uncommonly, one or more heart valves may be damaged by the blunt trauma, causing regurgitation in the heart valve. In addition, abnormal communication may be produced in the atrial or ventricular septum, causing atrial or ventricular septal defect, respectively. Chordae tendineae or papillary muscles (tissue structures supporting the mitral valve) may also be ruptured, and new heart murmur(s) corresponding to the damaged heart valve(s) or septal defect will be observed. Blood vessels in the pericardium or coronary arteries may be injured by the blunt trauma. Hemopericardium is often produced under these circumstances. When coronary arteries are severely damaged, the patient may develop angina pectoris or even a new heart attack. Needless to say, the most serious cardiac injury is a rupture of the atrial or ventricular wall, and it is invariably fatal. A variety of cardiac arrhythmias and various ECG abnormalities may also occur.

When suffering from significant valvular lesion(s) or septal defect resulting from blunt trauma, the patient develops various manifestations of CHF very rapidly.

In this case, an immediate surgical approach has to be undertaken, because the usual medical management has little or no effect. Likewise, surgical treatment has to be provided promptly for hemopericardium or cardiac rupture. One or more anti-arrhythmic agents may be necessary (see Table 6.2) for various cardiac arrhythmias.

Open (Penetrating) Trauma to the Heart

Open injuries to the heart are, of course, much more serious than closed trauma. Gunshot or stab wounds to the heart often result in sudden death, either because of hemopericardium or massive hemorrhage. When the victim is fortunate enough to survive, various structures in the heart are found to be severely damaged, and manifestations of acute CHF and/or cardiogenic shock are usually present. New heart murmur(s) is (are) heard as a result of valve damage or septal defect in the atrial or ventricular level, as seen in patients with blunt cardiac trauma. In addition, all types of cardiac structure damage resulting from blunt trauma to the heart can be expected, but the nature of the damage is, of course, much more serious. Immediate surgical treatment is essential. Bacterial endocarditis may occur when the contaminated wound is not well cleaned and treated.

SYPHILITIC HEART DISEASE

Syphilis (also known as "bad blood") is one of the most common venereal diseases, which occur primarily through sexual intercourse. The disease process involves many organs diffusely, including genital organs, reproductive system, skin, heart, blood vessels, and central nervous system. The primary lesion (called a "chancre") appears on the genital organs soon after sexual intercourse as a result of infection by treponema. Fortunately, the incidence of syphilis has declined in recent years because of a general improvement in the living standard, with better education of the general public in conjunction with the availability of penicillin. The therapeutic result of penicillin therapy is excellent. The most serious manifestations are involvement of the cardiovascular system and central nervous system (e.g., brain), which usually takes place approximately ten to thirty years after the appearance of the primary lesion, chancre. Many patients feel that their syphilis is cured completely when the chancre has healed. After a long latent period, however, cardiovascular and/or neurosyphilis appears. Certain individuals may not develop cardiovascular or neurosyphilis, even when proper treatment is not provided for the chancre. Syphilis involves men about three times more often than women, and cardiovascular syphilis is usually recognized between ages thirty and sixty. Blood tests for syphilis are positive in approximately 85 percent in untreated cases, whereas the fluorescent treponemal antibody absorption test (a more accurate test for syphilis) is positive in nearly 100 percent of cases.

The fundamental lesion of cardiovascular syphilis is aortitis (inflammation of the aorta), and aortic regurgitation occurs in approximately 10 percent of the untreated cases. In addition, syphilis may cause aortic aneurysm and the narrowing of the coronary ostia. In other words, aortic regurgitation, aortic aneurysm, and coronary ostial narrowing are the major complications of syphilitic aortitis. Cardiovascular syphilis commonly affects the ascending aorta, the arch, and the descending aorta, but the abdominal aorta is only rarely involved.

Clinical Manifestations and Diagnosis

Although the incidence of *aortitis* in cases of untreated syphilis has been estimated to be as high as 70 to 80 percent, there are no clinical manifestations as long as no complications develop. Nevertheless, syphilitic aortitis may be strongly suggested when there is dilatation of the ascending aorta, a tambour-quality ringing and accentuated A_2 in the absence of hypertension or atherosclerosis, a soft mid-systolic murmur at the base, retrosternal pain, and dyspnea. An additional finding, such as linear calcification of the ascending aorta, particularly at the root of the aorta and arch, is supportive evidence for the diagnosis. Chest X-ray, fluoroscopy, and echocardiogram will confirm the evidence of aortic root dilatation.

Aortic regurgitation is the most common complication of syphilitic aortitis. Clinical manifestations and various laboratory test results are essentially the same as those for rheumatic aortic regurgitation (see Chapter 11). However, the characteristic feature of aortic regurgitation of syphilitic origin is the absence of co-existing aortic stenosis or mitral valve disease. Saccular aneurysm is associated with aortic regurgitation in about 10 percent of cases. Many patients may be symptom free for many months or years. However, once the patient develops CHF, it soon becomes refractory to conventional medical treatment. Most patients die from severe CHF within two to five years unless surgical replacement of the aortic valve is carried out promptly.

The *aortic aneurysm* develops as a late complication about fifteen to thirty years following the initial infection with syphilis. Incidence of the aortic aneurysm is reported to be approximately a third as high as that of aortic regurgitation due to syphilis. About 50 percent of syphilitic aneurysms occur in the ascending aorta, 30 to 40 percent in the transverse arch, and 15 percent in the descending aorta. The abdominal aorta is involved in less than 5 percent. It is not uncommon to observe multiple aneurysms in the aorta.

Various clinical manifestations are greatly influenced by the location and size of the aneurysm. Symptoms and physical signs are produced by the aneurysm's compression of different organs and adjacent structures. For instance, aneurysm of the ascending aorta often causes compression of the pulmonary artery, the superior vena cava, or the right main bronchus (airway in the right lung), with predictable end results from involvement of each structure. In this circumstance, visible pulsation and dullness over the manubrium (the breastbone) and at the upper sternal border (first to third intercostal spaces), reduced BP in the right arm, and an aortic midsystolic murmur with palpable thrill commonly occur. Aneurysm of the aortic arch often produces cough, dyspnea, dysphagia (difficulty in swallowing), recurrent infection in the lungs, hemoptysis, hoarseness, edema of the face and neck, distended neck veins, and engorgement of veins in the upper chest. In addition, unequal pulses in the arms and unequal pupils in the eyes may occur. In contrast, the patient with aneurysm of the descending aorta is commonly symptom free unless the aneurysm is very large. The large aneurysm of the descending aorta may cause erosion of the ribs or spine, producing pain, which is usually aggravated by lying down. Visible or palpable pulsations are often noted medial to the left scapula. Aneurysm of the abdominal aorta frequently produces a pulsating mass in the upper abdomen with abdominal and back pain.

The most serious consequence of aortic aneurysm is its rupture. In the chest cavity, an aortic aneurysm frequently ruptures into the pericardial cavity, pleural cavity, bronchial tree, and esophagus. Aneurysm of the ascending aorta tends to rupture into the pericardial space or right pleural space, causing hemopericardium or hemothorax (bloody fluid accumulation in the chest cavity). The prognosis for syphilitic aortic aneurysm is grave, and the average life expectancy after the onset of symptoms is usually from a few months to six months. The surgical excision of the aneurysm is the treatment of choice, but symptomatic treatment toward the complications should be carried out even before surgery. Of course, a full course of antisyphilitic therapy with penicillin is mandatory.

The narrowing of the *coronary artery ostia* usually develops gradually and progressively as a complication. When chest pain is produced by syphilitic coronary ostial disease, the clinical finding is indistinguishable from ordinary angina pectoris. The development of a heart attack as a result of syphilitic coronary ostial narrowing is rare. Coronary ostial narrowing is often associated with syphilitic aortic regurgitation. Therefore, the possibility of coronary ostial disease should be raised whenever angina pectoris occurs in patients with syphilitic aortic insufficiency. The prognosis for coronary ostial disease is poor, and sudden death due to VF is not uncommon.

Management and Prognosis

A full course of antisyphilitic treatment with penicillin should be given to all patients with syphilitic cardiovascular diseases, including aortitis, aortic regurgitation, and aortic aneurysm. Conventional treatment for CHF is indicated when these patients develop CHF. For severe aortic regurgitation, a prosthetic valve is needed to replace the damaged aortic valve. The best surgical result can be expected before these individuals develop significant CHF. Surgical repair of an aortic aneurysm may be performed as indicated, but the surgical risk is generally high. For severe and symptomatic coronary ostial narrowing, CABS is indicated. It is extremely important to emphasize that syphilis can easily be prevented when the general public is adequately informed and highly motivated.

The status of the thyroid gland is closely related to cardiac function. Hyperthyroidism (thyrotoxicosis—increased function of the thyroid gland) is frequently associated with a variety of cardiac arrhythmias, particularly AF. In fact, thyrotoxicosis is the most common cause of AF among noncardiac disorders. In addition, cardiomyopathy may be produced by a long-standing hyperthyroidism. Hyperthyroidism should be treated with antithyroid drugs. When a tumor of the thyroid gland is found, it should be removed surgically. Myxedema (hypothyroidism—decreased function of the thyroid gland) commonly causes pericarditis and pericardial effusion. In addition, various cardiac arrhythmias may occur. Thyroid replacement with thyroid hormone is indicated for the treatment of myxedema. Pericardiocentesis may be necessary if the pericardial effusion is pronounced (see Chapter 13).

15

CARDIOPULMONARY RESUSCITATION (CPR)

Cardiopulmonary resuscitation (CPR) may be required when the cardiopulmonary system fails to provide adequate and effective function. CPR is indicated when the heart and/or lungs stop functioning suddenly and unexpectedly. The purpose of CPR is to restore normal functions of the heart and lungs so that the delivery of adequate oxygen to vital organs is reestablished and maintained. Cardiac arrest most commonly occurs during the first few hours of a heart attack. Remember that permanent brain damage is a common end result when CPR is not applied within four minutes, even if cardiac function is restored.

All medical as well as paramedical personnel must be fully capable of performing CPR. In addition, it is highly advisable for the general public to learn the proper technique for CPR because cardiovascular collapse is totally unpredictable. Full understanding of CPR is more urgently needed for family members of heart attack victims because the chance of cardiac patients' developing cardiovascular collapse is much greater than that of healthy individuals. The technique for CPR is relatively easy to learn, and CPR courses are given frequently by the local Heart Association, by many other medical societies, and in adult education programs.

INDICATIONS FOR CPR

CPR should be performed immediately when there is a sudden cessation of effective cardiopulmonary performance. In most medical institutions, particularly in the United States, the term *code blue* is commonly used to designate cardiopulmonary arrest. Cardiopulmonary arrest is usually manifested by (1) loss of consciousness, (2) loss of pulse, (3) loss of respiration, (4) loss of heart tones (sounds), and (5) loss of BP.

On whom should CPR be performed? Obviously, the answer is not a simple one; varying philosophical views may be involved. For example, CPR would seem inappropriate for patients with an incurable or terminal illness, such as terminal cancer, and for elderly patients with irreversible and terminal strokes. Thus, CPR should be aimed primarily at the patient in whom restoration of cardiopulmonary function will result in a potential for continuous productive life.

TEAM AND EQUIPMENT FOR CPR

CPR can be performed by one person, but it is preferable to have a team, especially in the hospital. There must be a standardized and well-organized team for CPR at every medical institution, and the team should be available instantly when cardiovascular collapse occurs. Each member of the team should be clearly aware of his or her assigned duty in the CPR process.

The following organization is recommended for CPR:

1. The senior physician or director of the CPR team assumes overall responsibilities and directs all necessary procedures and drug therapy.
2. The junior physician (or nurse) performs closed-chest cardiac resuscitation (massage) and artificial ventilation (respiration).
3. The junior physician starts the intravenous line for administration of various drugs.
4. The nurse has access to and prepares the required drugs, administers intravenous medications, and monitors heart rhythm and BP.
5. The laboratory technician may be available to perform all necessary laboratory tests ordered by physicians.

Of course, the organized teamwork for CPR is impossible to expect if cardiopulmonary collapse occurs outside a hospital. In this circumstance, whoever is available should initiate the necessary CPR until a more experienced medical or paramedical team arrives on the scene. In the hospital, certain equipment and various drugs (see Tables 6.2, 7.2, and 15.1) are necessary for CPR. For example, a cardioverter for DC shock is the most important equipment for terminating various rapid heart rhythms, particularly VF (Figure 3.5). An artificial cardiac pacemaker should also be available for the treatment of very slow heart rhythms, particularly complete A-V block (see Chapter 16). It is preferable to have equipment for artificial respiration. A tracheal tube (a plastic tube to be inserted in the windpipe) is essential for the establishment of an airway.

TABLE 15.1. Drugs Commonly Used in Cardiopulmonary Resuscitation.

Indication	Drug	Dosage
Asystole	Isoproterenol	200 mg-1000 mg IV or IC infusion of 2-12 mg/min
	Epinephrine	200 mg-1000 mg IV or IC infusion of 2-12 mg/min
	Calcium chloride	10 ml (10% solution) IV to a total of 30 ml
Bradycardia	Atropine	0.3-1.2 mg IV bolus
	Isoproterenol	IV infusion of 2-6 mg/min
Ventricular tachycardia/fibrillation	Lidocaine	50-100 mg bolus to a total of less than or equal to 300 mg
		IV infusion 2-4 mg/min
	Pronestyl	100-mg bolus to a total of less than 1000 mg
		IV infusion of 2-4 mg/min
	Dilantin	100 mg over 5 minutes Repeated to a total of less than 500 mg
	Propranolol	1 mg IV q̄ 5-10 min to a total of 5-10 mg

Reproduced with permission from Chung, E.K.: *Cardiac Emergency Care,* Second Edition, Philadelphia, Lea & Febiger Publishers, 1980.

TECHNIQUES AND INITIAL MEASURES

The purpose of the initial measures in CPR is to initiate and maintain ventilation of the lungs so that adequate amounts of oxygenated blood can be delivered to all organs. Thus, initial measures should include clearing an airway, initiating and maintaining respiration, and restoring blood circulation. A forceful blow should be delivered to the sternum (around the breastbone) with the heel of the hand, and it may be repeated once or twice if there is no response. A direct blow to the sternum can terminate VF and may restore normal heart rhythm. If the maneuver is not successful, however, one should immediately proceed to the next step.

The patient should be placed in a supine position. Place one hand behind the patient's neck and the other hand on the forehead (Figure 15.1). When the head is

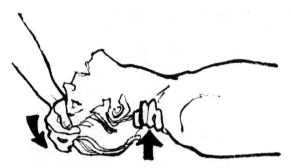

FIGURE 15.1. Head-tilt method of opening the airway. (Reproduced with permission from the *Journal of the American Medical Association* and the American Heart Association.)

tilted back, this maneuver lifts the tongue from the back of the throat so that the patient's airway will be fully open. During this maneuver, any obvious foreign body in the mouth and airway should be removed. In many patients, this maneuver alone may be adequate to restore breathing and to implement recovery from cardiopulmonary arrest.

Mouth-to-Mouth Resuscitation

While maintaining the backward tilt of the patient's head with one hand, pinch the nostrils closed with the other hand. Then, place the mouth over the patient's mouth, completely sealing it so that there is no leak of air (Figure 15.2). At the end of inspiration (breathing in), one should exhale (blow out) a larger than normal breath into the patient's mouth. If the technique is correct, a rise should be noted in the patient's chest. There should be no loss of air through the nose or mouth as

FIGURE 15.2. Mouth-to-mouth resuscitation. (Reproduced with permission from the *Journal of the American Medical Association* and the American Heart Association.)

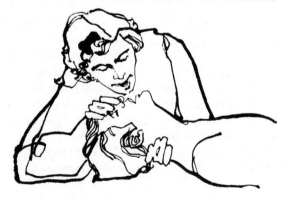

the lungs inflate. After inflation of the lungs, one should remove the mouth from the patient's mouth, allowing the patient's lungs to deflate. Air should be heard escaping from the lungs during that period.

Mouth-to-Nose Resuscitation

The principle of mouth-to-nose resuscitation is essentially the same as that of mouth-to-mouth resuscitation. In this technique, while maintaining the backward tilt with one hand, one should close the patient's jaw and seal the patient's mouth with the other hand. Then place the mouth over the patient's nose; after inhaling deeply, exhale into the patient's nose. Artificial respiration should be performed at a rate of twelve breaths per minute.

Problems with Artificial Respiration

If there is resistance to inflation of the lungs, a foreign body should be suspected in the airway. One should roll the patient onto his or her side and deliver a firm blow between the shoulder blades in order to dislodge the foreign body (e.g., a piece of meat). The patient's mouth and airway should then be explored for the foreign body. Another maneuver that has recently been popularized for the removal of a foreign body is the *Heimlich maneuver.* The Heimlich maneuver can be performed when the patient is either upright or supine. When the patient is upright, grasp him or her from behind, below the rib cage, with your fist against the patient's abdomen (Figure 15.3). If the patient is supine, place your hands, one on top of the other, on the patient's abdomen, between the rib cage and the navel (Figure 15.4). In both maneuvers, the hands are thrust quickly inward, against the patient's abdomen. The thrust increases the pressure within the large airway, and thus forces out the foreign body. As can be expected, vomiting may occur during CPR. Suction equipment should be available for that purpose. Gastric (stomach) distension is best handled by inserting an indwelling nasogastric tube (a kind of soft plastic or rubber tube). Recurrence of gastric distension may be prevented by intermittent epigastric pressure (pressure on the upper abdomen).

Closed-Chest Cardiac Massage

The next step in the initial resuscitative measures is the application of cardiac massage. Closed-chest cardiac massage is recommended in practically all clinical circumstances except when the patient is already in the operating room or when chest wounds preclude open-chest massage.

As far as technique is concerned, the patient's back must be placed on a firm surface. When the patient is on a soft surface such as a bed, a hard board should be placed under the patient's back. While standing alongside the patient, place the heel of one hand over the lower third of the patient's sternum. Only the heel of the

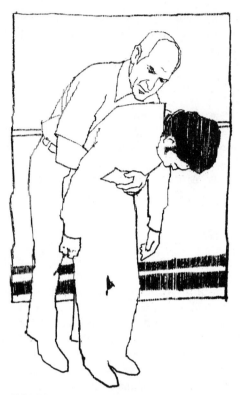

FIGURE 15.3. Heimlich maneuver (standing position). (Reproduced with permission from Henry J. Heimlich, M.D., and the *Journal of the American Medical Association* 234:398, 1975.)

hand should be in touch with the patient's chest. The other hand may rest on the first hand (Figure 15.5). The patient's chest should be depressed 1.5 to 2 in., and the pressure should be smooth and uninterrupted. Following compression, release the sternum, and ready the hand for the next compression. The duration of chest compression should be similar to that of relaxation. The chest compression should be about sixty times per minute, and it should be coordinated with artificial respiration. If only one operator is present, it is recommended that fifteen chest compressions be performed, followed by two quick artificial respirations. When two or more resuscitators are available, every fifth chest compression should be followed by a lung ventilation. In order to assess the efficacy of closed-chest cardiac massage, peripheral pulses (e.g., pulses on the neck or groin arteries) should be palpated periodically. When an indwelling arterial line (a small plastic tube) is placed in the artery, the contour of the pressure pulse obtained will be of value in assessing the efficiency of cardiac massage.

Although closed-chest cardiac massage is a safe procedure, one must not be

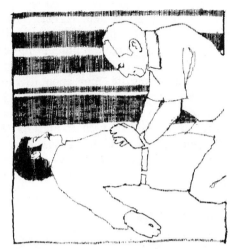

FIGURE 15.4. Heimlich maneuver (suspine position). (Reproduced with permission from Henry J. Heimlich, M.D., and the *Journal of the American Medical Association* 234:398, 1975.)

FIGURE 15.5. Two-rescuer cardiopulmonary resuscitation (CPR) consisting of artificial respiration and closed-chest cardiac massage. (Reproduced with permission from the *Journal of the American Medical Association* and the American Heart Association.)

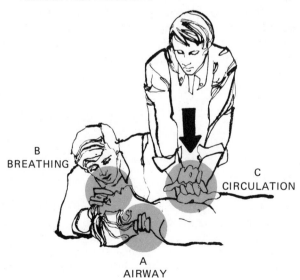

B
BREATHING

C
CIRCULATION

A
AIRWAY

overly vigorous in chest compression, particularly in children. Various complications may include fractures of the ribs and sternum, hemothorax, hemopericardium, pneumothorax (collapse of the lungs), bone marrow emboli, rupture of the stomach, lacerations of the liver and spleen, and rupture of the aorta. These complications usually occur primarily because of inappropriate application of cardiac massage. Various types of mechanical devices (some manual and some automatic) are available for closed-chest cardiac massage. In the hands of trained persons, these devices make cardiac massage easier and facilitate resuscitative efforts. However, these mechanical devices should never be used by inexperienced persons. Misapplication of these devices may result not only in ineffective resuscitation but also in further injury to the patient.

Evaluation of the Efficacy of the Initial Measures

During the initial measures of CPR, one must check for several signs that indicate the success or failure of the resuscitative efforts. Important signs include pulses in the femoral or carotid arteries, heart tones, spontaneous respiratory efforts, and palpable or recordable BP. Of course, one should also be alert to any change in the patient's neurologic status and in the status of consciousness.

When there is any evidence that resuscitative efforts have been successful, one may stop and observe the patient for several seconds. If the cardiovascular collapse is over, the patient should continue to be observed very closely, and the cause of the collapse should be investigated by a physician. When resuscitative efforts have been successful outside the hospital setting, the patient should be transported promptly to a nearby ER by ambulance or similar vehicle equipped with cardiovascular emergency equipment and a continuous monitoring system (see Chapter 3). If, however, there is no change in the patient's status, artificial respiration and cardiac massage must be continued. CPR should not be stopped for longer than five seconds. It is difficult to indicate when to stop CPR because many medicolegal as well as philosophical factors are involved.

SECONDARY MEASURES

In the hospital, if there is no response to the initial measures, a physician must act as follows while CPR is continued.

1. Quickly review the patient's chart to extract any pertinent information.
2. Obtain an ECG to assess the cardiac rhythm and to evaluate any abnormal finding such as recent heart attack, pulmonary embolism, and so forth.
3. Obtain an arterial blood gas analysis (e.g., the value of oxygen and CO_2 in the blood) to assess the acid-base balance and the adequacy of artificial respiration.

4. Obtain a blood sample for the determination of serum electrolytes (e.g., potassium, sodium, calcium, and chloride).
5. Establish an intravenous infusion site if one is not already available.

When these steps have been taken, further emergency treatment should be administered as indicated. For various cardiac arrhythmias, proper medication, DC shock, and artificial pacemakers may be required (see Chapters 16 to 18). Medications commonly used in CPR are summarized in Table 15.1.

TERMINATION OF CPR

There are two major reasons to terminate CPR. The first reason is failure to restore an appropriate rhythm and adequate pumping action in the heart. The second reason is evidence of severe and irreversible brain damage. Otherwise, CPR should be continued. Determination of the severity of brain damage is often difficult even for experienced physicians, and it can have medicolegal ramifications. By and large, severe brain damage is suggested by unconsciousness, lack of spontaneous movement, lack of spontaneous respiration, dilatation of pupils without response to light. For lay people, it is wise to continue CPR until medical personnel determine whether it should be continued or not.

CARE AFTER CPR

Following successful CPR, assessment of the underlying cause of the cardiopulmonary collapse is essential. Thus, every individual who has recovered from cardiopulmonary arrest must be closely observed and treated in the CCU for at least several days. When there is any abnormal heart rhythm, it should be treated with appropriate medications, DC shock, and artificial pacemaker (see Chapters 16 to 18). Likewise, underlying heart diseases (e.g., heart attack) should be treated accordingly. A careful and complete assessment of the degree of recovery should be part of post-CPR care. Particular attention should be directed to the patient's neurologic status (degree of brain damage). If there is any evidence of significant brain damage, a neurologic consultation is required. As a rule, all patients who have recovered from cardiopulmonary collapse by CPR should be observed for several weeks (at least two to three days in the CCU) to ensure their stability. During the observation period, emergency resuscitative facilities should be immediately available because cardiopulmonary collapse may recur, particularly in patients who have had a heart attack.

16

ARTIFICIAL CARDIAC PACEMAKERS

Artificial cardiac pacing is one of the most important and reliable ways to manage various cardiac arrhythmias, particularly slow heart rhythms. Until several years ago, the primary use for permanent artificial pacing was the treatment of complete A-V block (Figure 3.6), but the most common use at present is to treat sick sinus syndrome (SSS) (Figure 3.7). In addition, artificial pacing with overdriving rate (faster than usual pacing rate) is often a life-saving measure for refractory tachy-arrhythmias.

The artificial cardiac pacemaker functions in a manner very similar to that of the natural pacemaker; it initiates the electrical impulses generated by small batteries. The electrical impulses travel through small wires to the heart. The artificial pace-maker is timed to produce the electrical impulses (usually 70 to 72 beats/min.) just like the cardiac impulses initiated by the natural pacemaker (sinus node). In most cases, the heart is capable of pumping adequate amounts of blood under the control of an artificial pacemaker.

Approximately 250,000 people live with artificial cardiac pacemakers in the United States alone, and 25,000 to 40,000 (100,000 to 110,000, according to some reports) new patients will require artificial pacemaker implantation annually. Al-though it is difficult to know exactly how many people live with an artificial pace-maker, it is estimated to be at least 500,000 people worldwise. The total number of artificial pacemakers sold within the last twenty years is estimated to be approxi-mately 1.5 to 2 million. It is evident that artificial pacing can provide not only the prolongation of human lives but also significant improvement in the quality of life. Long-term administration of various drugs for slow heart rhythms is no longer necessary because of the availability of artificial pacemakers in most industrialized countries.

The fundamental principles for the utilization of an artificial pacemaker were established as early as 1932, and external cardiac pacing was introduced into clinical medicine in 1952. In 1957, temporary direct myocardial stimulation in the treatment of complete A-V block was introduced, and a transistorized, self-contained, implantable pacemaker for long-term correction of complete A-V block was established in 1960.

The average cost of the artificial pacemaker itself ranges from $2,000 to $3,000. The total cost for the implantation of a pacemaker, including the surgeon's fee, hospitalization, and various laboratory tests, is about $6,000 to $7,000 in most hospitals.

TYPES OF ARTIFICIAL PACEMAKERS AND ENERGY SOURCES

There are many types of artificial pacemakers manufactured by many different companies, but the most commonly used model is a demand ventricular pacemaker. The electrical circuit of this demand pacemaker senses the natural heartbeats. It shuts off the artificial pacemaker automatically when the natural heart rhythm is faster than the preset pacing rate (usually 70 to 72 beats/min.) and turns the artificial pacemaker on again when the natural heart rhythm becomes slower than the preset pacing rate. In this type of pacemaker, the tip of the wire is situated in the apex of the right ventricular cavity (Figure 3.8). Another kind of artificial pacemaker that used to be very popular until a decade ago is a fixed-rate pacemaker that produces constant electrical impulses at the preset rate. The most commonly used site for implantation of the pulse generator of the pacemaker is the right upper chest beneath the skin (Figure 3.8). Therefore, minor surgery is necessary for pacemaker implantation. The average size of the pulse generator (about 10 mm thick and 50 mm high) is comparable to that of a pocket watch (Figure 3.10), and it weighs around 45 g. In addition, the heart may be stimulated at various locations including the atria or coronary sinus (near the A-V junction). Although atrial or coronary sinus pacing is more physiologic (an effect similar to the natural normal heart rhythm), ventricular pacing provides adequate stimulation to the heart for sufficient blood circulation. Thus, in most clinical circumstances, a ventricular demand pacemaker is recommended. The proper selection of a specific type of artificial pacemaker will be made by an attending physician or surgeon according to clinical circumstances.

A newer pacemaker is a multiprogrammable pacemaker in which various pacemaker functions (e.g., pacing rate, energy output, sensitivity, refractory period) can be controlled and adjusted noninvasively after implantation. By adjusting these parameters, the pacemaker functions most suitably for a given patient and clinical conditions can be provided precisely. Even in the same patient, various pacemaker functions have to be changed from time to time in order to provide the best cardiac function. For example, a faster-than-usual pacemaker rate is often necessary for patients with SSS. Conversely, many patients with angina pectoris need a pacing rate slower than usual. Remember that clinical conditions may change from time to time even in the same patient, and various complications may occur at any time among cardiac patients.

The battery energy for various types of pacemakers today is a lithium source that replaced the old energy source—a mercury-zinc battery. Nuclear-powered pacemakers are also available for clinical medicine, but their use is not as popular as expected. The main reason for this is that there is no significant superiority in the nuclear pacemaker compared to the lithium energy source in terms of longevity, in addition to the various expected problems related to nuclear energy. It has been shown that a lithium battery lasts anywhere between ten and twelve years. The nuclear-powered pacemaker may last up to twenty years.

INDICATIONS (WHO NEEDS A PACEMAKER?)

Artificial pacemakers may be used only temporarily, but they are often implanted permanently. The former is termed "temporary or short-term artificial pacing," whereas the latter is termed "permanent or long-term artificial pacing." Temporary pacing is indicated when it is required for only a few days to a week (at times, two to three weeks) for transient bradyarrhythmias. In addition, temporary pacing is necessary for a few hours or days when a cardiac surgeon is not immediately available for permanent pacemaker implantation. Furthermore, a temporary pacemaker may be used as a prophylactic measure when a slow heart rhythm, particularly complete A-V block, is anticipated, especially in patients with recent heart attack. Customarily, a temporary artificial pacemaker is inserted by a cardiologist, but it may be inserted by a cardiac surgeon. A permanent artificial pacemaker is implanted by a cardiac surgeon under general anesthesia, and the surgical risk is very minimal. Indications for temporary as well as permanent pacing may vary slightly between medical institutions, and the specific indication for a given patient will be determined by the attending physician according to clinical circumstances. By and large, any symptomatic (e.g., syncope or near-syncope) slow heart rhythm (most commonly, SSS and complete A-V block) usually requires artificial pacing. Occasionally, an artificial pacemaker with an overdriving pacing rate is indicated for recurrent tachyarrhythmias refractory to conventional therapy (medications and/or DC shock).

During the insertion of a temporary pacemaker or implantation of a permanent pacemaker, the danger of provoking VF is always present; therefore, a cardioverter (DC shock) must be immediately available. In addition, various commonly used antiarrhythmic drugs (see Table 6.2) and drugs necessary for CPR (see Table 15.1) should be available. Common complications associated with artificial pacing are discussed next.

Malfunctioning Artificial Pacemakers

The malfunction of a pacemaker may be manifested by acceleration of pacing rate ("runaway pacemaker"), slowing of pacing rate, irregular pacing, and failure of cardiac capture and/or sensing (see Figure 16.1). The runaway pacemaker is a very rare complication in the demand pacemaker, but it is not uncommon in the fixed-rate pacemaker. An extremely rapid runaway pacemaker may produce a pacing rate faster than 1,000 beats/min. Fortunately, not every pacing stimulus is able to activate the heart in this circumstance, so that a very rapid heart rate usually does not occur. Slowing of the pacing rate develops progressively as a manifestation of malfunction in most modern pacemakers. Thus, far-advanced cases of malfunction are rather unusual today when there is adequate and periodic follow-up care. Failure of the cardiac capture and/or sensing by an artificial pacemaker may be

FIGURE 16.1. Artificial pacemaker malfunctions. A: Acceleration of the pacing rate ("runaway pacemaker"). B: Irregular and slow pacing. C: Failure of sensing and cardiac capture (arrows indicate P waves of sinus origin).

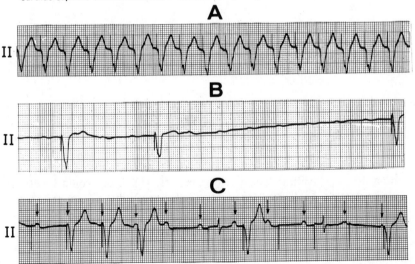

associated with acceleration or slowing of the pacing rate. Likewise, irregular pacing may be associated with the aforementioned other manifestations.

It should be noted that a failure of cardiac capture by an artificial pacemaker (a condition in which the artificial pacemaker stimuli fail to activate the heart) may be due to hyperkalemia (increased potassium content in the body), quinidine (or procainamide), edema, or fibrosis around the pacemaker electrode and advancement of underlying heart disease even when the pacemaker itself is in perfectly good condition.

Perforation of the Ventricles

Perforation of the heart, particularly the ventricles, may occur when a transvenous pacemaker catheter electrode is used, especially by an inexperienced physician. Perforation of the ventricles may be suspected when the following findings occur unexpectedly:

1. RBBB (Figure 9.9)
2. Recurrent contractions of the diaphragm
3. Pericarditis or pericardial effusion (see Chapter 13)
4. A pansystolic murmur due to rupture of the ventricular septum (see Chapter 8)

Other Findings

Other complications may include (1) electrode fracture, (2) infection, (3) thrombosis or embolism, (4) knotting of the pacemaker wire, and (5) various cardiac arrhythmias.

INTERFERENCE WITH ARTIFICIAL PACEMAKER FUNCTION

Function of the newer models is seldom interfered with by any electromagnetic source because of improved biomedical engineering. However, various interferences may occur when dealing with artificial pacemakers manufactured five to ten years ago.

The interference may be due to (1) electric shavers, (2) automobile motors, (3) motorcycles, (4) malfunctioning television sets, (5) direct contact with an ungrounded electrical appliance, (6) indirectly by proximity to equipment producing strong and rapidly fluctuating electromagnetic fields, (7) electric motors fitted with brushes and commutators, (8) a muscle stimulator for home use, (9) motor-operated beds, (10) electrosurgical and physical therapy equipment, and (11) DC shock.

It should be emphasized that commonly used weapon detectors in airports usually do not interfere with pacemaker function. Likewise, it is perfectly safe to ride commercial airplanes, trains, buses, and ships after pacemaker implantation.

FOLLOW-UP PACEMAKER CARE

Just like any other mechanical or electronic device or piece of equipment, the artificial pacemaker needs constant care. As described previously, complications and malfunctions may occur, although they are rare. The lithium battery that supplies the energy, like any other kind of battery, will wear out over a period of time and must be replaced. As the battery wears down, the pacemaker often slows down or fails to stimulate the heart, but it will *not* stop suddenly. When the pacing rate slows down, the physician or surgeon should be notified immediately. When the pacemaker or its battery needs replacement, a minor surgical procedure is required, but most newer pacemakers usually last ten to twelve years. The recommended aftercare of patients with artificial pacemakers is briefly described here.

What Does the Patient Have to Do?

Patients with a permanent pacemaker should check their pulse once or twice daily to be certain that the pacemaker's preset rate remains constant. When the patient's heart action entirely depends on the artificial pacemaker (called a "pacemaker-dependent patient"), the pacing rate should remain the same as the preset pacing rate (usually 70 to 72 beats/min.). However, most patients may have their own natural heartbeats from time to time, so that the actual heart (pulse) rate is often slightly different from the preset pacing rate. Therefore, the occasional occurrence of a slight irregularity of pulses (heartbeats) or a slightly faster-than-usual pulse (heart) rate is a perfectly normal finding after pacemaker implantation. When the pulse (heart) rate slows down, especially below 40 to 50 beats/min., the physician must be notified at once because the finding may indicate malfunction. Remember that the number of pulse beats per minute is the same as the number of times the heart beats. The best way to check pulse beats is to place the fingertips on a point at the inside of the wrist (radial pulse). The pulse beats should be counted for one full minute. If the patient is unable to count the pulse beats, someone else (e.g., a family member) should do it. When the pulse (heart) rate speeds up and remains fast (especially faster than 100 beats/min.), the physician should also be notified. Likewise, the physician should be notified when any new symptoms or signs (e.g., chest pain, dizziness, syncope, near-syncope, shortness of breath, wound infection, swelling of legs or ankles) occur.

Many patients require various medications (see Chapter 17) even after permanent pacemaker implantation. Thus, it is very important to continue to take prescribed medications. Remember that an artificial pacemaker regulates only the electrical activity of the heart; it by no means cures the underlying heart disease. It is important to remember that it takes about eight weeks for an artificial pacemaker to settle firmly in place. Therefore, sudden, jerky, or violent actions that may pull the arm away from the body should be avoided during the first eight weeks after pacemaker implantation. It is also advisable to avoid long reaches, especially over the head, if the pacemaker wires are through the veins (transvenous pacemaker). In addition, excessive pressure over the area of the pacemaker pulse generator should be avoided. It is perfectly safe to engage in ordinary daily activities, including taking showers or baths and engaging in sexual activity, after pacemaker implantation. The artificial pacemaker is completely protected against contact with water. Trips by automobile, airplane, bus, or train are perfectly safe. Remember again that the artificial pacemaker does *not* cure the underlying heart disease. Thus, excessive activity beyond the patient's physical limitations should be avoided. The physician should be consulted when the individual would like to engage in any extraordinary physical activity.

Every patient should carry an identification card at all times that contains the pertinent information about artificial pacemaker implantation. In case of an accident or unexpected hospitalization, this card will provide very important information to medical personnel. The identification card is also useful when traveling by air. Most airports now use antihijack devices that will detect the metal used in the artificial pacemaker. Needless to say, one can avoid the unnecessary inconvenience of being called back if the identification card is shown to airline personnel. It is essential to have periodic medical checkups following pacemaker implantation indefinitely (discussed shortly).

What Does the Physician Have to Do?

The patient should be fully instructed regarding usual daily care, including common signs of complications and malfunction, following pacemaker implantation and before discharge. The patient should be given an *identification card* indicating: (1) name, age, and sex of the patient; (2) date of pacemaker implantation; (3) names of the surgeon who performed the implantation and the physician who will follow up on pacemaker care after discharge; (4) name of the institution where the implantation was performed; (5) type, model, and serial number of the pacemaker and the manufacturer's name; and (6) a medical summary, including medications (optional).

Today, most pacemaker manufacturers provide the identification card coated with a plastic cover that is convenient for the patient to carry.

The *usual follow-up care* after pacemaker implantation is as follows: (1) *first visit* (one month after discharge): (a) check surgical wound; (b) detect any evidence of malfunction or complication; and (c) ask the usual pulse rate and whether there is any complaint, such as chest pain or syncopal episodes; (2) *routine visit* (every three to six months): (a) perform such procedures as ECG analysis; (b) if a sophisticated pacemaker follow-up device is available, various pacemaker functions will be assessed; (3) elective hospitalization if necessary for replacement of the pulse generator or battery; and (4) emergency hospitalization for replacement of a malfunctioning pacemaker.

Pacemaker follow-up procedures for each visit include the following: (1) Complete checkup of the patient's cardiac status and of the pacemaker implantation site and pacemaker functions. (2) Long ECG rhythm strips to check the pacing rate and to compare with the preset pacing rate. (3) A 12-lead ECG (at least once or twice a year) to detect any unsuspected or new ECG abnormality. (4) When the patient's own natural rhythm returns from time to time (a rather common occurrence) following implantation of a demand pacemaker, certain maneuvers, such as reducing the patient's own natural heart rate by carotid sinus stimulation (massage of the side of the neck) or by edrophonium chloride (Tensilon) injection, or by accelerating the pacing rate with an induction coil (magnet), should enable one to check the function of the pacemaker. Of course, various pacemaker functions can easily be assessed when a specially designed device is available. (5) Ask about any unusual or new complaints, such as chest pain or fainting episodes. (6) Arrange elective or emergency hospitalization as needed.

In addition to ECG analysis, *chest (sometimes abdomen) X-ray films* are taken following pacemaker implantation as follows: (1) before discharge; (2) six to nine months after discharge; (3) yearly thereafter; and (4) immediate radiographs when malfunction is suspected. In addition, check the position of the pulse generator and lead (wire) system (malposition, twisting, angulation, rotation of electrode or pulse generator should be checked); and check the state of the battery in order to detect any early sign of malfunction.

In the past five to ten years, many medical institutions have set up *artificial pacemaker follow-up clinics* to examine all patients with permanent pacemakers. A sophisticated device for follow-up care is available at these pacemaker clinics so that various pacemaker functions can be evaluated precisely. In addition, there are pacemaker follow-up laboratories (not affiliated with medical institutions) at various locations throughout industrialized countries. These commercial laboratories can provide similar pacemaker follow-up care, but all patients with pacemakers *must* be seen by their physician periodically. Furthermore, *transtelephonic pacemaker follow-up care* (evaluation of pacemaker functions utilizing a specially designed device by long-distance telephone) is also available in certain areas.

17

MEDICATIONS
FOR HEART DISEASES

Most drugs have two names: a generic or chemical name and a brand or trade name. Many drugs are manufactured by several different pharmaceutical companies; therefore, a particular drug may appear in stores under several different brand names even though it has only one chemical name. It is extremely important that people take only those medications prescribed specifically for them. No one should try any drug prescribed for someone else even if that individual seems to have a very similar, if not identical, heart condition.

Two or more different medications may be prescribed in combination, and frequent adjustments in the dosage of each drug may be necessary. When two or more drugs are given together, the actions of each drug may be increased or decreased. Periodic blood tests are required in order to maintain an ideal therapeutic blood level of certain drugs. For instance, the determination of the prothrombin time (the degree of coagulability—stickiness) is essential when anticoagulants are prescribed. Thus, it is mandatory to be examined by a physician periodically during long-term drug therapy. Some drugs are given by intravenous or intramuscular injection, but most drugs for long-term therapy are taken by mouth. In life-threatening conditions (e.g., cardiac arrest), however, certain drugs (e.g., epinephrine, isoproterenol) can be applied directly into the heart.

Although it is not always possible, every patient should preferably remember the names and dosages of medications he or she is taking. Remember that most drugs have various actions—some desired, some undesired. The undesired actions are called side effects, or adverse effects, and serious side effects are often manifestations of toxicity (poisoning). It is important to emphasize that serious side effects or toxicity may occur even with a very small dosage when an individual has an unusual or very sensitive reaction to a drug. In serious cases, sudden death may occur in this circumstance. The best example of this is "penicillin shock" (death or near-death following administration of penicillin). This type of drug reaction is a severe form of allergy. When any unusual or allergic drug reaction is present, this fact should be clearly and precisely indicated on the identification card. This identification card should be carried by the patient at all times so that physicians and other medical personnel may be informed immediately when any drug therapy becomes necessary. Of course, serious side effects or toxic reactions often occur when large amounts of any drug are taken. When these side effects are serious enough to disturb the patient's health or life-style, the medication has to be discontinued. Needless to say, the physician must be informed when a side effect occurs so that proper medical advice can be provided. It is foolish to discontinue any medication or to change the dosage without consulting the physician. A feeling of well-being by no means indicates that the prescribed drug is no longer necessary. In fact, many cardiac patients may maintain ideal health in this circumstance simply because of various actions of the drugs. It can be said unequivocally that no cardiac drug is safe unless constant medical advice is provided. Taking heart medications without a physician's guidance is extremely dangerous, and even death may occur in severe cases.

DIGITALIS ("HEART PILLS")

Digitalis is one of the oldest and most commonly used drugs today; it is better known as "heart pills." Digitalis is extracted from the foxglove plant, and the drug is primarily used to increase the pumping action of the heart. Thus, digitalis is an essential medication in the treatment of CHF. In addition, digitalis is also very useful in reducing the heart rate or terminating rapid heart actions, particularly AF.

Digitalis is the generic name of the foxglove plant. Therefore, all drugs extracted from the foxglove plant are commonly referred to as "digitalis." Today, the most commonly used digitalis preparation is called "digoxin" (Lanoxin), whereas a less commonly used digitalis is "digitoxin." Digitalis is also available as a liquid suitable for intravenous or intramuscular injection and for oral use by children. When the clinical situation is very urgent, digitalis (in liquid form) is administered by intravenous injection. Digoxin is available in a liquid form and in tablets. In addition, the manufacturer produces digoxin tablets in different strengths (dosages). For instance, a white digoxin tablet contains 0.25 mg, whereas a yellow tablet contains 0.125 mg. A green digoxin tablet that contains 0.5 mg is also available. Remember that too much digitalis is much more serious than too little digitalis, because the drug produces significant side effects and even death when the patient develops digitalis toxicity (see Table 17.1). The usual maintenance dosage of digoxin is 0.25 mg daily. Common methods of digitalization are shown in Table 6.1. Some individuals may require a very small amount of digitalis, while others may need a larger than usual dosage. Therefore, the required dosage varies considerably among people. It should be stressed that digitalis is no longer beneficial to the patient when digitalis intoxication (poisoning) is produced (see Table 17.1).

DIURETICS

Diuretics have been discussed fully in Chapter 6.

ANTIARRHYTHMIC AGENTS

A variety of heart diseases is frequently associated with cardiac arrhythmias. This is particularly true in patients with recent heart attack. On the other hand, various arrhythmias may also occur in apparently healthy individuals. Depending upon the

TABLE 17.1. Manifestations of Digitalis Intoxication.

Symptoms	Common	Uncommon
Gastrointestinal	Anorexia, nausea, vomiting	Abdominal pain, constipation, diarrhea, hemorrhage
Cardiac	Worsening of congestive heart failure, ventricular premature contraction, paroxysmal atrial tachycardia with block, nonparoxysmal AV junctional tachycardia, AV block, sinus bradycardia	Atrial fibrillation, atrial flutter, ventricular tachycardia, ventricular flutter, sinus arrest, SA block, atrial premature contraction, AV junctional premature contraction
Visual	Color vision (green or yellow) with halos	Blurring or shimmering vision, scotoma, micropsia or macropsia, amblyopia
Neurologic	Fatigue, headache, insomnia, malaise, confusion, vertigo, depression	Neuralgia, convulsions, paresthesia, delirium, psychosis
Nonspecific	— —	Allergic reaction, idiosyncrasy, thrombocytopenia, gynecomastia

Reproduced from Chung, E.K.: *Cardiac Emergency Care,* Second Edition, Philadelphia, Lea & Febiger, 1980.

type of cardiac arrhythmia as well as clinical circumstances, the therapeutic approach varies considerably. By and large, no active treatment is necessary for occasional extra heartbeats or any transient arrhythmia, especially in healthy people. On the other hand, immediate application of a defibrillator (DC shock) is a life-saving measure for VF (see Figure 3.5).

When any clinically significant arrhythmia occurs, one or more antiarrhythmic agents (drugs that regulate heartbeats) are indicated. Selection of a specific anti-arrhythmic agent will be determined by the physician, depending on the type of arrhythmia and clinical circumstances. Certain drugs (e.g., lidocaine) are only given by intravenous injection or infusion, whereas others (e.g., quinidine, procainamide, propranolol) may be available in intravenous liquid form as well as oral tablets. Many patients with heart disease have to take one or more antiarrhythmic medications for months, years, or even indefinitely.

The most commonly used intravenous antiarrhythmic agent in the treatment of ventricular tachycardia (see Figure 9.4) is lidocaine (Xylocaine). For long-term oral antiarrhythmic therapy for a variety of abnormal heart rhythms, quinidine is most commonly used. Common antiarrhythmic agents are summarized in Table 6.2. It may be necessary to determine the blood level of the antiarrhythmic agent from time to time for the best therapeutic approach and for the prevention of possible toxicity. It should be remembered that every antiarrhythmic agent may cause a variety of side effects and toxicity (see Table 6.2). In addition, some individuals may be unusually sensitive to a certain medication. Therefore, every patient must be followed by a physician very closely during antiarrhythmic drug therapy.

ANTIANGINAL DRUGS

Some drugs possess the capability of reducing the work load imposed on the heart, leading to improvement of symptoms in patients with angina pectoris. These medications are called "antianginal drugs." The work load the heart must perform can be reduced in several ways, including lowering the BP, slowing the heart rate, and reducing the resistance the blood vessels offer to blood circulation. The most commonly used antianginal drug is nitroglycerin (NG), which has been fully discussed in Chapter 3.

The most commonly used oral antianginal drug is propranolol (Inderal), which is available in tablets of varying doses. Inderal may be taken in a dosage of 10 to 40 mg, three to four times daily by mouth, with or without the intermittent use of sublingual NG (0.3 to 0.4 mg). In advanced cases, much larger amounts (60 to 80 mg, three to four times daily) of Inderal may be needed under close medical supervision. The proper dosage of Inderal has to be determined by a physician according to therapeutic results and the severity of angina pectoris. Of course, CABS should be seriously considered when the patient requires large amounts of Inderal and/or frequent usage of NG. Propranolol is also an extremely valuable drug in treating many other cardiovascular disorders, including hypertension, a variety of cardiac arrhythmias, and IHSS (see Chapter 12). Other antianginal drugs include various forms of nitrates, such as Isordil, Sorbitrate, and Cardilate; these medications can be used in conjunction with sublingual NG and/or oral propranolol.

All of the aforementioned antianginal drugs may cause side effects. Headache is the most common complaint immediately following sublingual administration of NG, and dizziness is not uncommon. Similar side effects are observed when oral nitrates are used. Propranolol often causes significant slowing of the heart rate and shortness of breath. Propranolol may predispose to CHF when cardiac function is already considerably deteriorated. Hypotension may also occur in some patients when an antianginal drug is used. Propranolol should not be used in patients with slow heart rate, CHF, or bronchial asthma.

When angina pectoris is clearly due to coronary artery spasm (narrowing of the coronary artery resulting from spasm), NG may be injected into the coronary artery itself, especially during coronary arteriography or during a provocative test (e.g., using ergonovine maleate). Intracoronary injection of NG is often effective. In addition, various calcium antagonists, such as nifedipine, diltiazem, and verapamil, are effective to prevent and treat chest pain due to coronary artery spasm (some of these agents are still investigative drugs).

VASODILATORS

Vasodilators are medications that have the capability of dilating blood vessels. Vasodilator therapy in the treatment of CHF is actually an extension of conventional drug therapy, which primarily consists of digitalization and diuretic therapy. Vasodilators provide a very important therapeutic approach to both acute and chronic CHF. This is particularly true when CHF does not respond satisfactorily to conventional treatment. Vasodilators improve heart function by increasing cardiac output and/or diminishing venous return, reducing congestion in the lungs, and lowering oxygen requirements of the heart muscle. Vasodilator therapy is often ideal for CHF due to coronary artery disease, because these agents reduce oxygen demand and improve blood circulation.

Commonly used vasodilators include nitroprusside (Nipride), phentolamine (Regitine), hydralazine, prazosin (Minipress), isosorbide dinitrate, NG, and pentaerythritol tetranitrate. Some vasodilating agents such as Nipride and Regitine are administered by intravenous infusion, while others such as Minipress are given by mouth. Certain agents like isosorbide dinitrate are available in oral, sublingual, and chewable tablets. Intravenous infusion of vasodilators (e.g., Nipride) is a very rapid and effective way of attaining clinical improvement, but it is essential to have continuous invasive monitoring of pressures in the various heart chambers and measurement of cardiac output. Selection of a specific vasodilating agent and a route of administration will be made by a physician according to clinical circumstances.

ANTIHYPERTENSIVE DRUGS

Antihypertensive drugs were discussed fully in Chapter 5.

ANTICOAGULANTS (BLOOD-THINNING DRUGS)

Although there is a significant controversy among physicians regarding the use of anticoagulants, some doctors use various drugs in different cardiovascular disorders. Common indications for blood thinners include thromboembolic phenomena in various organs (e.g., pulmonary embolism). Anticoagulants have the capability of reducing the coagulability of blood (clotting). The beneficial effects of blood thinners have to be weighed against the complications, particularly bleeding episodes.

There are different types of anticoagulants—some for intravenous injection, and others for oral use. When a rapid blood-thinning effect is desired, such as in the early stages of heart attack or pulmonary embolism, heparin is administered intravenously. In general, intravenous heparin is given for three to ten days and is followed by oral warfarin (e.g., Coumadin or Dicumerol) for weeks to months. The exact dosage and duration of anticoagulant therapy will be determined by a physician depending upon blood test results (e.g., prothrombin time) and clinical circumstances. It is very important to have frequent blood tests to monitor the ideal therapeutic blood level. Of course, every patient has to be closely observed by a physician during anticoagulant therapy. When the prothrombin time and the required daily dosage of Coumadin or Dicumerol become stable during long-term anticoagulant therapy, the blood test may be performed every four to six weeks under a physician's close medical guidance.

When excessive amounts of anticoagulants are administered, there will be bleeding from various organs and tissues. The most common bleeding sites are in the mouth around the gums while brushing the teeth and in the urine, causing hematuria. Therefore, the physician has to be notified at once when any evidence of bleeding is discovered by the patient or a family member during long-term anticoagulant therapy. Aspirin and/or dipyridamole (Persantine) are mild blood thinners. Any type of anticoagulant is, of course, contraindicated when there is any bleeding disorder or peptic ulcer.

MEDICATIONS FOR SHOCK AND CARDIAC ARREST

Treatment for cardiogenic shock and cardiac arrest has been fully discussed in Chapters 7 and 15. Medications commonly used for shock and cardiac arrest are summarized in Tables 7.2 and 15.1.

BLOOD LIPID-LOWERING MEDICATIONS

Medications commonly used to reduce blood fat contents include clofibrate (Atromid-S) and cholestyramine (Questran). Stomach discomfort and indigestion are the most common side effects of these drugs, and a variety of cardiac arrhythmias may also be produced.

MEDICATIONS TO REDUCE MYOCARDIAL INFARCTION (HEART ATTACK) SIZE

There has been much talk and literature in recent years regarding limiting MI size, but overall success is less than impressive. Nevertheless, a number of different medications have been shown effective in reducing the size of the damaged heart muscle secondary to heart attack when the drugs are given soon after the onset of MI.

The most effective medications in reducing infarction size are beta-blocking agents. Propranolol (Inderal) is administered intravenously in a dosage of 0.1 mg/kg, divided into three equal doses at five-minute intervals under careful monitoring. The intravenous administration of Inderal is followed one hour later by oral doses of 20 to 80 mg, every six hours. Other commonly used agents are nitrates. NG can be given by intravenous infusion (10 μg/min. with stepwise increases of 10 μg/min.) or sublingually (0.3 to 0.6 mg). In addition, various agents, including hyaluronidase, glucose-insulin-potassium solution, and corticosteroids, have been tried with varying degrees of success. Furthermore, intraaortic balloon counterpulsation and reperfusion (e.g., CABS) have also been tried. Further experience and investigations are required in order to evaluate the true efficacy of these therapeutic approaches in reducing MI size.

ANTIPLATELET DRUGS

Recent medical studies have shown that some medications may interfere with platelet aggregation and consequently may influence blood clotting so that heart attack may be prevented. Platelet-inhibiting agents include aspirin, beta-blocking

284

agents (e.g., propranolol), clofibrate (Atromid-S), dipyridamole (Persantin), and sulfinpyrazone (Anturane).

Favorable, but not conclusive, investigative results using a combined therapy of aspirin and Persantin have been briefly described in Chapter 3. Recently, an even more striking therapeutic achievement with Anturane has been reported. Sulfinpyrazone (Anturane), which has been known as a drug to treat gout, is reported effective to prevent sudden death in the early high-risk period (the first seven months after a heart attack). The efficacy of Anturane (200 mg, four times daily) for the prevention of cardiac deaths was studied in 1,558 patients with previous heart attacks for a twenty-four-month period. In this investigation, a 32 percent reduction of cardiac mortality with a 43 percent reduction of sudden death was most impressive. The mechanism of Anturane in preventing sudden death among heart attack victims seems due to a suppression of fatal ventricular arrhythmias (e.g., VF) rahter than—as in the original hypothesis—to preventing platelet-mediated phenomena. Unfortunately, Anturane was not effective in protecting against new heart attack. At any rate, Anturane seems to be the most effective agent in preventing sudden death in the first two to seven months after a heart attack. This drug is still an investigative agent (other than in its usage for gout) that requires further evaluation for a definitive conclusion.

18

ELECTRIC-SHOCK TREATMENT FOR ABNORMAL HEART RHYTHMS

It has been well documented that an electric shock causes momentary depolarization (activation) of the majority of heart muscle fibers, thereby terminating various tachyarrhythmias and allowing the sinus node to be reestablished as the primary pacemaker. Today, such electric-shock treatment is recognized as the best therapeutic approach to a variety of serious tachyarrhythmias, particularly VF (Figure 3.5).

Alternating current was used until two or three decades ago, but at present, only DC shock is used because of its many superior features. The first successful defibrillation in humans was performed in 1947. Today, the efficacy of electric-shock treatment for a variety of tachyarrhythmias has been well estabished. DC shock equipment is readily available at every medical institution throughout the world. In addition, portable DC shock equipment is also available in most ambulances and all mobile CCUs. Valuable contributions by Lown and his co-workers have been well recognized, and some DC shock equipment is named after him—called the "Lown Cardioverter." In general, DC shock equipment is often called the "cardioverter," the "defibrillator," the "DC defibrillator" or the "DC cardioverter," interchangeably.

It has been shown that about 90 percent of the cases of AF (Figure 9.2) are successfully converted to sinus rhythm, whereas 95 to 97 percent of cases of ventricular tachycardia (Figure 9.4) can be terminated by DC shock. It has also been shown that ninety out of hundred patients with AF refractory to large doses of quinidine could be converted to sinus rhythm by DC shock. Without a doubt, electric cardioversion has been found to be much safer and more effective than various antiarrhythmic drugs. For successful cardioversion, it is very important to apply the procedure properly, and all possible contraindications should be eliminated. It should be emphasized that DC shock may not only be ineffective for digitalis-induced arrhythmias but also may be fatal, since VF or standstill (arrest) may be induced by electric shock. Thus, when treating digitalis-induced arrhythmias, DC shock may be attempted only as a last resort, after all other available measures have been exhausted.

There has been a remarkable new development by a team of doctors and scientists at Johns Hopkins University in Baltimore, and favorable therapeutic achievements have been demonstrated after in-depth experimental studies in the past twelve years. The new electronic device—called a "minidefibrillator" or "automatic implantable defibrillator"—is implanted under the skin of the abdomen and attached to the heart by two electrodes—one through the veins to the right atrium and the other to the apex (tip) of the right ventricle. This minidefibrillator senses the onset of VF (Figure 3.5) and automatically delivers the electric shock (700 volts) to the heart to terminate the arrhythmia and restore sinus rhythm. The size of the new device is comparable to that of a cigarette pack, and it weighs about 250 g (9 oz). The electric shock can be delivered in 15 to 20 seconds after the initiation of VF, and a conscious patient feels a sharp tingling sensation from the shock. When VF persists and normal heart rhythm is not restored by the first electric shock, this minidefibrillator commands up to three more shocks. The device has a capacity of delivering as many as one hundred electric shocks during the three-year life of its lithium batteries. The expected cost of this minidefibrillator is approximately $5,000. The way the automatic minidefibrillator works is somewhat comparable to how an artificial cardiac pacemaker works. If this new electronic device is found to be effective and safe, and if it becomes available in clinical practice, many cardiac patients, particularly those recovered from heart attack(s), can have protection against VF outside the hospital so that sudden death may be prevented.

TECHNICAL CONSIDERATIONS, PREPARATIONS, AND PRECAUTIONS

Maintenance care is necessary to be certain that DC shock equipment is in good working condition. In general, the electrical integrity of the equipment should be checked every month by biomedical engineering personnel. Paddles must be large enough to stimulate most of the heart muscle fibers simultaneously. Otherwise, small paddles may deliver high electric-current density in a localized pathway, causing heart muscle damage. For external DC shock, anterior and posterior paddles are ideal, but two anterior paddles are an alternative. Anterior and posterior paddles are preferable because the patient lies on the flat posterior paddle and only the anterior one needs to be held by the operator (a physician or nurse). This method is an important safety measure, particularly with equipment in which one paddle is grounded. The anterior-posterior paddle position is said to lower the amount of electrical energy necessary for electric-shock treatment considerably in comparison to using two anterior paddles.

As a rule, food should be withheld for at least several hours before applying DC shock (except for emergency treatment) in order to avoid vomiting. Induced transient amnesia (loss of memory) is necessary during application of DC shock (except for emergency treatment), and the amnesia can easily be produced by intravenous injection of diazepam (Valium) in a dosage of 5 to 10 mg. General anesthesia or premedication is unnecesary. The duration of action of Valium is only 3 to 4 min., and additional doses may be given, if necessary, within a few minutes after the first injection. The treatment room where DC shock will be applied should be fully equipped for continuous cardiac monitoring (e.g., heart rhythm) and full CPR facilities, including all cardiac emergency medications and an artificial cardiac pacemaker. Recording of specific ECG leads should be possible, as needed, before, during, and after electric-shock treatment. Before DC shock treatment, a short heart rhythm strip (lead V_1 or II) should be recorded in order to confirm the underlying heart rhythm, so that it will be obvious when normal heart rhythm is restored after electric-shock treatment. Paste (ECG paste is commonly used) should be applied liberally to the patient and rubbed well into the skin to reduce electrical resistance. It should be certain that no part of the patient's skin is in direct contact with the metal of the trolley or the bed on which he or she is lying. No one should touch the patient, the bed, or any equipment to which the patient is attached at the moment of applying DC shock.

Amounts of electrical energy required for DC shock vary considerably depending upon the type and nature of the arrhythmia and clinical circumstances. By and large, a very small amount of energy (5 to 10 wsec. [watt seconds]) is necessary when treating atrial flutter (see Figure 9.2). For treatment of AF, slightly larger amounts of energy (50 to 100 wsec.) may be needed. When dealing with a life-threatening arrhythmia, such as VF (see Figure 3.5) 200 to 400 wsec. should be applied. When the first shock is ineffective, additional shocks with progressively larger amounts of energy may be applied once or twice consecutively, if necessary. The exact amounts of energy discharged will be determined by a physician according to clinical circumstances. Because of the danger of provoking serious cardiac arrhythmias with DC shock in patients who are taking digitalis, smaller than usual energy should be delivered. DC shock should be avoided if possible when an individual is taking digitalis.

For elective cardioversion, all types of digitalis preparations should be withheld for at least twenty-four to forty-eight hours before electric-shock treatment. If the shock treatment cannot be postponed in patients who are taking digitalis, 100 to 250 mg of diphenylhydantoin (Dilantin) should be given by intravenous injection before DC shock. Alternatively, 50 to 75 mg of lidocaine (Xylocaine) or 50 to 100 mg procainamide (Pronestyl) may be injected intravenously in place of Dilantin. These medications may reduce the incidence of serious arrhythmias considerably in this circumstance.

Since the incidence of thromboembolic phenomena is relatively high in certain high-risk groups, anticoagulants may be beneficial before and after DC shock. Anticoagulant therapy is highly recommended for patients with recent heart attack, cardiomyopathies, RHD, artificial heart valves, a previous history of thromboembolic phenomena and for elderly people. Many physicians recommend anticoagulant therapy at least a few days to one week before DC shock and three to four weeks after shock treatment under these circumstances. The true efficacy of the routine use of anticoagulant therapy for DC shock treatment is not certain. After the termination of tachyarrhythmia by DC shock, the 12-lead ECG should be recorded. The ECG should be monitored at least for the next twenty-four hours. In addition, BP should be measured every half hour until it becomes stable and reaches the control value before shock treatment. A chest X-ray film may be taken within twenty-four hours to exclude the possibility of pulmonary edema, especially when a high-energy-level shock is applied. Even when normal heart rhythm is restored by DC shock, various medications may be needed thereafter.

EMERGENCY SHOCK TREATMENT

Emergency shock treatment is indicated for the termination of acute tachyarrhythmias, particularly life-threatening ventricular tachycardia or VF (Figures 3.5 and 9.4). The term *code blue* is commonly used to designate cardiopulmonary arrest, in which VF is the most common underlying rhythm disorder. Immediate application of DC shock is the only reliable life-saving measure in the treatment of VF. When the clinical circumstance is extremely urgent, premedication for transient amnesia is not needed. Thus, 100 to 200 wsec. of DC shock can be applied directly. If the arrhythmia persists, DC shock with increased energy (200 to 400 wsec.) should be applied immediately. Of course, all necessary CPR measures should be provided if indicated. On the other hand, if the clinical situation is not extremely urgent, small amounts (5 to 10 mg) of Valium may be injected intravenously in order to induce a transient amnesia immediately before the application of DC shock.

ELECTIVE CARDIOVERSION

The term *elective cardioversion* is used when electric-shock treatment is applied as an elective procedure to terminate chronic tachyarrhythmias, particularly AF (see Figure 9.2). Elective cardioversion is indicated when a restoration of sinus rhythm is considered definitely beneficial to the patient. By and large, a restoration of sinus rhythm after termination of tachyarrhythmias is considered to be beneficial for most patients for the following reasons: (1) an improvement of CHF and an increase in exercise tolerance are expected during sinus rhythm because of an increment in cardiac output; (2) it is easier to control and maintain the ideal heart rate during sinus rhythm; and (3) the incidence of thromboembolic phenomena is reduced during sinus rhythm.

CONTRAINDICATIONS OR NONINDICATIONS FOR ELECTRIC-SHOCK TREATMENT

One of the most important aspects in considering the indications for electric-shock treatment is the probability of restoration of normal heart rhythm and its maintenance for a reasonable period of time. In general, a heart that is difficult to convert to sinus rhythm is also difficult to maintain in sinus rhythm.

In the following clinical situations, electric-shock treatment is either contraindicated or not indicated:

1. Digitalis toxicity and/or hypokalemia (low potassium ion content in the body)
2. Severe mitral regurgitation and/or marked enlargement of left atrium
3. AF or flutter with advanced or complete A-V block causing a slow heart rhythm
4. Chronic AF with duration of five years or longer
5. Immediately before valvular surgery
6. Recurrence of AF or flutter during adequate digitalis and quinidine therapy
7. SSS (Figure 3.7)

A final decision as to the indications versus the contraindications for electric-shock treatment will be made by a physician according to the clinical circumstance and the type and nature of a given cardiac arrhythmia.

COMPLICATIONS OF ELECTRIC-SHOCK TREATMENT

Various complications can be reduced to minimum or even avoided in most instances when the patient is properly selected and the procedure properly applied. In general, complications are directly related to technical errors during the procedure, severity of atrial damage, and improper use or overdose of antiarrhythmic drugs. A major technical error is failure to synchronize the electrical discharge with the R-wave (tip) of the QRS complex. Excessive energy setting may cause serious cardiac arrhythmias.

Various complications related to the use of electric-shock treatment are summarized as follows:

1. DC shock may unmask digitalis-induced arrhythmias (see Chapter 17), and the procedure may cause VF or cardiac arrest in some cases, especially in patients with advanced heart disease.
2. Serious ventricular arrhythmias may be provoked when a high energy setting is used.
3. Slow and unstable heart rhythm may follow DC shock because preexisting complete A-V block or SSS may be unmasked by the procedure.
4. DC cardioversion may induce new atrial tachyarrhythmias (e.g., AF), but cardioversion-induced atrial tachyarrhythmias can be terminated by an additional DC shock in most cases.
5. The occurrence of thromboembolic phenomena, particularly strokes in elderly individuals or patients with a previous history of thromoembolic phenomena, within twenty-four to forty-eight hours following DC shock is not uncommon.
6. Repeated DC shocks or high-energy electric discharge may cause damage to the heart muscle.
7. Superficial burns of the skin under the paddle may be induced by repetitive applications of DC shock, especially when jelly (paste) is not sufficiently applied.
8. Electric shock with a high energy setting may cause malfunction of the artificial pacemaker in certain models (see Chapter 16).

FOLLOW-UP CARE AFTER ELECTRIC-SHOCK TREATMENT

Digitalis and one or more antiarrhythmic medications (see Table 6.2) are often necessary in many patients with chronic cardiac arrhythmias, even after restoration of sinus rhythm by DC shock, in order to prevent a recurrence of the arrhythmia. When ventricular tachycardia or VF is terminated by DC shock, intravenous infusion of lidocaine (Xylocaine) is indicated for twenty-four to forty-eight hours (a few days to a week in some cases) in order to prevent these tachyarrhythmias. One or more oral antiarrhythmic agents may be required thereafter for weeks, months, years, or even indefinitely when the danger of recurrence of these ventricular arrhythmias is great. An artificial cardiac pacemaker is indicated when a slow and unstable heart rhythm occurs after termination of any rapid heart rhythm. Appropriate antiarrhythmic drugs (see Table 6.2) are, of course, indicated when any new cardiac arrhythmia is provoked by DC shock. Some high-risk individuals may require anticoagulant therapy for weeks or months after the termination of cardiac arrhythmias by DC shock. While electric cardioversion is highly successful, at least momentarily, the number of patients who remain in sinus rhythm is disappointingly small, particularly when AF is treated. In addition, any type of cardiac arrhythmia has a tendency to recur after the termination by DC shock. Therefore, it is extremely important for every patient to have periodic medical checkups, especially during antiarrhythmic drug therapy and/or anticoagulant therapy.

19

DIET AND THE HEART

There are many millions of people, especially in the United States, who are trying to stay on some form of diet program. Many people are diet conscious without considering their actual purpose. In addition, some slender and even underweight individuals, especially young females, try to lose weight because they misjudge that they are overweight. In fact, some extreme cases may refuse to eat any type of food because they are afraid of gaining weight. In this circumstance, severe malnutrition with extreme emaciation will be the end result, and the condition may become so serious as to cause death. This life-threatening and self-abusing physical and emotional illness is called "anorexia nervosa"; it must be treated vigorously in a hospital under the care of a good medical-psychiatric team.

It is rather hazardous to try to stay on any form of restricted diet program without proper medical guidance. When unbalanced diets are eaten, various forms of malnutrition and vitamin deficiencies may be produced needlessly. Therefore, it is essential to receive proper instruction regarding any form of restricted diet program from a physician, and the purpose of the special diet should be clearly understood. The risk-benefit ratio of a special diet program should be carefully evaluated by the physician.

There is no single diet program that is suitable for everyone. Thus, it is best to prescribe a specific diet for a special medical reason. This should be done by a qualified dietitian under a physician's guidance. Nevertheless, there are many standardized diet programs designed for different clinical circumstances. Commonly used diet programs may include "low-fat (low-cholesterol) diets" (see Table 3.3), "mild sodium-restricted diets" (1,800 calories), and low-calorie diets (see Tables 3.9 and 19.1). Of course, patients with diabetes mellitus must use the "diabetic diet" (see Table 3.10). For all individuals with hypertension and/or CHF, daily salt intake must be reduced considerably. Overeating is by all means detrimental to health for all cardiac patients and individuals with known risk factors.

On the other hand, there is no point in perfectly healthy, slender, and physically active individuals without any known risk factors staying on special restricted diet programs. However, it should be stressed that a self-determined "perfectly healthy condition" should be thoroughly evaluated beforehand by a physician. This evaluation should include all necessary tests (e.g., exercise ECG testing, blood tests to determine cholesterol and triglycerides).

SATURATED VS. UNSATURATED FATS

There are three different types of fats: saturated fats, polyunsaturated fats, and monounsaturated fats. Saturated fats are closely related to the development of atherosclerosis, which frequently leads to heart attack and stroke. Saturated versus unsaturated fats were fully discussed in Chapter 3.

CHOLESTEROL AND TRIGLYCERIDES

Cholesterol and triglycerides are normally found in the blood. When the blood content of these fats (lipids) is increased, the risk of heart attack and stroke increases considerably. The relationship between these fats and the development of heart attack was fully discussed in Chapter 3.

Most of the fats in the blood are combined with proteins—called "lipoproteins." The lipoproteins are classified into two types—low-density and high-density. It has been shown that individuals whose blood contains a higher percentage of high-density lipoprotein molecules have less chance of developing atherosclerosis and heart attack than those with a greater percentage of low-density lipoprotein molecules.

In many individuals, both cholesterol and triglyceride levels are elevated in the blood. In many others, the blood contents of cholesterol may be elevated while those of triglycerides may be normal, or vice versa. In the medical literature, hyperlipemia or hyperlipidemia (elevated fat or lipid contents in the blood) is classified into five types. In type I hyperlipidemia or hyperlipemia, cholesterol is only slightly elevated whereas triglyceride is markedly elevated. In type II, cholesterol is increased but triglyceride is normal. In type III, both cholesterol and triglyceride levels are elevated. In type IV, cholesterol may be normal, but the triglyceride level

TABLE 19.1. Low-Calorie Diets.

	800 kcal	1000 kcal	1200 kcal	1500 kcal
Milk (nonfat, skimmed, or buttermilk)	2 cups	2 cups	2 cups	2 cups
Eggs, any way but fried	One	One	One	One
Breads, enriched or whole grain*	½ slice	1 slice	2 slices	3 slices
Meat, fish, or poultry, any way but fried**	4 oz.	5 oz.	6 oz.	6 oz.
Fats and oils, butter, margarine, mayonnaise, or oil	None	3 tsp.	5 tsp.	6 tsp.
Vegetables, raw (salads) (1 serving = ½ cup)	2 servings	2 servings	2 servings	2 servings
Vegetables, cooked green, yellow, or soup (1 serving = ½ cup)	2 servings	2 servings	3 servings	3 servings
Starch, potato, etc.	None	None	None	1 serving
Fruit, unsugared (½ cup)	3 servings	3 servings	3 servings	3 servings
Artificial sweeteners	As desired	As desired	As desired	As desired

*May substitute ½ cup cooked cereal or 1 cup dry prepared cereal for 1 slice bread.
**May substitute ½ cup cottage cheese or 3 slices (3 oz.) cheddar cheese for 3 oz. meat.

is increased. In type V, the triglyceride level is markedly elevated, but the cholesterol level may be elevated in varying degrees. Type II and IV hyperlipidemia (hyperlipemia) is common in our practice, whereas types I, III, and V are relatively uncommon. The functions of these lipids were discussed in Chapter 3.

The blood lipid levels should be checked once a year unless the values are extremely high. Detailed descriptions of the method of determining blood lipid levels are found in Chapter 3. Individuals who have normal blood lipid levels should try hard to maintain their desirable body weights (see Table 3.4) by eating sensible diets and with regular physical exercise in order to maintain their normal blood lipid levels. When blood lipids are found to be elevated, caloric intake and consumption of animal fats should definitely be reduced.

DIET PROGRAMS

There is no single diet program suitable for every patient's needs. By and large, cardiac patients have to restrict the intake of salt and animal fats (saturated fats), with reduced caloric intake. A similar diet program is recommended for all individuals with known risk factors (see Table 3.1).

Normal Diet

The three major energy sources in foods are fats, carbohydrates, and protein. The most common carbohydrates are sugars and starches, whereas proteins yield energy and contain nitrogen, which is indispensable for life. Fats provide energy and are the most concentrated source of calories. In addition, alcohol also provides calories. Minerals and vitamins are contained in foods in small amounts, and they are essential to maintain normal body function. In healthy individuals with a stable body weight, caloric intake should be the same as caloric expenditure. For example, the caloric requirements in a 70-kg man engaged in moderate activity are about 2,500 to 2,800 cal/day. In the average American diet, 15 percent of these calories are derived from protein, 45 to 50 percent in the form of carbohydrates, and the remaining 35 to 40 percent from fat. Of course, physically active individuals require many calories (as much as 3,500 to even 6,000 cal/day) to meet the body's demands.

Low-Cholesterol and Low-Fat Diet

A low-cholesterol and low-fat diet is essential for all patients with CAD and individuals with obestiy and/or elevated lipid contents in the blood. As a rule, the intake of food containing large quantities of saturated fats and cholesterol should be minimized or avoided (see Table 3.2). For example, the intake of egg yolks, well-marbled beef or pork, bacon, ham, lamb, cream, and milk products with a large butterfat content, such as butter and cheese should be reduced. In addition, the intake of shellfish (lobster, oyster, shrimp) should also be significantly reduced. Furthermore, overeating is undoubtedly detrimental because it hastens the development of coronary atherosclerosis, especially when the individual is physically inactive and/or obese. Since most foods in the United State and many European countries have a high content of saturated fats and cholesterol, with many calories, the diet factor considerably influences the high incidence of heart attack, even in young individuals. In place of these Western diets containing large quantities of animal fats, a variety of Asian foods, containing large amounts of vegetables, carbohydrates, and fish, are highly recommended for all cardiac patients.

Various organ meats such as brain, heart, kidney, and liver, are high in cholesterol. These meats, therefore, should be avoided as much as possible. In addition, solid vegetable shortenings should not be used because hydrogenation elevates the saturation of fats. Instead, polyunsaturated fats (a fat of vegetable origin, such as margarine) should be used. All cardiac patients should limit meats of four-legged animals whenever possible, and they should eat more fish and poultry (without skin) for protein intake. Since marbled beef contains fat diffusely throughout the meat, the fat cannot be removed. This is why marbled beef or pork is bad for cardiac patients. Whenever possible, visible fat should be trimmed from the meat before cooking and eating, and the skin should be removed from poultry. In order to eliminate animal fats, soup should be kept in the refrigerator to cool off, and hardened fats (animal fats) floating on top of the soup should be removed before eating. Skim milk is always preferable to ordinary homogenized milk.

As far as methods of cooking are concerned, barbecuing and broiling are highly effective in reducing the fat from meat, fish, or poultry. The animal fat will drain from roasted or baked meat, and it can be discarded. In addition, the remaining fat can easily be removed from the meat later, when it has hardened through refrigeration. Regarding salad dressings, lemon or vinegar dressing is a good choice. Salad dressings such as Italian, French, or oil and vinegar are also acceptable, providing vegetable oil (e.g., corn oil) has been used in the dressing. Cardiac patients should avoid cream cheese, sour cream, or whipped cream. A commonly used low-cholesterol and low-saturated-fat diet is summarized in Table 3.3, whereas cholesterol contents of common foods are listed in Table 3.2. Many other special diet programs for cardiac patients can be obtained from the local Heart Association, a local Medical Society, or the dietary department of most hospitals.

The value of a low-cholesterol and low-fat diet for healthy individuals without any known risk factors as a preventive measure is not certain. The risk-benefit ratio should be carefully weighed. A physician should be consulted if a healthy individual is interested in any special diet as a preventive measure. In addition, there is no clear evidence that lowering the blood cholesterol level of individuals over the age of 65 will reduce their risk of having a heart attack or a stroke. Therefore, it is *not* justified to prescribe a low-cholesterol and low-fat diet for elderly people.

Low-Salt Diet

An average American diet contains about 10 g of sodium chloride per day, and many individuals eat foods containing more sodium than they need. Sodium chloride is the chemical name for table salt, which is 40 percent sodium. In many Asian countries, soy sauce is commonly used for cooking a variety of foods or making pickles, and it is often added after the food is served. The soy sauce contains a large quantity of salt. The excessive sodium is excreted in the urine in healthy individuals as long as the kidneys and other organs function normally. Thus, there is no harmful effect of extra sodium content in foods for healthy people. However, excessive sodium is unquestionably harmful to cardiac patients with CHF and/or hypertension. In certain individuals, a large intake of sodium may elevate BP, whereas reducing the amount of sodium in the diet of individuals with hypertension may help to lower the BP, as well as to increase the efficacy of anti-hypertension medications. In fact, the mild restriction of salt intake alone is often effective to lower the BP to a normal level in patients with mild to moderate hypertension. For obese and hypertensive people, weight reduction by means of low caloric intake is, of course, a very important therapeutic approach.

Remember that abnormal kidney functions caused by CHF lead to sodium and water retention in the body, edema, congestion in various organs, increased venous pressure, and weight gain. In this circumstance, the amount of sodium and water retention due to CHF can be reduced considerably simply by decreasing the intake of salt. Of course, various diuretics will be effective to reduce or prevent sodium and water retention in patients with CHF. A low-sodium diet with diuretic drug therapy may be used simultaneously in advanced CHF. By and large, rigid restriction of sodium is not necessary for patients with mild CHF, primarily because a diet in which salt is markedly restricted is quite an unpleasant experience for most individuals. Fortunately, rigid restriction of sodium intake may not be necessary in many patients because of the availability of effective oral diuretics. Nevertheless, it is wise for all cardiac patients with CHF to avoid obviously salty foods (e.g., bacon, ham), and they should not add salt after food is served. These measures can reduce daily salt intake by as much as 5 g. It is rather foolish to add salt to food without tasting it, although some people have this bad habit. It should be stressed that many restaurants in the United States prepare various foods that are obviously salty. This is particularly so of soup served in low- to middle-class restaurants. Remember also that some foods and liquids that do not taste salty may contain large amounts of sodium. For convenience, many cardiac patients prefer to take oral diuretics rather than eating a diet with a rigid restriction on sodium.

When CHF is not well controlled with a slight restriction on salt intake and/or oral diuretic therapy, however, more rigid restriction of sodium is required. For most cases of advanced CHF in this circumstance, only a mild restriction (2 to 4 g of sodium chloride/day) of salt intake is indicated. Thus, a mild sodium-restricted diet with 1,800 cal (see Table 3.9) is the most commonly used diet program for patients with CHF. When CHF is not controlled with the aforementioned measures, a stricter low-salt diet containing only 0.5 to 1 g sodium has to be prescribed. Needless to say, these low-salt diets with a rigid restriction on sodium result in food that most people cannot tolerate for a long period of time. Careful and skillful preparation of low-salt diets, assisted by a qualified dietitian, is essential in making the food palatable and nutritious. It is very important to recognize the patient's preference for certain specific substances of low-salt food and his or her intolerance or dislike of certain other items. This is especially true when dealing with elderly people and individuals with long-standing heart disease. In order to prevent nutritional and vitamin deficiency, supplementary multi-vitamins or vitamin B complex should be given to individuals with poor appetite and poor food intake, especially the elderly. The degree of salt restriction in the diet will be determined by a physician according to the severity of CHF and/or hypertension and the response to treatment provided. Salt substitutes are available for those who are unable to eat a very restricted low-salt diet, but they are not very popular. Most of these salt substitutes contain potassium, which may cause adverse effects in some cardiac patients with CHF.

Low-Caloric Diet (Weight-Reducing Diet)

For obese people, weight reduction is definitely the first and most important step in preventing a variety of serious complications, including heart attack and/or stroke. Desirable body weights according to height and body frame are summarized in Table 3.4, but most people should know whether they are overweight or not. Simple weight reduction alone is often effective in controlling high BP and diabetes. It is necessary to reduce the intake of foods to below caloric requirements. The intake of 500 kcal/day less than the required calories is often sufficient to lose weight—as much as 0.5 kg/week. Caloric requirements vary considerably depending upon various factors, including the age, degree of physical activity, occupation, the character of the individual, and the urgency of the need for weight reduction. A physician will determine precisely a daily caloric intake for a patient according to the clinical picture, but low-calorie diets with 800 to 1,500 kcal will be satisfactory in most clinical circumstances (see Table 19.1). Remember that the caloric requirements of a healthy 70-kg man engaged in moderate activity range from 2,500 to 2,800 cal per day. Supplementary vitamins are highly recommended for patients on low-calorie diets of less than 1,200 kcal.

It is essential that all patients who engage in low-calorie diet programs be closely supervised by a physician, and a periodic medical checkup is mandatory. Going on a low-calorie diet without medical supervision is rather dangerous. Complications such as weakness, postural hypotension (reduction of BP upon standing or sitting), ulcerative colitis (inflammation and ulceration of the large intestines), nutritional and vitamin deficiency, and mental depression may occur, especially during rapid weight reduction. A physician should be consulted immediately when any complication is observed.

Diet with Water Restriction

In general, it is not necessary to restrict the water intake of most patients with CHF. Thus, there is no problem in ingesting water, as much as 2 to 3 liters/day. When the patient suffers from severe and far-advanced CHF, however, the fluid intake may be reduced to 500 to 1,000 ml/day. In addition, frequently small feedings are recommended in order to prevent fatigue and shortness of breath in this circumstance.

Diabetic Diet

The diabetic diet will be discussed briefly here, because many cardiac patients have diabetes mellitus (commonly called "sugar diabetes"), and because diabetes is one of the common risk factors for premature atherosclerosis and heart attack. A proper diabetic diet stablizes body weight at ideal or near-ideal levels, minimizes hyperglycemia (excessive sugar in the blood and body), and protects against hypoglycemia (insufficient sugar in the blood and body) in diabetic patients requiring insulin injections. Thus, an appropriate diet program is the first and most important step in therapy for diabetes mellitus. Recently, diabetic diet programs have been altered somewhat by lowering saturated fat intake with a concomitant increase in polyunsaturated fat content in order to delay or prevent the development of atherosclerosis. The proper diabetic diet program has to be designed for the individual by a dietitian and prescribed by a physician.

At first, the optimal caloric requirement has to be determined. Basal metabolic requirements are about 22 kcal/kg/day, and rough estimates of additional caloric requirements for sedentary, moderately active, and very active individuals will be 30, 50, and 100 percent of the basal metabolic requirements, respectively. When the diet program is designed for weight gain or weight reduction, a proper caloric adjustment has to be made accordingly. In fact, a low-calorie diabetic diet of varying degrees is commonly designed because 60 percent or more of diabetic patients (especially adult-onset diabetics) are overweight. Conversely, a high-calorie diabetic diet is required for thin, wasted, insulin-dependent diabetic patients, particularly children. The minimal protein requirement for adequate nutrition is approximately 0.9 g/kg/day, whereas the recommended carbohydrate content of the diabetic diet is 40 to 50 percent of total calories. The remaining calories are derived from fat. The degree of dietary restriction varies considerably depending upon the severity of the diabetes and the degree of overweight or underweight. For instance, a simple caloric restriction is often sufficient for asymptomatic and obese diabetic patients. On the other hand, most symptomatic patients with advanced diabetes mellitus must stay on a stricter diet program. These individuals must be fully familiar with the diabetic diet with the exchange list technique.

Fundamentally, the caloric requirements and the desired distribution of fat, carbohydrate, and protein should be determined first. The *exchange lists* are groups of measured foods of the same caloric value that can be substituted in a detailed diabetic meal plan. Foods are divided into six groups or exchanges. For instance, various vegetables are listed in one group, whereas fats are listed in another. Various foods in any one group can be substituted or exchanged for other foods in the same group because of their equal caloric value.

The six major exchange lists are as follows:

List 1: Milk exchanges (including nonfat, lowfat, and whole milk)

List 2: Vegetable exchanges (including all vegetables except starchy vegetables)

List 3: Fruit exchanges (including all fruits and fruit juices)

List 4: Bread exchanges (including bread, cereal, pasta, starchy vegetables, and prepared foods)

List 5: Meat exchanges (including lean meat, medium-fat meat, high-fat meat, and other protein-rich products)

List 6: Fat exchanges (including polyunsaturated, saturated, and monounsaturated fats)

In each group of the exchange lists, an exchange is approximatly the same in terms of its calories and amounts of carbohydrates, proteins, and fat. Each exchange also contains similar amounts of minerals and vitamins. Since the foods of each exchange provide a special nutritional value, no one exchange group can supply all the nutrients necessary for a well-balanced diet. It is essential to combine all six listings in order to supply adequate nutritional needs. A diabetic diet with an appropriate caloric requirement can be specifically designed for an individual by a qualified dietitian under the supervision of a physician. A recommended diabetic diet (1,800 cal) is described in detail in Table 3.10.

It is important to remember that so-called diabetic food available on the market does not necessarily mean that the food is prepared for diabetic patients. Remember also that a label advertising "diabetic food" does not mean that the food can be eaten in unlimited amounts. A dietitian or physician should be consulted before eating any foods labeled "sugar-free" or "fat-free" in the supermarket.

Liquid Protein Diet

There have been numerous medical reports of sudden death associated with the use of extremely low-calorie protein diets, particularly those based on liquid protein products. Most deaths have been considered to be due to serious ventricular arrhythmias, particularly VF. In a recent medical report, all victims were obese women, ranging in age from twenty-five to fifty-one, who had lost an average of 83 lb after remaining on a liquid predigested protein diet for two to eight months. Of course, the purpose of the women following the liquid protein diet was to reduce body weight very rapidly.

Most of these low-calorie protein diets are either of modified proteins or hydrolysates (of collagen or gelatin) of extremely low nutritional quality. Most of the products are sold over the counter in pharmacies, grocery stores, and health food stores. As emphasized repeatedly, a low-calorie diet or any type of weight-reducing diet is often hazardous to health in the absence of careful supervision by medical personnel trained in their use. This is more so when weight reduction is very rapid regardless of the method used, and it is often suicidal. Obviously, sudden death associated with the liquid protein diet typifies the preceding statement. Greater than usual precautions are required for cardiac patients because life-threatening ventricular arrhythmias may be easily provoked by the liquid protein diet.

SUGGESTIONS FOR GOOD EATING HABITS

- The purpose of any special diet program has to be understood clearly before engaging in that program.

- All special diet programs have to be designed by or in consultation with a dietitian, and they must be prescribed by a physician.

- Any special diet program in the absence of adequate and constant medical supervision is hazardous, because a nutritional imbalance with a deficiency of vitamins and/or minerals may be produced, and even death may result.

- Low-calorie protein diets should be avoided unless under the strict supervision of a physician. Sudden death has occurred during or immediately after the liquid protein diet program.

- No single diet program is perfectly suitable for every patient. Thus, the ideal diet program has to be designed on an individual basis.

- A low-cholesterol and low-saturated-fat diet with low caloric intake is highly recommended for all cardiac patients, especially those with obesity, elevated blood contents of cholesterol and/or triglycerides, hypertension, and known CAD. In addition, low-salt diets are mandatory for individuals with high BP and/or CHF.

- Average American foods contain a large quantity of cholesterol, saturated fats, and high calories. Foods containing large amounts of cholesterol, and saturated fats should be avoided whenever possible. Bacon and ham are the worst foods for cardiac and hypertensive patients because of their extremely high contents of animal fat and salt.

- Visible fat should be removed from meats before cooking and before eating. Dripping fat should be discarded before serving or eating. Cardiac patients should eat less fried foods; instead, roasted, broiled, baked, and boiled meats are highly recommended.

- Ordinary cooking methods such as barbecuing and broiling are very effective in reducing the fat from meat.

• Any fat that hardens by refrigeration after cooking is an animal fat that should be removed. For example, fat hardens on top of soup during refrigeration and should be skimmed off.

• In place of meats of four-legged animals, cardiac patients should eat more fish and poultry (without skin).

• Polyunsaturated fat (vegetable fat) should be used more often for cooking and dressings.

• Overeating is unequivocally harmful to many cardiac patients and individuals with various risk factors, particularly obesity and high blood contents of cholesterol and/or triglycerides.

• When people feel hungry, they should eat more vegetables, salads, and fruits.

• Various soups served in restaurants tend to contain large amounts of salt. When the soup is obviously salty, it should be avoided. Likewise, any food that seems salty should be avoided. Remember that some foods that do not seem salty may still contain a large quantity of salt.

• When ground beef is going to be used, it is advisable to select beef that looks lean (without much fat) first, and then have a butcher grind the meat. Thus, you will be certain of the type of meat used in your cooking. When meat is already ground (prepackaged) in a supermarket, it is impossible to determine the nature of the meat.

• It is foolish to add table salt to food before tasting it. In fact, adding salt is not advisable for cardiac patients, especially those with CHF and/or high BP.

• A variety of Asian foods are good for cardiac patients because their contents of animal fats and cholesterol are generally low. On the other hand, various Asian foods tend to contain large amounts of salt because of soy sauce, which is commonly used in cooking.

• Remember that all types of alcoholic beverages contain considerable calories. Therefore, caloric intake should be carefully calculated during a low-calorie diet program when drinking an alcoholic beverage. For instance, an average beer contains 120 cal, whereas an average cocktail contains 150 cal.

• The true value of any special diet program for a perfectly healthy individual without risk factors is uncertain. Likewise, the value of a low-fat, low-cholesterol diet for people over sixty-five years of age is not clearly documented.

• During any low-caloric diet program, supplementary vitamins and/or minerals are recommended under medical supervision.

SUGGESTIONS FOR MEALS AWAY FROM HOME AND ALCOHOLIC BEVERAGES

When eating meals away from home, the same precautions, rules, and diet programs have to be followed closely whenever possible. In a restaurant, a regular customer may ask for specially cooked foods that are required for a specific diet program. Likewise, common special diets are available at various hotels, on commercial airlines, and trains. It is perfectly acceptable to request a special diet under these circumstances rather than jeopardize the diet program and even one's health.

It is important to eat regularly at the expected time, especially for the diabetic patient. Excessive alcohol consumption should be avoided because any alcoholic beverage contains significant calories and will jeopardize the diet program of individuals on low-calorie diets. More importantly, alcohol depresses the heart function considerably for individuals with known heart disease. The depressive effect of alcohol for patients with CHF and significant heart damage is usually very marked. Nevertheless, moderate alochol consumption (e.g., one to two medium-strength cocktails) is acceptable for many cardiac patients as long as heart function is evaluated as adequate by a physician. Alcohol consumption should be stopped immediately when significant symptoms occur, and a physician should be consulted. In addition, alcohol may trigger abnormal heart rhythm, and it tends to elevate the fat content of the blood.

During travel, an adequate resting period is extremely important. Furthermore, unnecessary emotional stress, anxiety, or any unusual excitement should be avoided, especially when the travel is related to one's business or occupation. Emotional stress is bad for cardiac patients in many ways. Any vigorous physical activity or sexual activity should be avoided within two to three hours after a meal and/or alcohol consumption. Remember that many people tend to have a very irregular life-style with extraordinary activities while traveling. Thus, a physician must be consulted before taking a trip so that a serious outcome can be prevented.

20

SEX AND THE HEART

By and large, sexual activity should be avoided during the first two months after a heart attack, but various factors significantly influence sexual activity. The time at which the cardiac patient is permitted to resume sexual activity must be determined by a physician after a full evaluation including an exercise ECG test. More than 80 percent of heart attack victims can resume sexual activity without any serious risk. The remaining 20 percent, with more serious heart damage, may have to limit their sexual activity according to their individual cardiac capacity. The general outline regarding sexual activity after a heart attack has been described in Chapter 3. Although the primary concern is with sexual activity among heart attack victims, the same instructions and advice should be provided to every patient with any type of heart disease (e.g., RHD, myocarditis, cardiomyopathies).

NORMAL RESPONSES TO SEXUAL ACTIVITY

The energy expenditure during sexual activity can be determined using a concept of METs (measured in metabolic units) as well as caloric requirements, and it can easily be compared with all common physical activities (see Table 3.6 and 3.11). In addition, the energy expenditure in each physical activity can also be compared with the energy expenditure in an exercise ECG test (see Tables 3.12 and 3.13). One MET is the energy expenditure per kilogram of body weight per minute of a subject sitting quietly in a chair in a comfortable room. (One MET is comparable to 1.4 cal/min. for a 70-kg man.) The average man who has recovered from an uncomplicated heart attack has a maximal physical capacity of 8 to 9 METs. The maximal energy expenditure during sexual activity is shown to be about 5 METs, which is comparable to 6 cal/min. Therefore, usual sexual activity is allowed when the individual is able to perform physical activity of 6 to 8 cal/min. without experiencing significant symptoms, abnormal heart rate or BP response, or abnormal ECG response by an exercise ECG test (see Table 3.12 and 3.13). The expected normal responses to sexual activity include a transient elevation of BP, increase in heart rate and respiration, and a feeling of warmth, especially during orgasm. When a rapid heart rate (more than 120 beats/min.) and/or rapid breathing lasts more than thirty minutes after sexual intercourse, a physician should be notified. Likewise, a physician should be informed when significant symptoms (e.g., chest pain, shortness of breath) occur during or after sexual intercourse.

WHEN TO RESUME SEXUAL ACTIVITY

Although instruction regarding the exact timing of resumption of sexual activity may vary slightly from physician to physician, most cardiac patients may be able to return to their accustomed sexual relations within four to eight weeks after a heart attack. Of course, the patient must feel well before considering any sexual activity, and the individual should be free of any significant cardiac symptoms, particularly chest pain, shortness of breath, and extreme fatigue. In addition, the functional (physical) capacity of a given individual has to be carefully evaluated by a physician before he or she is permitted to resume sexual activity. In a practical sense, any individual who can climb two flights of stairs or walk a city block briskly may be able to resume his or her usual sexual activity. Ambulatory (Holter monitor) ECG is very useful in order to assess the nature of any symptoms an individual experiences, particularly chest pain or palpitations, during sexual activity. The exact timing of the resumption of sexual activity after a heart attack will be influenced by numerous factors, including the patient's age, general health, extent of heart damage, speed of recovery, and the status of sexual activity before the heart attack. By and large, three major symptoms, including chest pain, shortness of breath, and palpitations, prevent sexual activity. In addition, sexual activity is often prevented by unnecessary fear in the patient and/or spouse and by anxiety or depression.

SEXUAL RELATIONSHIP—METHODS, FREQUENCY, AND PARTNER

As far as the coital position is concerned, the cardiac patient should take the position that is the most comfortable and requires the least workload. Cardiac patients should be instructed to perform sexual intercourse in positions in which they will not support their body with their arms for sustained period of time. For the first few times after discharge from the hospital, it may be wise to spend more time in foreplay; it may not be necessary to achieve orgasm. On the other hand, the patient should not be afraid of achieving orgasm if he or she feels comfortable, without any significant symptoms during coitus. As a rule, sexual activities should be resumed very gradually as the individual's health, particularly cardiac status, permits. Most middle-aged or older patients are satisfied with sexual activity about once or twice a week, but the coital frequency largely depends upon sexual habits before the heart attack.

In order to minimize the cardiac work load of the patient during sexual intercourse, a position in which the spouse can undertake most of the activity is suitable. Thus, three coital positions are generally recommended. They include (1) sitting facing each other on a wide chair or armless chair, low enough for the feet to rest on the floor; (2) the supine position, with the spouse on top; and (3) lying on the side in the face-to-face position.

The room should be quiet with a comfortable temperature. The patient should be free of any symptoms and should not be tired. Sexual activity should be avoided within two to three hours after meals and/or alcohol consumption. It may be advisable to go to bed earlier than usual when sexual activity is planned, so that the cardiac patient will have sufficient time to rest after the activity.

A sexual relationship with a new partner or someone other than the spouse is said to be hazardous to cardiac patients because it tends to cause overexcitement, leading to an excessive cardiac work load. In addition, extramarital sexual relations often cause anxiety, guilt, and fear of detection, and all these emotional problems are undesirable. Sudden death has been reported among cardiac patients during or immediately after sexual activity with an extramarital partner or a new sex partner. The term *coital death* has been used under these circumstances.

NG may be taken sublingually just a few minutes before sexual activity in order to prevent angina, or a long-acting nitrate may be taken about fifteen minutes before the activity. If any symptoms occur during or immediately after coitus, the activity, of course, should be stopped immediately, and a physician should be consulted for further advice. Sexual abstinence is not necessary for most cardiac patients. It is advisable not to become pregnant after a heart attack, but to use means other than oral contraceptives.

FACTORS REDUCING LIBIDO (SEXUAL DESIRE)

There are numerous factors that may reduce libido in cardiac patients. The most common cause is a simple misconception. Namely, many people believe that sexual activity might cause another heart attack or even death. Proper instructions usually eliminate this misconception. Sexual activity may be disturbed by anxiety and depression, which are not uncommon soon after discharge from the hospital. Again, these emotional difficulties may be improved gradually with proper medical and psychological guidance. Of course, certain cardiac patients experience a loss of libido as a result of poor heart function due to severe cardiac damage. Sexual activity will improve as cardiac function improves with proper medical and/or surgical treatment.

It is important to remember that many commonly used drugs may inhibit sexual performance. For example, various antihypertensive drugs and central nervous system depressants (e.g., narcotics, alcohol, tricyclic antidepressants) frequently reduce sexual performance. Among antihypertensive medications, guanethidine, reserpine, clonidine, propranolol, and methyl dopa are well known to reduce sexual performance. When any question is raised regarding possible drug effects on sexual desires, a physician should be consulted. When poor sexual experience is considered to be based on any emotional or psychological reason, a psychologist, psychiatrist, or sex therapist may be consulted if necessary.

21

PHYSICAL ACTIVITY, EXERCISE, AND THE HEART

More than 15 to 20 million health-conscious Americans are estimated to participate in some form of regular physical activity, and jogging or running is probably the most popular form of exercise today. There are at least one hundred marathon races of 26.2 miles annually in the United States. Yet there is no direct evidence of the efficacy of these regular physical activities for the prevention of CAD, although there are many indirect beneficial effects for various cardiac functions. The quality of the life-style of cardiac patients seems to improve considerably through the aid of a properly designed exercise program, but unfortunately the exercise per se does not seem to prolong the life span of the patients.

In general, a regular physical exercise program improves blood circulation throughout the body; the lungs, heart, other organs, and muscles work together more efficiently. Thus, known beneficial effects of a regular physical exercise program include lowering of the resting heart rate, lowering of the heart rate and systolic BP during exercise, improvement of maximal cardiac output and maximal oxygen consumption, and rapid return to normal heart rate after exercise. Consequently, many cardiac patients with angina pectoris or previous heart attack may be able to do more and more physical activity progressively, without experiencing chest pain, shortness of breath, or excessive fatigue. There is good evidence that collateral circulation improves considerably with a proper physical exercise program in patients with CAD. Even healthy individuals who exercise can handle physical stress better, so that they are able to perform a variety of physical activities more efficiently without being tired. A regular physical exercise program is also very desirable for psychological well-being and is beneficial for relaxation, sound sleep, and releasing tension.

It is important to remember that any individual (even a healthy person) who is planning to participate in a vigorous or competitive exercise program or sport should be fully evaluated by a physician beforehand in order to make certain that he or she is physically fit for a given program. Another very important precaution before engaging in an exercise program is that the work load during physical activity should not be beyond the individual's physical limitations as determined by the exercise ECG test.

As can be expected, there are some undesirable effects and complications related to various exercise programs. They may include heat stroke, frostbite, various types of musculoskeletal injury including fractures, marked fatigue, near-syncope or syncope, cardiac arrhythmias, development of a new heart attack, and even death. Thus, the risk-benefit ratio of a given exercise program should be carefully weighed, and a physician should be consulted whenever necessary. A properly selected exercise program after careful medical evaluation can minimize or prevent various undesirable effects and complications related to a variety of physical activities. Physical activities after a heart attack have been described in Chapter 3.

EXERCISE PROGRAMS FOR HEALTHY PEOPLE

Although there is no direct and conclusive evidence to prove that physical exercise prevents the development of atherosclerosis and other related consequences, such as heart attack and stroke, many indirect beneficial effects of a proper physical exercise program are well known. Various well-designed exercise programs not only provide enormous psychological and/or emotional satisfaction and well-being to many individuals, but physical capacity is also reported to increase as much as 33 percent in both healthy people and cardiac patients.

As expected, there is no exercise program best suited to every individual. Therefore, the best exercise program for enjoyment and health has to be selected in consultation with one's physician. Unless the chosen exercise program provides a person with pleasure and enjoyment, it is extremely difficult to continue the exercise for a long period of time. Remember that all beneficial effects of the exercise program will disappear very quickly when the individual stops the exercise. Unfortunately, many people start various exercise programs with enthusiasm at the beginning, but they often drop out because convincing subjective or objective beneficial effects may not be evident during the first one or two months of the program. This may lead to discouragement and disappointment in some people, but the regular exercise program will provide a more satisfying and rewarding experience progressively as one continues the program faithfully for a long period of time. Remember that any exercise program should become a lifetime commitment.

Precautions and Preparations

It is essential to have a complete medical checkup, including exercise ECG testing, before engaging in any exercise program in order to prevent undesirable consequences, including sudden death. Self-claimed "perfect health" may not mean a healthy person from a medical viewpoint. A complete medical evaluation is especially critical for high-risk individuals (e.g., obese people, individuals with high blood cholesterol or triglycerides, a family history of sudden death or heart attack), even if they feel perfectly healthy. When the physical capacity is determined by a physician, a suitable exercise program will be chosen, but the exercise work load should not exceed the person's physical limitations. Physical limitations can be determined easily by the exercise ECG test using an exercise protocol (see Table 3.12) expressed by amounts of METs (metabolic unit showing energy expenditure). Any exercise program that requires an exercise work load beyond one's capacity will obviously be hazardous to health. Periodic medical checkups with repeated exercise ECG tests are necessary to determine the progression of physical capacity as the individual participates in the exercise program regularly. Thus, the suitability of the exercise program as well as its effectiveness for the individual can be assessed. Preferably, one should be able to perform the selected exercise program year-round without interruption. It is important to wear proper clothing and footwear for an exercise program, and temperature and humidity should be in comfortable ranges. It is hazardous when the weather is too cold or hot and when the humidity is too high. When the weather is undesirable, heat stroke or frostbite may occur, and even life-threatening consequences may result in extreme cases.

As repeatedly emphasized, sudden exercise is hazardous to health. Therefore, during a warming-up period, mild exercise such as calisthenics are highly recommended. Calisthenics can provide a good preparation before engaging a regular exercise program by providing various motions of the head, neck, torso, hips, arms, and legs. In general, a warming-up period should last at least three to five minutes or even longer. Likewise, sudden cessation of physical activity may be hazardous after vigorous exercise, and thus a gradual decrease of such activity ("cooling-down" or "cooling-off") is recommended. Tapering off the exercise program should end exertion prior to a warm shower (neither cold nor hot). Any physical exercise should be avoided soon after a heavy meal and/or alcohol consumption. In addition, any vigorous physical exercise will be harmful when the individual is unusually tired or has just recovered from any significant illness. It is rather foolish and hazardous to push to a high exertional intensity when under severe emotional tension, because serious ventricular arrhythmias may be provoked in this circumstance. Remember that physical exercise will by no means cure a tired feeling or emotional stress. It is inadvisable to push oneself to the point of complete exhaustion, leading to the development of unnecessary complications (e.g., near-syncope or syncope).

Various recommended exercise programs include brisk walking, jogging, swimming, bicycling, and mild popular sports (e.g., tennis without intense competition). Some sports, like push-ups and weight lifting, are not recommended for most people. High motivation with great enthusiasm is necessary for a continuous and regular exercise program, and the exercise should be performed at least three times weekly for thirty minutes. Once-a-week exercise programs (e.g., weekend golfers) do not provide sufficient beneficial effects to health other than enjoyment and pleasure.

Intensity of Exercise

People cannot predict their physical capacity (limitation) until they actually participate in any exercise program. Therefore, it is extremely important to estimate one's physical capacity before engaging in any type of exercise program, even for healthy people. It is rather hazardous to participate in a vigorous exercise program or competitive sport blindly, without knowing one's limitations. For the determination of physical capacity, a progressive multistage exercise (stress) ECG test is considered the best established, practical approach. Ideally, however, direct observation with possible ECG monitoring during an actual exercise program or sport is superior to exercise ECG testing; needless to say, that is rather impractical and often impossible. The multistage exercise ECG test is performed most commonly by using a motor-driven treadmill (less commonly, by using a bicycle ergometer), and a standard exercise protocol is used (see Table 3.12).

In most medical centers, the exercise ECG test is terminated when the individual's heart rate reaches 85 to 90 percent of the age-adjusted, predicted maximal heart rate, or when the individual develops significant symptoms (e.g., chest pain) or significant ECG abnormalities (including cardiac arrhythmias), whichever comes first. The maximal or submaximal heart rate is faster in young people than in older individuals. For example, 90 percent submaximal heart rate in young people (age twenty to twenty-nine) is 175 beats/min., whereas it is 160 beats/min. in older individuals (age sixty to sixty-nine). In middle-aged people (age forty to fifty-nine), 90 percent submaximal heart rate ranges from 164 to 168 beats/min. The initial speed of the treadmill is 1.7 mph with a flat level (no grade or 0 grade, meaning no incline or slope) for the first three minutes during a warming-up period. Following this warming-up period, the exercise work load is increased progressively every three minutes with a constant speed (3.0 mph) by the treadmill but a progressive increment of 4 percent grade (slope or incline) in each stage (see Table 3.12). The treadmill becomes progressively steeper as the stage of the exercise work load increases.

Most young people and even many physically active middle-aged individuals may be able to complete a full seven-stage exercise protocol without any problem. A full course of the exercise protocol takes twenty-one minutes (three minutes for each stage). When an individual can complete the full seven-stage exercise protocol without any difficulty, his or her physical capacity is estimated as capable of tolerating any physical activity requiring the energy expenditure (exercise work load) of up to 16 METs. Remember that 1 MET means the energy requirement of a subject sitting quietly in a chair. Physically more active young people in top condition may be able to perform an additional exercise work load during the exercise ECG test (stages 8 and 9 are optional) beyond the capacity of the average healthy person.

The exercise work load a given individual is able to perform during the exercise ECG test can be expressed as METs (the metabolic units that express the energy expenditure). When an individual's physical capacity is determined by using the concept of METs during the exercise ECG test, a physician can select an exercise program or physical activity that requires no greater work load than the individual's maximal capacity. For example, if a person completed stage 4 of the exercise protocol without any problem, the energy expenditure (exercise work load) was 8 METs. This test result means that the individual may be able to participate in a physical activity that requires not more than 8 METs. The energy requirements during various physical activities and during the exercise ECG test can easily be compared using the METs concept (see Tables 3.11 and 3.12). When an individual's physical capacity is measured to be 8 METs by the exercise ECG test, he or she should be able to participate in a variety of physical activities, including walking (5 mph), jogging (5 mph), cycling (12 mph), badminton (competitive), tennis (average singles), canoeing (5 mph), and water skiing (see Table 3.11). The energy expenditure for running varies considerably, depending upon speed. For instance, running at 6 mph requires only 10 METs, whereas intense running at 10 mph needs at least 17 METs. Of course, a physically active individual in top condition who has completed a full seven-stage exercise protocol without any difficulty should be able to participate in any common sport or exercise program without any problem, because the exercise work load during the exercise ECG test is 21 METs (high-speed running requires only 17 METs). As a rule, most recreational games or sports should initially be undertaken at an energy requirement that does not exceed 50 percent of the calculated maximal work load for the duration of a given game or sport. In general, a 50 percent metabolic requirement usually elicits 60 to 75 percent of the maximum heart rate response.

It should be noted that some individuals with hard-driving personalities (so-called Type A personality) have a tendency to become competitive during any type of game or sport. When there is intense competition involved, the energy expenditure varies considerably, because emotional and psychological energy requirements are difficult to determine. By and large, any intense and competitive sport should be avoided by middle-aged or older people when their life-style has been sedentary, because an excessive work load will be required beyond one's physical limitation, which is hazardous to health. Sudden death has been reported during intense and competitive single tennis games among middle-aged executives and physicians who are apparently healthy. People should be instructed to count their pulse rate from time to time to make certain that it is not more than 75 percent of the maximal heart rate.

When an apparently healthy individual seems to have a history of palpitations, irregular or skipped heartbeats or any other cardiac symptom, or a family history of sudden death or heart attack, a Holter monitor ECG is highly recommended. This device can register any transient or occasional abnormal heartbeats or rhythms so that the underlying cause for palpitations and other symptoms can be determined and a proper management can be provided (see Chapter 24). Thus, an appropriate type of exercise program can be recommended by a physician, and proper medical advice can be given accordingly.

Duration of Exercise

The relative values of frequency-intensity-duration of various exercise programs are difficult to assess. Some people prefer jogging around the house or using a stationary bicycle or playing tennis, squash, or handball. Personal preferences significantly influence the ratio of the frequency, intensity, and duration of an exercise. By and large, however, a sufficient exercise work load requires at least twenty-five to thirty minutes of the exercise program (not including warming-up and cooling-off time) at a relatively high intensity in order to improve physical fitness and to supply various beneficial effects. In general, thirty to sixty minutes are recommended for each session of an exercise program depending upon the type of physical activity.

Frequency of Exercise

Improved fitness with beneficial effects can be expected when an individual engages in a proper exercise program at least twice a week. Many authorities recommend an exercise program three to five days/week (evenly spaced rather than consecutive days). Once-a-week physical activity (e.g., the weekend golfer or jogger) is not considered sufficient.

Type of Physical Activity

In general, any exercise program that involves the use of large muscles with rhythmic and repetitive motion (isotonic or dynamic physical activity) is highly recommended. Thus, physical activities that are generally recommended include brisk walking, hiking, jogging, running, bicycling, swimming, and various common games or sports. Strength-building isometric activities such as weight lifting are not recommended for cardiovascular health benefits. It is important to select an activity of exercise program that is enjoyable, providing the selected program is suitable for cardiovascular health benefits. If an individual cannot enjoy the exercise program, it will be impossible to continue for a long period of time. Competitive and very intense sports or games are not recommended for middle-aged or older people unless they have been physically active since childhood.

Regarding golf (one of the most popular recreational activities in America), its energy requirement varies considerably depending upon the way it is played. For example, only 2 to 3 METs are required when one rides in a power cart, but 4 to 5 METs are necessary when one carries the golf clubs (see Table 3.11). A more extreme example is that running at 6 mph requires only 10 METs, while vigorous running at 10 mph requires at least 17 METs. A proper exercise program has to be selected according to the participant's preference, and maximal physical capacity is determined by the exercise ECG test. It is interesting to note that a social dance (e.g., a fox trot), table tennis (Ping-Pong), badminton (singles), tennis (doubles), and a golf game (carrying clubs) have almost identical energy requirements (4 to 5 METs).

PHYSICAL ACTIVITIES AND EXERCISE PROGRAMS FOR CARDIAC PATIENTS

A proper exercise program and physical activity are even more crucial for cardiac patients, particularly those who have just recovered from a heart attack, because excessive work loads beyond their physical capacity will be extremely hazardous and may cause sudden death. Yet a proper and continuous exercise program will definitely be beneficial for many cardiac patients and individuals with various risk factors, especially being overweight and having high blood contents of lipids.

Physical Activities in the Hospital after a Heart Attack

Even on the first day, patients with a mild heart attack may be allowed to sit up for a short period of time, and even to get out of bed to use a bedside commode. Self-cleansing and feeding are usually allowed within twenty-four to forty-eight hours for victims of uncomplicated and mild heart attacks. Physical activity is progressively increased thereafter as long as the patient is free of any significant symptom(s) and vital signs and ECG findings are stable. Detailed descriptions regarding management and physical activities during hospitalization after a heart attack are found in Chapter 3.

Physical Activities of Heart Attack Victims after Discharge from the Hospital

Proper physical activity is extremely important for heart attack victims after discharge from the hospital because close medical supervision and continuous monitoring are no longer available. An excessive exercise work load will be unquestionably hazardous to health, and even sudden death may occur in this circumstance.

In many medical centers, a modified exercise ECG test with a low-level exercise work load is performed just before discharge in order to determine the patient's functional (physical) capacity. The modified low-level exercise ECG test is designed to provide the work load that requires approximately 70 percent of the predicted maximal heart rate. Initially, the patient walks on the flat level of treadmill (grade 0) at 1.2 mph for the first three minutes. After this warming-up period, the grade is increased by 3 percent every three minutes at the same speed (1.2 mph) for the next six minutes. If the patient is able to tolerate the aforementioned work loads, he or she can continue the treadmill exercise for another three minutes at a slightly faster speed (1.7 mph) at the same grade (6 percent). When an individual can complete the entire low-level treadmill exercise ECG test for twelve minutes, he or she is estimated to be able to participate in any physical activity requiring not more than 3.3 METs. In place of the low-level treadmill exercise ECG test, a standard exercise ECG protocol (see Table 3.12) may be used for the same purpose. In a practical sense, the exercise ECG test is terminated when the patient develops any significant symptoms, marked ECG abnormalities, or significant cardiac arrhythmias or when the maximal heart rate reaches 120 beats/min. (some physicians push up to 130 beats/min.)—whichever occurs first.

When the maximal physical capacity of a patient is determined through the METs concept, a proper activity that requires less than the maximal exercise work load tolerated will be selected by a physician (see Tables 3.11 and 3.13). Customarily, the functional capacity of cardiac patients is classified according to the New York Heart Association criteria (see Table 3.13 and Chapter 6). Functional class II patients can do all ordinary physical activities without symptoms, but they become symptomatic during extraordinary activities. On the other hand, functional III patients become symptomatic even with ordinary physical activities. For example, cardiac patients in a functional class I category can perform an exercise work load of at least 10 METs, whereas functional IV patients are unable to perform any exercise at all (1 MET exercise work load). Functional II patients perform an exercise work load of up to 6 METs, while the patient with functional III can perform an exercise work load of only up to 3 METs. Most heart attack victims are allowed to participate in any physical activity that requires less than 3.5 METs (see Table 3.11) during the first three to six weeks after a heart attack. This means that ordinary self-care and ordinary housework (e.g., making the bed, dressing, undressing, washing hands and/or face, showering; see Table 3.11) are allowed during this recovery period. Of course, physical activity will gradually be increased during the recovery period. Just before returning to work or engaging in any exercise program, an exercise ECG test and a Holter monitor ECG test are mandatory.

Return to Work

Although the exact timing of when the heart attack victim is able to return to work is difficult to determine, most patients who have recovered from a mild heart attack without major complications should be able to return to their former occupations within two to three months. Today, most relatively sedentary desk jobs require an energy expenditure of not more than 3 to 4 METs, which can be tolerated by most cardiac patients. Detailed descriptions are found in Chapter 3.

Exercise Prescriptions for Cardiac Patients

Again, no exercise prescription is perfectly suitable for every cardiac patient. It is mandatory for all cardiac patients to evaluate their functional capacity precisely by performing the exercise ECG test before engaging in any type of exercise program. When the functional classification is determined according to the New York Heart Association criteria (see Table 3.13), a physician will select a suitable exercise program. The exercise work load required for the program should not be more than the maximal physical capacity of the patient expressed in METs. There are various kinds of exercise programs, sports, and games that may require almost identical energy expenditures (exercise work loads; see Table 3.11). Thus, a suitable exercise program or sport can be selected according to individual preference under a physician's guidance. In addition to the exercise ECG test, an ambulatory (Holter monitor) ECG is also definitely indicated before engaging in any exercise program to make certain there is no significant cardiac arrhythmia, especially during physical activity. When significant cardiac arrhythmias are recorded on the Holter monitor ECG, proper management should be provided in conjunction with reevaluation of the entire cardiac status. Any exercise program has to be postponed when clinically significant cardiac arrhythmias persist.

As far as the nature and type of exercise program are concerned, again an isotonic or dynamic physical activity is recommended for cardiac patients. Of course, the intensity and duration of the program should be minimal at the beginning, and the work load should be increased gradually under close medical supervision. The exercise work load of cardiac patients is such that the maximal heart rate should not be faster than 120 beats/min. during a peak exercise period. Of course, physical activity should be terminated immediately when any symptom (e.g., chest pain) occurs, and a physician should be notified for further medical advice. For chest pain, NG may be taken sublingually. Competitive sports are not recommended for cardiac patients because an extraordinary energy expenditure may be required. Subjects with "hard-driving" personality (type A personality) should be very careful to avoid any competition during sports or games. The same precautions and preparations described for healthy people have to be observed even more carefully. Any exercise program or intense physical activity should be avoided two to three hours after a meal and/or alcohol consumption. Likewise, no exercise is recommended when the patient feels very tired or when there is any cardiac symptom. Similarly, any physical activity is very hazardous when the weather is very cold or hot and when the humidity is very high. Although there is no exercise prescription best suited to every cardiac patient, the recommended exercise program for heart attack victims following discharge from the hospital is summarized in Table 21.1. In this table, the first section contains the short-term exercise program for the first two months after a heart attack, and the second section explains the long-term exercise program for up to twenty weeks after a heart attack.

TABLE 21.1. Cardiac Rehabilitation Home Exercise Program.

SHORT-TERM PROGRAM FOR THE FIRST 2 MONTHS AFTER THE CORONARY INCIDENT[a]

Week	Activity
1-2	In-hospital exercise regimen
3	Walk 5 minutes at leisurely pace (¼ mile) once per day
End of 3[b]	Return to hospital for 1st follow-up visit
4	Walk 5 minutes at leisurely pace (¼ mile) 2 times per day
5	Walk 10 minutes at leisurely pace (½ mile) once per day
6	Walk 10 minutes at leisurely pace (½ mile) once per day
7	Walk 15 minutes at leisurely pace (¾ mile) once per day
8	Walk 15 minutes at leisurely pace (¾ mile) once per day
End of 8[c]	Return to hospital for 2d follow-up visit

LONG-TERM PROGRAM TO BEGIN AFTER THE FIRST 2 MONTHS THAT FOLLOW THE CORONARY INCIDENT

Week	Activity
9	Walk 20 minutes at leisurely pace (1 mile) once per day
10	Walk 20 minutes at moderate pace (1-1/3 miles) once per day
11	Walk 30 minutes at moderate pace (2 miles) once per day
12	Measure a 1-mile distance with car. Walk to point and back (total of 2 miles) in 40 minutes. Pulse at end should be less than 115 beats/minute[d]
13-14	Measure a 1.5-mile distance. Walk to point and back (3.0 miles) in 60 minutes
15-16	Measure a 2-mile distance. Walk to point and back (4.0 miles) in 72 minutes
17-19	Measure a 2-mile distance. Walk to point and back (4.0 miles) in 60 minutes (15-minute/mile pace)
20[e]	Measure a 2-mile distance. Walk to point and back (4.0 miles) in 56 minutes (14-minute/mile pace, just below a slow jog)

[a](Adapted from John L. Boyer, M.D., San Diego, California.)
[b]Objectives of 1st follow-up visit are: (1) evaluation of risk factor modification; (2) evaluation of current activity and physical therapy exercise program; (3) evaluation of medication regimen; (4) dietary consultation; (5) brief cardiovascular history and physical examination; and (6) 24-hour Holter monitoring.
[c]Objectives of 2d follow-up visit are: (1) same as objectives 1-5 above; (2) submaximal stress test; and (3) if patient is *not* planning to participate in gym program, instruct in long-term home walk program.
[d]The individual is taught to check his own pulse rate. He is not to advance to the next stage (as from week 1-2 to week 3-4) unless the immediate post-exercise rate is less than 115 per minute.
[e]Continue in this stage indefinitely.
Reproduced with permission from Fletcher, G.F.: "Exercise and the Heart" *(Current Problems in Cardiology).* Chicago: Year Book Pub., Inc., Vol. 4, Number 3 (June, 1979).

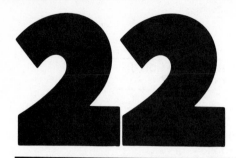

SMOKING
AND THE HEART

Today, everyone has some knowledge that cigarette smoking is harmful to health in many ways; there is even a warning statement about the dangers of smoking printed on every package of cigarettes. The harmful effects of smoking affect all organs and systems, including the heart, lungs, kidneys, nervous system, gastrointestinal system, and peripheral blood vessels (e.g., small blood vessels in the arms and legs). As repeatedly emphasized (see Chapter 3), cigarette smoking is one of the major risk factors for early development of atherosclerosis and CAD. In recent medical literature dealing with heart attack victims under forty years of age, heavy cigarette smoking was considered the sole major risk factor.

When one or both parents smoke, this bad habit directly or indirectly often influences their children to smoke sooner or later. When a family member or colleague at work smokes, other people have to inhale the smoke-filled air. This indirect smoking is also bad for health. Among other things, because of the harmful effects to health of indirect smoking, all commercial airlines and many restaurants provide a choice of seating arrangements between smoking and nonsmoking. Various other risk factors (e.g., overweight, high blood contents of cholesterol or triglycerides) are also frequently present in heavy smokers.

Various harmful effects of cigarette smoking are primarily due to nicotine, tar, and carbon monoxide. It has been shown that more than 85 percent (up to nearly 100 percent) of the chemical compounds inhaled during cigarette smoking will be retained in the lungs. Thus, those who smoke pipes or cigars will have less harmful effects, because these smokers seldom inhale as deeply as cigarette smokers do. The actual value of the filtered cigarette, however, is uncertain in terms of the degree of filtering of chemicals accomplished during smoking. When an individual inhales during smoking, these substances will enter the bloodstream, and they will eventually damage various organs and systems. Some of these chemicals will damage the inner layers of the blood vessels, particularly coronary arteries, and this event naturally predisposes to early development of CAD. Cigarette smoking increases the blood lipid contents and the stickiness of blood platelets, leading to thromboembolic phenomena in various organs and to heart attack or stroke. When the inner layer of the blood vessels is damaged or narrowed, increased contents of blood lipids, of course, will further speed up the development of heart attack and stroke very rapidly.

When small arteries and veins are involved in the extremities, blood circulation to the legs and/or arms will be considerably reduced. In advanced cases, marked reduction of blood to the extremities may lead to gangrene (necrosis or dead tissue), which often necessitates amputation of the involved extremity. This peripheral vascular disease is called "Buerger's disease"; it is considered directly related to cigarette smoking. When Buerger's disease is recognized in the early stage, the patient may improve markedly simply by not smoking anymore.

Effects of Nicotine

It is a well-known phenomenon that the aftereffects of nicotine will constrict blood vessels, leading to interference in blood circulation. This constricting effect of nicotine further deteriorates the functions of the diseased heart when the coronary arteries are already narrowed and when the heart muscle is significantly damaged. Consequently, the heart has to pump harder to increase blood circulation in order to supply sufficient oxygen and nutrients to various organs and tissues. Of course, the extra work load caused by nicotine is very difficult, even impossible, for the heart to carry when its functional capacity is already significantly reduced. When the degree of constriction by nicotine becomes severe, especially in patients with angina pectoris and previous heart attack, cigarette smoking itself may cause severe chest pain and even a second heart attack in certain cases.

In addition, nicotine causes the elevation of certain chemical substances, called catecholamines, in the bloodstream. The increased level of blood catecholamines often produces rapid heart rate, extra heartbeats, and sometimes irregular heart rhythm. This effect is, of course, harmful to cardiac patients.

Effects of Carbon Monoxide

Cigarette smoking creates a constant level of carbon monoxide, a poisonous gas, in the bloodstream. This poisonous gas quickly combines with hemoglobin in the blood, and consequently the oxygen supply throughout the circulation will be reduced. When this occurs, the insufficient oxygen supply to the heart muscle due to carbon monoxide will further impair cardiac functions when the heart is already damaged, particularly in patients with CAD.

Effects of Tar

Tar is a substance that accumulates in the lungs after smoking. It forms a brown, sticky mass containing chemical compounds that are responsible for the production of primary lung cancers (95 percent of such cases are heavy smokers). Tar does not seem to have a significant effect on cardiac function directly.

Other Effects of Smoking

Cigarette smoking increases the contents of blood lipids and the stickiness of blood platelets, leading to an increasing incidence of blood clot formation in various organs. The synergistic effects of smoking and birth control pills for the early development of blood clots and heart attack in many young to middle-aged women are well known. The fact that cigarette smoking often predisposes to Buerger's disease has been stressed. In addition to lung cancers, cigarette smokers frequently develop chronic bronchitis, emphysema, and many other chronic lung diseases. The common term *cigarette cough* is very familiar to the general public, and this chronic cough is usually a manifestation of the chronic bronchitis (irritation and inflammation of airways in the lungs) of heavy smokers. When any chronic lung disease persists for a long period of time, right ventricular function gradually deteriorates, leading to right ventricular failure (see Chapter 6). The term *chronic cor-pulmonale* is used when right ventricular failure develops as a result of various chronic lung diseases, particularly emphysema. In addition, the incidence of peptic ulcer (stomach ulcer) and other gastrointestinal disorders seem to increase among heavy smokers.

THE RELATIONSHIP BETWEEN SMOKING AND HEART DISEASE

The relationship between smoking and heart disease is briefly summarized as follows:

23

ALCOHOL
AND THE HEART

Although alcohol has been a part of human life in many aspects for hundreds of thousands of years, it is also known that alcohol has many harmful effects on various organs and systems. In particular, the toxic effects of alcohol to the liver, heart, nervous system, and gastrointestinal system have been well recognized. It has been estimated that there are at least 10 million alcoholics in America alone, and their life-styles have been jeopardized in many ways, especially in terms of their health, family relationships, and jobs. There are also numerous indirect harmful consequences. For instance, approximately 2.5 million arrests or criminal cases are estimated to be alcohol-related events in the United States, and there are about 25,000 alcohol-related traffic fatalities annually. Furthermore, some medical reports indicate that about 50 percent of all adult bone fractures are related to alcohol, and approximately 15,000 alcohol-related homicides and suicides occur annually. Deaths related to alcohol directly or indirectly are difficult to estimate because so many other factors may be involved in many diseases and accidents.

As far as economics are concerned, about $2 billion is necessary for health and welfare annually in the United States, whereas $3 billion is spent on property damage and medical expenses related to alcohol. Moreover, at least $10 billion is wasted through industrial accidents and absenteeism in America. Alcoholism involves people at all social levels—white-collar as well as blue-collar workers, poor and rich, educated or uneducated, even the very highly educated. Although numerous people enjoy drinking alcohol at home and at parties, and although it appears indispensable even at high-level national and international gatherings, excessive alcohol consumption is unequivocally harmful to health and is even life-threatening in many cases. Of course, some psychosocial benefits (to relieve daily tension and for entertaining) are a well-known value as long as health is not jeopardized and alcohol does not cause any other undesirable consequences. This can be avoided by limiting the amount of alcohol consumption.

The term *social drinker* is difficult to define because people's tolerance to alcohol without suffering various undesirable consequences and harmful effects varies considerably. Alcohol's effects on body functions depend upon various factors, including amounts of alcohol ingested, duration of regular or habitual alcohol consumption, the individual's threshold (tolerance) to alcohol and status of general health, and especially the presence or absence of preexisting diseases involving the heart, liver, and gastrointestinal tract. Thus, it is difficult to say that alcohol is good or alcohol is bad in every case, because moderate amounts of alcohol consumption, if they do not cause these undesirable effects in healthy people, will not be harmful. Various harmful effects to health are usually enhanced when alcohol is ingested without eating. This is one of the reasons why severe cases of advanced alcoholism are less common in Asia than in Western countries, because Asian people usually drink alcohol with some food (usually protein).

That liver cirrhosis is a common occurrence among alcoholics is well known, but alcohol-induced harm on heart function is equally important to recognize. Namely, excessive alcohol consumption may cause beriberi (a heart muscle disease from vitamin B_1 deficiency), alcoholic cardiomyopathy, a variety of cardiac arrhythmias, reduction of the pumping action of the heart (particularly in cardiac patients), and elevation of BP (especially in hypertensive patients). In addition, chronic alcoholics eventually develop irreversible brain damage leading to delirium tremens (in this condition the patient becomes delirious and disoriented; this is associated with convulsions, frequently leading to death in advanced cases), and some alcoholic patients develop esophageal varices (dilatation and bulging of the food tube connecting the mouth and stomach) that often rupture, leading to death. Alcohol also causes elevation of triglycerides in the blood; thus it is more harmful to individuals who already have a high triglyceride level.

It is important to remember that alcohol contains significant calories (8 oz of beer contains 120 cal; one cocktail has 150 cal). Therefore, any individual who follows a low-calorie diet program should be careful about drinking alcoholic beverages. Recently, peripheral skeletal muscle damage (e.g., predominantly involving the proximal girdle muscles) due to alcohol, comparable to alcoholic cardiomyopathy, has been reported. By and large, it is not necessary for most cardiac patients to maintain total abstinence as long as their general health and cardiac functions are not disturbed by alcohol consumption. That is, one or two "regular-sized" cocktails, 8 oz of wine, or two cans of beer per day are acceptable as tolerated by the individual under medical guidance. It should be kept in mind, however, that all cardiac patients should refrain from engaging in any type of extraordinary or intense physical activity, vigorous dancing, or sexual intercourse within two or three hours after a meal and/or alcohol consumption.

<hr>

EFFECTS OF ALCOHOL
AND CARDIOVASCULAR DISORDERS

The term *alcoholic heart disease* is used to designate all types of cardiac disorders, including alcoholic cardiomyopathy, beriberi heart disease, "holiday heart syndrome," and so forth.

Alcoholic Cardiomyopathy

Medical studies indicate that an intake of 60 oz or more of ethyl alcohol per month (e.g., an average daily intake of 2 oz, or roughly 30 cc of alcohol, equivalent to about 5 oz of 80-proof whiskey, 16 oz of ordinary table wine, or five 12-oz cans or bottles of ordinary beer) increases the risk of producing toxic changes in the heart muscle. In general, relatively high blood levels of alcohol (80 to 100 mg/100 ml) are necessary before evidence of impaired pumping action can be demonstrated in healthy individuals with normal hearts. Of course, the depressive action of alcohol on the heart muscle is much greater in cardiac patients, even at lower blood alcohol levels. Thus, it can be said that the quantity of alcohol necessary to depress cardiac function is smaller in the presence of heart disease and/or a history of chronic drinking over a long period of time. It has been demonstrated at autopsies that abnormal changes frequently occur in the heart muscle (as much as 90 percent in some studies) of chronic alcoholics even when clinical evidence of heart disease is not diagnosed before death. Furthermore, abnormal heart functions (e.g., reduced pumping action) are often documented by various cardiac tests among alcoholics in the absence of clinical evidence of heart disease. Thus, it can be concluded that alcohol causes definite toxic effects on heart muscle and eventually leads to alcoholic cardiomyopathy when large amounts of it are ingested for a long period of time. Alcoholic cardiomyopathy and beriberi heart disease were discussed fully in Chapter 12.

"Holiday Heart Syndrome"

The term *holiday heart syndrome* has become popular among physicians recently. It describes a variety of cardiac arrhythmias experienced by a group of healthy individuals after brief drinking sprees. Since this particular alcohol-induced event occurs more frequently during holidays and weekends, such terminology seems appropriate. Extra heartbeats and AF are most common. In holiday heart syndrome, a variety of abnormal heart rhythms is most likely to be provoked by the release of adrenalinlike substances (adrenalin is a hormone secreted by the adrenal glands). Abnormal heartbeats and rhythms often disappear upon stopping drinking. Otherwise, digitalis and/or antiarrhythmic agents (e.g., propranolol, quinidine; see Table 6.2) may be required for a short duration. The heart is found to be normal in individuals with holiday heart syndrome, but the chance of developing more serious cardiac arrhythmias will be greater in cardiac patients when they drink alcohol excessively.

Relationship to Heart Failure

As mentioned earlier, excessive alcohol consumption definitely causes depression of the heart muscle functions, so that its pumping action will be reduced even in healthy people. This alcohol-induced myocardial depression is found to be more pronounced among cardiac patients who already have considerable reduction of the heart's pumping action. It has been shown that consumption of more than 2 oz of alcohol per day (e.g., 5 oz of 80-proof whiskey per day) will cause significant myocardial depression in cardiac patients. Thus, all cardiac patients should not drink any more than two cocktails of 80-proof whiskey, 8 oz of table wine, or two bottles (12 oz) of ordinary beer per day. When the patient suffers from significant CHF, one cocktail or one 12-oz beer will be adequate. Of course, no alcohol is allowed for patients with advanced CHF and for those who develop more serious symptoms after drinking. It is strongly advised that all cardiac patients and their families consult their physicians before alcohol consumption is resumed.

Relationship to High Blood Pressure

It has been shown that rapid consumption of alcohol causes dilatation of blood vessels, which may reduce BP, but at the same time, alcohol-induced acceleration of the heart rate may raise BP. These two effects usually cancel each other out so that no significant BP change is observed in most instances. However, consumption of large amounts of alcohol, in excess of 60 cc per month (more than 2 oz of alcohol or 5 oz of 80-proof whiskey a day), may result in a significant elevation of BP if ingested over a long period of time. Alcohol-induced hypertension is often more pronounced in individuals with a family history of high BP. Of course, BP may rise readily when the individual is already hypertensive. Thus, alcohol consumption should be limited to less than two cocktails, 8 oz of wine, or two bottles of beer per day for all hypertensive patients and those with a strong family history of high BP. It is preferable to check BP from time to time in these individuals after drinking, especially when they experience any significant symptoms. Again, a physician should be consulted before these individuals start any alcoholic consumption.

Relationship to Coronary Artery Disease

Although some medical reports suggest that alcohol consumption may have a protective mechanism against heart attack and death from CAD in certain cases, this finding should be interpreted with extraordinary care. There are many physicians who do not concur this view. It is extremely important to weigh the risk-benefit ratio carefully. Any possible beneficial effect of alcohol to health will quickly disappear when excessive amounts of it are ingested. Excessive alcohol consumption is absolutely harmful to health, particularly to cardiovascular function. Remember also that alcohol consumption often causes elevation of the blood triglyceride level. The relationship of alcohol consumption to physical activity was discussed in Chapter 21.

Relationship to Various Drugs

Alcohol and drugs may react differently—some synergistically and some antagonistically. Therefore, it is important for the patient to ask a physician whether any drugs he or she is taking may have an unusual reaction when mixed with alcohol. As a rule, many sedatives and tranquilizers have synergistic actions with alcohol.

Cardiomyopathy Due to Arsenic-Contaminated Beer

In 1900, a major epidemic (over 6,000 cases with more than 70 deaths) of cardiomyopathy due to contamination of beer with small amounts of arsenic was reported. Acute and severe CHF was said to be the major clinical picture, and most deaths were the result of severe CHF. For a discussion of cardiomyopathy due to cobalt-contaminated beer, see Chapter 12.

PREVENTION AND MANAGEMENT OF ALCOHOLISM

Various problems related to chronic and excessive alcohol consumption have to be handled very carefully by a well-organized team of physicians, psychiatrists, psychologists, social workers, involved family members, patients themselves, and many others. In order to handle multiple problems related to alcoholism, there are many medical and psychiatric institutions as well as organizations for long-term treatment. For example, Alcoholics Anonymous is a private group consisting of former alcoholics as well as present alcoholics who meet together regularly. In addition, there are many other similar organizations, some sponsored by federal, state, or city government; some others are sponsored by private organizations. For instance, Metro Atlanta Recovery Residences Inc. (MARR Inc.) in Atlanta, Georgia, is a rehabilitation institution for chronic alcoholics who are not yet ready to return to an alcohol-free life. This rehabilitation center is closely coordinated with the Georgia Mental Health Institute, and the fee for participants is $125 per week. The residents include lawyers, ministers, professors, physicians, nurses, and office managers. Classes and meetings occupy the free time of the residents, and formal therapy sessions are held three times a week by visiting counselors. Residents discuss various problems with the counselors. Fortunately, most of the residents are able to join the outside world after months of therapy. Interestingly enough, the decision to leave the institution is made jointly by the resident, his/her housemates, and staff members of MARR Inc. If a resident breaks the rule against using drugs or alcohol, expulsion is said to be automatic. The Navy's Alcohol Rehabilitation Service in Long Beach, California, is another well-known institution where many high-ranking officers and politicians, as well as their families are treated.

PRACTICAL ADVICE TO CARDIAC PATIENTS

• It is difficult to say whether alcohol is "bad" or "good" for every individual, but excessive alcohol consumption is certainly harmful in many aspects.

• The harmful effects of alcohol depend upon various factors, including the amount of alcohol intake, the duration of alcohol consumption, the individual's threshold (tolerance) to alcohol, general health, and various preexisting diseases, particularly cardiac disorders.

• Alcohol is said to protect against heart attack in certain cases, but this view is not uniformly accepted by most physicians.

• Harmful effects of alcohol to the cardiovascular system are as follows:

1. Excessive alcohol intake causes various cardiac arrhythmias even in healthy people—called "holiday heart syndrome."
2. Excessive alcohol intake tends to elevate BP, particularly in hypertensive patients.
3. Excessive alcohol intake depresses the pumping action of the heart, particularly in cardiac patients.
4. Excessive alcohol intake tends to elevate the blood triglyceride level.
5. Excessive alcohol intake for a long period causes cardiomyopathy, which often leads to CHF. Death is the ultimate outcome in advanced cases.
6. Beriberi heart disease is often found in chronic alcoholics.

• Absolute abstinence from alcohol is not necessary for most cardiac patients, but no more than two cocktails or two bottles of beer are recommended as tolerable per day.

• In patients with significant CHF and/or serious cardiac arrhythmias, only one cocktail or one beer is recommended. In severe CHF, of course, no alcohol is allowed.

- Remember that alcohol may dull perception of chest discomfort in cardiac patients. Thus, the severity of chest pain is often underestimated. Use of alcohol for angina pain is absolutely harmful. Alcohol is by no means a substitute for NG.

- A physician should be notified when any symptom (e.g., chest pain) occurs during or after drinking.

- Cardiac patients should not drink alcohol when they experience any cardiac symptom.

- For hypertensive patients and those with a high blood triglyceride level, alcoholic intake should be minimized. At most, two drinks are enough for these people.

- No extraordinary or vigorous physical activity, including sexual intercourse or dancing, is allowed for cardiac patients within two or three hours after alcohol intake.

- In order to stop heavy and chronic drinking, various medical and mental health institutions, as well as private organizations, are available; but a proper education, strong will power, and high motivation are absolutely necessary for the best therapeutic approach.

24

COMMONLY USED TESTS
FOR HEART DISEASES

There have been remarkable developments and advancements in biomedical engineering in the past two or three decades in terms of diagnosis and treatment of various cardiovascular disorders. The availability of many valuable cardiac tests in America and other countries enables physicians to make a correct diagnosis and to provide proper treatment. Various cardiac tests provide information regarding not only the anatomical structures of the heart and related organs or tissues but also the functions of the heart. These test results have to be interpreted and evaluated in conjunction with clinical history and physical findings.

Various diagnostic tests include noninvasive and invasive cardiac tests. A noninvasive test is one performed without using a knife or needle, so that it can be accomplished without any tissue injury or bleeding. On the other hand, invasive diagnostic tests are performed by using a knife and/or needle, so that minimal tissue injury and/or slight bleeding cannot be avoided. In various invasive cardiac tests, one or two catheters (long, thin, flexible plastic tubes) are introduced into various cardiac chambers and large blood vessels connected with the heart through a vein or artery in the arm or groin by way of a small incision. Consequently, invasive cardiac tests usually require a short hospitalization (a few days), and some risks are involved. Since many noninvasive cardiac tests can provide essential diagnostic information in a variety of clinical circumstances, time-consuming, expensive, high-risk, invasive diagnostic tests can often be avoided today.

Common noninvasive diagnostic cardiac tests include (1) Electrocardiogram (commonly known as "EKG" or "ECG"); (2) exercise (stress) electrocardiogram (exercise ECG test); (3) ambulatory (Holter monitor) electrocardiogram (Holter monitor ECG test); (4) chest X-ray (chest roentgenogram); (5) echocardiogram; (6) phonocardiogram; (7) vectorcardiogram (commonly known as "VCG"); and (8) myocardial imaging.

Common invasive cardiac tests include (1) cardiac catheterization, (2) coronary arteriography, (3) hemodynamic monitoring, (4) His bundle ECG, and (5) other electrophysiological studies. In addition, various blood tests and urine tests are often performed on cardiac patients. Carotid sinus stimulation (massage of the side of the neck below the jaw) is frequently applied when dealing with various tachyarrhythmias for diagnostic as well as therapeutic purposes. A renal arteriogram (visualization of the kidney arteries on X-ray films after dye material is injected into the aorta) and an intravenous pyelogram (visualization of kidney structure on the X-ray films after dye material is injected through the vein) are necessary in some patients with high BP when hypertension is considered to be due to possible kidney disease or renal artery stenosis.

ELECTROCARDIOGRAM (ECG)

The ECG is unquestionably the most essential and the most common diagnostic test for every kind of heart disease (and also for many noncardiac disorders). In addition, an ECG is obtained even in healthy individuals for multiple purposes, including preoperative evaluations (e.g., before an appendectomy), screening for life insurance applications, screening for certain job applications, and so on. It is almost a general rule to obtain at least one or two ECG tracings for any individual who is hospitalized, regardless of the reason for the hospitalization. Most periodic medical checkups of healthy people as well as of individuals with illness (particularly suspected or known cardiovascular disorders) include an ECG. The ECG is probably the test most commonly performed in medical practice today.

The ECG is a graphic recording of the electric events of the heart during each heartbeat. The routine ECG includes a 12-lead system that actually records each electrical event from 12 different points. The 12 ECG leads include 6 extremity leads and 6 chest (precordial) leads. Each electrical event coincides with the mechanical event of the heart, and each heartbeat is felt as a pulse (e.g., radial pulse). The ECG registers the P wave (atrial depolarization), the QRS complex (ventricular depolarization), and the T wave (ventricular repolarization) (see Figures 2.1 and 9.1). The ECG is recorded on special ECG paper using an ECG machine. The electric activities generated by the heart are transmitted to the machine through wires connected to small metal plates that are placed on the skin of the arms, legs, and chest using a special ECG paste for best conduction of the electric currents.

The primary value of the ECG is to diagnose heart chamber enlargement, heart attack, and various cardiac arrhythmias (see Figures 3.4 and 9.2 to 9.9). In addition, the ECG can register myocardial ischemia (inadequate oxygen supply to the heart muscle in patients with angina pectoris), myocarditis, pericarditis, various electrolyte imbalances, various drug effects and toxicity, ventricular aneurysm, pulmonary embolism, central nervous system disorders, and so forth. The ECG is also useful in evaluating artificial pacemaker function versus malfunction (see Chapter 16 and Figure 16.1). Many forms of modified ECGs (e.g., Holter monitor ECG; exercise ECG test; continuous ECG monitoring in the CCU, operating rooms, recovery room, and the ER) are equally valuable for diagnosis as well as treatment. ECG abnormalities and cardiac arrhythmias have been discussed elsewhere (see Chapters 3 to 6 and 9 to 18).

EXERCISE (STRESS) ECG TEST

The exercise (stress) ECG test is one of the most popular and important noninvasive cardiac tests today. It has two main purposes: (1) diagnosis of CAD and (2) assessment of functional (physical) capacity. Another reason to perform the exercise ECG test is to evaluate the nature of various cardiac arrhythmias; certain abnormal heart rhythms may be provoked or abolished by physical exercise. An exercise ECG test can help determine the proper therapeutic approach. As a rule, cardiac arrhythmias, particularly those of ventricular origin that are provoked or aggravated by exercise, are clinically serious, and the underlying problem is often CAD.

Until two decades ago, Master's two-step test (the patient goes up and down two wooden steps; the duration and amount of exercise are determined by the patient's age and body weight) was the standard method for the exercise ECG test, but this test has been replaced by modern methods using a motor-driven treadmill or a bicycle ergometer (stationary bicycle). The Master's two-step exercise test has been abandoned because it is not reliable enough to detect an early or mild stage of CAD (meaning a high incidence of false negative tests). In the United States the treadmill exercise ECG test is much more popular than the bicycle exercise ECG test. On the contrary, the bicycle exercise ECG test is very popular in Europe. The amounts and duration of exercise work loads are determined primarily by the patient's age, status of heart disease, and functional capacity. The younger and healthier the individual, the heavier a work load is required.

For the treadmill exercise ECG test, a standard exercise ECG protocol (see Table 3.12) is used, and the exercise work loads are progressively increased every three minutes. Special equipment for continuous ECG monitoring with a motor-driven treadmill is used, and the test is performed by a specially trained technician under the direct supervision of a physician (see Figure 4.3). Before the actual exercise ECG test, a 12-lead resting ECG is obtained to make certain there is no major ECG abnormality to prevent the test. In addition, the physician who will supervise the test examines the patient briefly in order to ascertain the patient's suitability (in physical and cardiac terms) for the test. In the exercise ECG laboratory, all necessary equipment (e.g., DC cardioverter) and commonly used cardiac drugs for CPR must be available, because there is a certain risk (two to three heart attacks per 10,000 and one sudden death per 10,000 tests) involved. The test should be fully explained to the patient beforehand, including the entire procedure and possible risks, and an informed consent form should be obtained before the test is performed. Since certain drugs may influence results, the attending physician who ordered the test should be consulted before the exercise ECG test if necessary.

During the warming-up period, the patient walks on the flat surface (0 grade or no angle or incline) of the treadmill at a very slow speed (1.7 mph) at stage 1 for three minutes. Following this warming-up period, the exercise work loads are increased by elevating the angle of slope or incline up to a 4 percent grade at a faster speed (3.0 mph) at stage 2 for three minutes. After stage 2, the speed of the treadmill remains the same, but the angle of slope is increased with a 4 percent grade in each stage every three minutes until 85 to 90 percent of the predicted maximal heart rate is reached or significant symptoms (e.g., chest pain, marked shortness of breath, severe fatigue), ECG abnormality, significant cardiac arrhythmias, or abnormal BP response (excessive elevation or any reduction) occurs—whichever happens first. The physician who supervises the test will determine when to terminate the exercise ECG test. The standard exercise protocol consists of seven stages for completion, and it takes twenty-one minutes for a full seven-stage course (see Table 3.12). Many young people and even healthy older individuals are able to complete the full seven-stage exercise protocol, and some physically active young people can exercise even beyond stage 7 (stages 8 and 9 are optional; see Table 3.12). Of course, many older people and cardiac patients are unable to complete a full seven-stage exercise protocol, depending upon their degree of physical fitness and/or the severity of their heart disease.

The diagnosis of CAD can be made by recognizing abnormal ECG changes (e.g., S-T segment depression of elevation due to myocardial ischemia) shown on the exercise ECG test (see Figure 4.4). In other words, many coronary patients may have adequate oxygen supply to the heart muscle in the resting state in spite of narrowed coronary artery(ies), and accordingly, the resting 12-lead ECG may be entirely normal. As soon as the exercise work loads are increased beyond the physical limitation of these patients by the exercise ECG test, however, oxygen and blood supply to the heart muscle is no longer adequate because of narrowed coronary artery(ies). The inadequate oxygen and blood supply to the heart muscle causes ECG abnormality(ies) (e.g., S-T segment depression or elevation due to myocardial ischemia—inadequate oxygen supply to the heart muscle) shown on the exercise ECG (see Figure 4.4). As with any other laboratory test, false positive (abnormal test results in the absence of CAD) or false negative (normal or negative test results in spite of definite CAD) results occur occasionally. In addition, the exercise ECG test provides very important information regarding the status of functional capacity. The functional capacity (physical limitation) of a given individual (healthy persons as well as cardiac patients) can be estimated with reasonable accuracy judging from the exercise work loads (energy expenditures) required during the exercise ECG test. In fact, the exercise ECG test is required for certain job applications or activities that require extraordinary physical fitness in order to evaluate people's physical (including cardiac) condition. In addition, some life insurance companies request the exercise ECG test for screening purposes.

Exercise work loads (energy expenditures) are expressed as METs (metabolic units), and the exercise ECG test result can be adapted easily to various physical activities, including ordinary daily activities , recreational activities, sports, or games (see Tables 3.11, 3.12, and 3.13). The determination of functional capacity is extremely important for cardiac patients, particularly heart attack victims, before they return to daily activities after discharge from the hospital, any rehabilitation or exercise program (see Table 21.1), resume sexual activity, and before they return to work (see Chapters 20 and 21). When the exercise ECG test result is equivocal or difficult to interpret, radioisotope study (myocardial imaging) is indicated.

AMBULATORY (HOLTER MONITOR) ELECTROCARDIOGRAM

It can be said that the ambulatory (Holter monitor) ECG is probably one of the most commonly used noninvasive diagnostic cardiac tests today, and it is essential to document any cardiac arrhythmia that occurs only transiently or intermittently. The term *Holter monitor ECG test* is used because the test was invented by Doctor Holter (a scientist [physicist] but not a physician) as early as 1949. It is rather difficult and often impossible to record certain cardiac arrhythmias that occur only transiently, because a routine 12-lead ECG has the capability to record cardiac electrical activity for only ten seconds.

The Holter monitor equipment is a small, portable, tape recorder (comparable in size to a camera or a small, transistorized radio) attached to 2 or 3 ECG leads and electrodes taped to the chest. The patient can carry it on a shoulder strap during all kinds of daily activities at home, at work, and even during various recreational activities and sexual intercourse. The patient is encouraged to participate in a variety of physical activities (except for bathing or swimming) so that certain types of cardiac arrhythmias related to particular physical activities can be reproduced. In addition, the patient is instructed to write down briefly his or her physical activities every hour or so, especially when any symptom (e.g., dizziness, chest pain, palpitations, shortness of breath, near-syncope, or syncope) occurs. From this record, the patient's physical activities and symptoms can be correlated with any particular cardiac arrhythmia recorded on the Holter monitor ECG. Consequently, a precise diagnosis of a given cardiac arrhythmia can be made, and proper treatment can be provided. The Holter monitor ECG is particularly valuable for heart attack victims who progressively increase their physical activities after discharge from the hospital. The exercise ECG test and the Holter monitor ECG are performed frequently on heart attack victims during their first six months after discharge from the hospital.

As for the technical aspects of the Holter monitor ECG, the electrical activities of the heart are recorded on magnetic tape via wires and electrodes connected to the patient. After twenty-four hours of recording, the magnetic tape recording is played back by a specially trained technician via a Holter scanner to reproduce the actual ECG on ordinary ECG paper. It takes an experienced cardiologist only a few minutes to interpret the Holter monitor ECG after a completion of the scanning. Remember that various complaints and symptoms may or may not be related to actual cardiac arrhythmias. When suspected cardiac arrhythmias are not recorded on the Holter monitor ECG, the test may be repeated periodically if necessary. The patient is instructed to perform a particular physical activity during the Holter monitor ECG test when a certain symptom (e.g., palpitations, chest pain) is said to be related to any specific activity (e.g., sexual intercourse).

CHEST X-RAY

The chest X-ray (roentgenogram) is one of the oldest and most commonly used tests in medicine; it certainly is indispensable in detecting various abnormalities, including structures and functions of the heart, lungs, and bones. A routine chest X-ray takes two films, including P-A (posterior-anterior) view and lateral (side) view. When information on any specific heart chamber enlargement or related structures is desired, a cardiac series (four X-ray films of the heart and lungs taken from four different angles or views) is obtained. The enlargement of certain chambers is particularly obvious on the chest X-ray film after the esophagus is filled with barium (the patient swallows barium just before the X-ray film is taken), because the barium-filled esophagus is displaced by the chamber enlargement (particularly left artrial enlargement).

Chest X-ray films provide information regarding the degree of heart chamber enlargement (if any); abnormal location of various structures, including large blood vessels connected to the heart; calcification on the heart valve(s) or other parts of the heart; pericardial effusion; degree of heart failure (if any); and many other abnormalities in the heart and lungs. A chest X-ray is particulary valuable for patients with congenital heart diseases and valvular heart diseases (see Chapters 10 and 11). However, chest X-rays have no value in the diagnosis of angina pectoris or heart attack, although they are indispensable when various complications (e.g.,

CHF) occur. Sometimes, fluoroscopy (the radiologist examines cardiac and pulmonary structures and functions such as calcification, pericardial effusion, and motion of the heart through X-ray by inspection without taking an actual photo) is performed in the darkroom of the X-ray laboratory when necessary. Any abnormality in bone structures (e.g., fracture of the ribs), of course, will be detected by a chest X-ray.

ECHOCARDIOGRAM

The echocardiogram is a relatively new noninvasive cardiac test, but it has become extremely popular in the past decade for diagnosing a variety of heart diseases. The principles of the echocardiogram is somewhat comparable to that used in sonar detection of submarines. Since various structures of the heart (both normal and abnormal) behave differently when ultrasonic waves pass through them, the diagnosis of various cardiac diseases can be made. In particular, such cardiac abnormalities as mitral valve prolapse syndrome (see Chapter 10), IHSS (see Chapters 10 and 12), cardiac tumors (see Chapter 14), and pericardial effusion (see Chapter 13) are diagnosed very accurately by an echocardiogram. In addition, abnormal valve structure or motion, calcification of the valve(s), various chamber enlargements, and status of pumping action can be recognized and assessed with reasonable accuracy. A special device is used for the echocardiogram, which is taken by a specially trained technician under the direct supervision of a cardiologist. The test is painless and simple, and it is harmless to pregnant women and their fetuses. An echocardiogram is usually recorded on special paper, but it can be taken on movie film.

PHONOCARDIOGRAM

The phonocardiogram is a recording of heart sounds, and it is not as popular as other noninvasive diagnostic tests today. A special device has the capability of magnifying heart sounds and heart murmurs, and it produces a graphic recording of these sounds. By evaluating the exact nature and timing of different heart sounds and murmurs, a variety of heart diseases can be diagnosed. Thus, the phonocardiogram is especially useful for diagnosing various valvular and congenital heart diseases (see Chapters 10 and 11).

VECTORCARDIOGRAM

The vectorcardiogram is closely related to the ECG; actually, the former is a modified ECG. Instead of using 12-lead ECG recordings, the vectorcardiogram is a recording of the electrical activity of the heart from three-dimensional views: horizontal (superior to inferior), frontal (anterior to posterior), and sagittal (lateral or side). The vectorcardiogram is recorded in loop form with a special camera on photographic paper (Polaroid film is commonly used). It has been said that a vector-cardiogram provides more diagnostic information than the ECG in certain cardiac abnormalities.

MYOCARDIAL IMAGING

Myocardial imaging (nuclear scanning or radioisotope study of the heart) is a new cardiac test that is considered a noninvasive test although it includes an injection into the arm vein to administer a radioactive isotope. Myocardial imaging has the capability to detect heart muscle damage from heart attack; it can also identify areas of myocardial ischemia.

When small amounts of a radioactive isotope chemical (e.g., thallium) are injected into the arm vein, this radioactive material migrates to the heart muscle. Healthy and damaged heart muscle absorb different amounts of the radioactive material, so that the test result enables physicians to diagnose CAD even when other diagnostic test results are equivocal. Special equipment is utilized for myocardial imaging, and the finding is registered on photographic paper or film. Myocardial imaging can be performed while a patient is in a resting state, but the test is commonly performed in conjunction with the exercise ECG test. Myocardial imaging is especially valuable when the exercise ECG test result is equivocal or difficult to interpret because of various preexisting ECG abnormalities or drug effects (e.g., digitalis) in patients with suspected CAD.

A similar radioisotope study is performed to detect pulmonary embolism. This is called a "lung scan"; a radioactive material is injected into the circulation of the lungs, and areas of the lungs containing blood clots are visualized in this study.

CARDIAC CATHETERIZATION
AND CORONARY ARTERIOGRAPHY (ANGIOGRAPHY)

Cardiac catheterization is an invasive test that requires hospitalization for a few days. Cardiac catheterization is required when the diagnosis is not certain from various noninvasive cardiac tests and, more importantly, when cardiac surgery is planned. The decision on indications versus nonindications for cardiac catheterization has to be made carefully by a cardiologist, who often consults a cardiac surgeon and other cardiologists. Before cardiac catheterization, an informed consent form is obtained because there is a slight risk involved with the test (a mortality rate of 0.3 percent). Of course, the entire test procedure and possible risks should be explained to the patient and family members before cardiac catheterization.

In the technique of cardiac catheterization, a small incision is made into the vein in the groin area or in the crease of the elbow after local anesthesia is administered (the skin made numb by injecting an anesthetic). Cardiac catheterization is performed in the catheterization laboratory, which is fully equipped with special medical devices for the test, an X-ray machine, a special movie camera, monitors for continuous ECG and hemodynamic data, a defibrillator, an artificial pacemaker, and all commonly used cardiac drugs (see Table 6.2). The catheterization team consists of a cardiologist (the head of the team) specially trained in this field, a cardiac nurse(s), an assistant physician(s) (commonly, cardiology fellows), and a specially trained technician(s). As soon as the small incision is made into a vein, a small catheter is inserted in the vein and is slowly pushed into the heart. Depending upon medical indications, one or two catheters are inserted. During manipulation of the catheter(s) into the heart, a cardiologist will constantly observe the direction and location of the catheter under a fluoroscope (seeing through the object with an X-ray machine). As soon as the catheter has reached the desired location in the heart, a chemical (dye) is injected into the catheter, and the dye reaches the various heart chambers and large blood vessels connected with the heart. When CAD is suspected or present, particularly when CABS is scheduled, the dye is also injected into the coronary arteries (see Figure 4.5). X-ray movie films can be taken continuously or intermittently during the entire procedure of cardiac catheterization and coronary arteriography.

Blood samples can be taken through the catheter from different locations of the heart chambers and large blood vessels in order to determine the amount of oxygen in the blood. In addition, pressures in the heart chambers and large blood vessels are measured, and the degree of various valve abnormalities and congenital cardiac lesions (if any) will be demonstrated. Furthermore, the status of the pumping action can be evaluated by recognizing the motion of the entire heart during each heartbeat. Remember that two or more cardiac lesions often coexist. For instance, coronary artery stenosis may involve many arteries, and it may coexist with one or more heart valve lesions.

When the X-ray movie films are developed, the cardiologist will review them with all involved physicians and cardiac surgeons to determine the precise nature of the heart disease and the exact location and degree of valve lesions, the narrowing of coronary arteries, and/or congenital cardiac defects. If necessary, it is possible to make a photograph of any segment of the X-ray movie film (see Figure 4.5). By doing so, an exact diagnosis as well as the proper therapeutic approach will be determined. It is absolutely essential to perform cardiac catheterization when any surgical correction is planned, and coronary arteriography is indispensable before CABS.

HEMODYNAMIC MONITORING

Hemodynamic monitoring is the measurement of pressures in various heart chambers and large blood vessels and the determination of oxygen contents in blood samples obtained from these chambers and blood vessels. Thus, hemo-dynamic monitoring is commonly performed when dealing with very sick cardiac patients, especially those suffering from recent heart attack. These measurements provide very important information for the best therapeutic approach, especially during the first few days following a massive heart attack. In general, two types of catheter are inserted into the heart via a vein with the same technique as cardiac catheterization. Measurements through a catheter located in the pulmonary artery (see Figures 1.1 and 1.2) provide valuable information regarding the degree of CHF and the amount of blood filling the left pumping chamber. BP determination can be made precisely through a catheter placed in an artery of an arm or leg. Blood samples, of course, can easily be obtained through this catheter for the measure-ment of oxygen content or any other necessary tests.

Remember that hemodynamic monitoring is *not* required for every patient with heart attack. It is indicated only for heart attack victims with extensive heart muscle damage, often associated with serious and life-threatening complications such as heart failure and cardiogenic shock. Hemodynamic monitoring is usually carried out in the CCU or any intensive care area with similar facilities.

HIS BUNDLE ELECTROCARDIOGRAPHY

A routine 12-lead ECG cannot provide every detail of the electrical events of the heart, but the recording of electrical events can be carried out by inserting electrodes into the heart chambers. This intracardiac ECG is commonly called a "His bundle ECG" because various intervals and the conduction time of cardiac impulses between various locations can easily and precisely be measured by recognizing the His bundle potential (an electrical event generated by the His bundle or common bundle; see Figure 1.3). The His bundle is a segment of the con-duction pathway located just below the A-V node connecting the atria and the ventricles; in a way, it functions as a bridge to transmit electrical impulses from upper to lower heart chambers.

The basic technique of inserting an electrode catheter and equipment is essen-tially the same as for cardiac catheterization, and the His bundle ECG is usually performed in the cardiac catheterization laboratory. The same precautions should be followed for the His bundle ECG, and a small risk is involved. A consent form is required before performing the test, and procedures should be explained to the patient in detail. The His bundle ECG is recorded on photographic paper by a special recorder. Various electrical events shown in the His bundle ECG enable physicians to understand the exact mechanism of cardiac arrhythmias, the exact site(s) of heart block and the exact origin of any cardiac impulse formation. When these parameters are available, a proper therapeutic approach can be provided. Besides the His bundle ECG, there are many other types of electrophysiologic studies that can be performed in modern medical centers.

CAROTID SINUS STIMULATION

When dealing with various tachyarrhythmias, carotid sinus stimulation is often necessary for the differential diagnosis as well as for treatment, because different responses to this procedure are expected depending upon the nature and origin of the arrhythmia. Carotid sinus stimulation is performed by a physician massaging the side of the patient's neck below the jaw (around the area where the pulse of the neck artery is felt) with one or two fingers. Carotid sinus stimulation requires no instrument or device, and the massage should be done on only one side at a time. Atrial tachycardia (Figure 9.2) is often terminated by carotid sinus stimulation, whereas ventricular tachycardia (Figure 9.4) does not respond to the procedure.

BLOOD TESTS

A variety of blood tests are performed in cardiac patients depending upon the nature of their heart disease and the drugs they are taking. In patients with recent heart attack, blood tests to determine the contents of enzymes are always performed for the diagnosis of heart attack itself as well as for assessment of heart muscle damage (see Chapter 3). Blood tests to determine the values of cholesterol and triglycerides are commonly performed on cardiac patients as well as on healthy people (see Chapter 3). Contents of hemoglobin or hematocrit is often measured in patients with various heart diseases, because the values may be abnormally low (meaning anemia) or abnormally high (meaning polycythemia), depending upon the nature of cardiac disease. For example, most patients with SBE (see Chapter 13) have significant anemia, whereas various congenital cardiac lesions are often associated with polycythemia (see Chapter 10). In addition, long-standing anemia often leads to CHF. Furthermore, white blood cell counts are often elevated in patients with bacterial infection (see Chapter 13). In diabetic patients, the determination of blood sugar is, of course, essential.

When anyone is taking an anticoagulant, periodic blood tests (e.g., pro-thrombin time) should be performed. The determination of blood urea nitrogen (BUN) is indicated when kidney functions are considered abnormal, because BUN often rises in this circumstance. Remember that various kidney diseases commonly cause high BP, and CHF is frequently produced by a long-standing hypertension. Thus, BUN must be measured in patients with high BP, kidney diseases, and/or CHF, so that a proper diagnosis can be entertained and adequate treatment provided.

MISCELLANEOUS

Urinalysis (a urine test) is one of the routine laboratory tests performed on every patient. Various urine tests provide important information for the diagnosis of a

340

variety of cardiac and noncardiac diseases. For instance, the presence of blood in the urine often indicates various kidney diseases and some cardiac diseases. Diabetic patients usually show glycosuria (sugar in the urine). Proteinuria (protein in the urine) is often present in patients with kidney disease and some heart disease. The presence of white blood cells in the urine often indicates infection or inflammation of the kidneys (e.g., pyelonephritis), and many hypertensive individuals have various kidney problems. In hypertensive patients, a renal arteriogram and an intravenous pyelogram are performed when high BP is considered a result of kidney disease or renal artery stenosis.

25

CORONARY BYPASS SURGERY

Increasing numbers of cardiac patients receive various types of cardiac operations today because of improved surgical techniques with more sophisticated equipment and instruments, in conjunction with well-established surgical indications for a variety of cardiac disorders and minimal mortality rates. In particular, coronary artery bypass surgery (CABS) has become the most commonly performed major operation in the United States today; more than 70,000 bypass surgeries are performed annually. In addition to CABS, different types of surgery are also indicated for patients with CAD when they develop major and life-threatening complications such as ventricular septal defect or papillary muscle rupture or dysfunction (rupture or dysfunction of the tissue structure supporting the mitral valve). When complete A-V block develops as a complication of a heart attack, most patients require permanent artificial pacemaker implantation (see Chapter 16). The surgical approaches to various congenital cardiac anomalies and valvular heart diseases have been discussed in Chapters 10 and 11.

Less commonly performed cardiac surgery may include removal of cardiac tumors, repair of various cardiac traumas, aneurysmectomy (resection of a ventricular aneurysm), various surgical approaches to malignant or drug-resistant cardiac arrhythmias, pericardiectomy (resection of a portion of the pericardium), myocardial infarctectomy (resection of the damaged heart muscle due to heart attack), and repair of cardiac rupture (see Chapters 13 and 14). Cardiac transplantation is performed in selected patients at selected medical centers as a last resort, but it is still considered experimental surgery by many physicians (see Chapter 26).

It is extremely important to remember that the indications versus nonindications for any type of cardiac operation have to be carefully considered because the surgical approach does not necessarily guarantee a favorable outcome in every case. In addition, certain surgical risks (although generally minimal) cannot be ignored. Thus, every cardiac case has to be evaluated with extreme care by a competent cardiologist and a cardiac surgeon before any cardiac surgery is attempted. If necessary, medical or surgical consultation may be obtained by the cardiologist for further evaluation. In addition, the patient or family members may request another medical opinion regarding the proposed cardiac surgery from another physician.

CORONARY ARTERY BYPASS SURGERY (CABS)

Remarkable achievements have been accomplished in the field of CABS (see Figure 3.9) in the past decade, but a primitive surgical approach to CAD was attempted as early as 1929. In most modern countries, CABS can be performed in the majority of modern teaching institutions, such as university hospitals. Although indications for CABS differ slightly among physicians, the surgery is performed primarily on patients who experience considerable angina in spite of full medical treatment, especially young individuals (below age fifty). This is true whether the patient suffers from angina with or without previous heart attack. Although CABS is indicated primarily to improve the quality of life for patients with CAD by eliminating or reducing angina attacks, recent medical experience indicates that bypass surgery can also prolong the patient's life in many cases. This is so for relatively young patients with advanced CAD, such as triple-vessel or left main coronary artery lesions. Sudden death from VF in patients with advanced CAD is considered preventable in significant numbers through bypass surgery.

Recent medical reports indicate that angina is eliminated completely after CABS in at least 60 percent of the cases with CAD. Furthermore, considerable improvement of angina (it may not be complete relief from pain) is observed in at least 90 percent of the cases. CABS is performed by removing a saphenous vein (a large vein running the length of each leg) from the leg; the vein is sewn into the heart, bypassing the segment of artery that has narrowing or blockage (see Figure 3.9). Thus, the function of the leg vein for blood circulation in the heart artery is somewhat comparable to a detour on a highway that bypasses an obstruction (e.g., a traffic accident or area under construction) on the road. When the bypass operation is successful, blood circulation to the heart muscle through the bypassed graft will be restored.

It should be stressed that the underlying CAD process (see Figure 2.2) and atherosclerosis cannot be cured or prevented by CABS. By the same token, the development of a new heart attack cannot be prevented even after CABS. The graft of the CABS remains open in 70 to 80 percent of the cases after five years, but the degree of opening of the bypass graft is uncertain beyond five or six years. There is a strong possibility, however, that the duration of the graft patency (opening) will increase progressively in the near future in view of rapidly improving medical and surgical techniques and knowledge.

It is essential to have a coronary arteriogram (visualization of the coronary arteries on X-ray movies after a dye is injected into the heart—a part of cardiac catheterization; see Figure 4.5 and Chapter 24) before considering CABS, so that the exact site and degree of narrowing or blockage of the coronary artery(ies) can be clearly identified. Many other necessary noninvasive cardiac tests (see Chapter 24) are often performed before coronary arteriography. Until recently, CABS usually involved up to four or five coronary arteries; not uncommonly, however, six vessels are bypassed with favorable results today.

Preparations for CABS

Although the diagnosis of CAD can be made on clinical grounds in conjunction with various noninvasive cardiac tests (e.g., 12-lead ECG, exercise ECG test, myocardial imaging) as well as blood tests (for recent heart attack) in most cases, the exact site and degrees of stenosis or obstruction in the diseased coronary artery(ies) are impossible to ascertain without performing coronary arteriography. Thus, it is essential to perform coronary arteriography before attempting coronary artery bypass surgery. In a way, the evaluation of a coronary arteriogram before CABS is comparable to studying a road map before taking a trip.

Before CABS is scheduled, the entire surgical procedure with possible risks should be fully explained to the patient and family members. It is also a good idea to discuss briefly the usual cost involved with CABS and related tests. When the patient is fully satisfied with the information, an informed consent form must be signed by the patient and witnessed by the physician or surgeon. In addition, it should be certain that the cardiac condition is at its optimal state, under the circumstances, and that all the complications (e.g., CHF, cardiac arrhythmias) are under control. Sufficient amounts of blood suitable for transfusion (in the patient's blood type, of course) should be ready before surgery. Furthermore, all necessary equipment and devices as well as commonly used cardiac drugs for CPR should be available in the operating room (see Chapters 15 to 18).

For CABS, the chief cardiac surgeon is assisted by a well-organized team consisting of assistant surgeons, anesthesiologists, specially trained surgical nurses, and technicians who will operate a heart-lung machine and electronic equipment for continuous monitoring of the patient throughout surgery. A cardiologist should also be available for consultation whenever necessary. As a rule, CABS is scheduled ahead of time, and it is performed as an elective operation in most cases. Therefore, most patients require two different hospitalizations—one for diagnostic purposes, including coronary arteriography (for several days), and another for CABS (for about ten days). It is rather uncommon to perform CABS as an emergency operation. When CABS is planned for patients with recent heart attack, it is a general policy to wait about two or three months.

Technical Aspects of CABS

Needless to say, surgical technique greatly influences the outcome of CABS and the incidence of various complications related to the operation, including perioperative MI and even death. At present, the saphenous vein graft technique is a standard method of CABS, and it was introduced in the late 1960s. Less commonly, CABS is performed using an internal mammary artery (an artery supplying blood to a portion of the anterior chest) in place of a saphenous vein but in a similar manner. At times, a saphenous vein graft and an internal mammary artery graft are performed in the same patient, especially when many coronary arteries have to be bypassed simultaneously.

The saphenous vein is a large vein that runs the length of each leg, and it can be removed for CABS because other veins can take over its role in blood circulation to the leg. The saphenous vein is removed from the leg, and it is carefully examined for suitability for CABS. One end of the removed vein is attached to the aorta, and the other end is attached beyond the area of blockage or narrowing in the coronary artery (Figure 3.9). CABS may involve only one artery, but the bypass graft is often performed on four or five coronary arteries (rarely up to six arteries). After the patient is fully anesthesized (with general anesthesia), he or she is connected to the heart-lung machine. The heart-lung machine takes over the functions of both the heart and lungs during the entire operation. The machine removes carbon dioxide from the blood, adds oxygen, and pumps the blood through the body for proper circulation.

The patient's chest is opened, and the heart is stopped by briefly applying two electrodes. Now the surgeon begins CABS. The saphenous vein, after removal and careful testing for suitability, is attached with sutures (stitching material as fine as a human hair)—one end to the aorta and the other to the coronary artery beyond the point of narrowing or blockage (see Figure 3.9). When CABS is completed, the heart-lung machine is disconnected from the patient. The patient's own heart beating is restored. Now blood circulation to the heart muscle is carried out through the graft that bypassed the diseased coronary artery. After the patient's chest is closed, he or she is transferred to the recovery room for close observation. It takes about three to six hours to complete CABS, but it will take longer when many coronary arteries are bypassed and/or when serious complications occur. Following CABS, the patient is observed in the surgical cardiac (intensive) care unit, where continuous monitoring is used for immediate detection and management of possible postoperative complications. The average length of stay in the hospital is approximately ten days, but it varies considerably depending upon the degree of CAD and the presence or absence of major complications.

Indications of CABS

CABS has become a standard therapeutic approach for refractory stable (chronic) angina pectoris (angina in spite of all available medical treatment) and unstable

345

(crescendo) angina pectoris (increasing intensity, frequency, and/or duration of angina, and angina even at rest) in the past decade. In addition, CABS is indicated for patients who experience considerable angina that interferes with a desired life-style in spite of full medical treatment following recovery from a heart attack. Less critical indications of CABS are as follows. Many physicians recommend CABS for young patients with minimal or mild angina pectoris who have significant stenosis (70 percent or more narrowing), or obstruction of the left main coronary artery, double or triple vessels, or the proximal portion of the left anterior descending artery (see Figures 1.4 and 2.2). In addition, CABS is often recommended for Prinzmetal's angina (atypical or variant angina) when a coronary arteriogram documents that the angina is due to persistent marked stenosis or obstruction in the coronary arteries. Furthermore, even in asymptomatic patients, CABS is recommended when the coronary arteriogram, which is performed because of a markedly positive exercise ECG test (see Figure 4.4), reveals significant stenosis or obstruction of the left main coronary artery, or double or triple coronary arteries. By and large, CABS is more frequently performed on younger individuals than on elderly patients.

Various indications for coronary artery bypass surgery are briefly summarized as follows:

1. Unstable angina pectoris
2. Stable angina pectoris that interferes with a desired life-style in spite of full medical treatment
3. Significant angina after recovering from a heart attack in spite of full medical treatment.
4. Young patients with significant stenosis (70 percent or more narrowing) of left main, triple-vessel, double-vessel, or proximal portion of the left anterior descending artery with or without significant symptoms
5. Markedly positive (abnormal) exercise ECG test with minimal exercise work loads (less than 70 percent of the predicted maximal heart rate)
6. Refractory (drug-resistant) ventricular arrhythmias associated with known advanced CAD (a rare indication)

Complications Associated with CABS

Like any other major operation, CABS can be attended or followed by certain complications. In general, the risk of death related to CABS is only 1 to 3 percent, but it may be as high as 20 percent or even higher when dealing with older patients or individuals with advanced multivessel or left main coronary artery lesions. Of course, surgical mortality rates will be higher when there are various preoperative major complications (e.g., CHF, cardiogenic shock, serious cardiac arrhythmias) and/or when the patient has suffered a massive heart attack. One of the most serious complications is the occurrence of a new heart attack during or immediately following CABS. This is called "perioperative MI," and its incidence is reported to be 5 to 15 percent. It is difficult to predict which patient will develop the perioperative MI, although the chances of such a complication occurring will be greater in patients with advanced multivessel CAD. When a new heart attack occurs during or soon after CABS, the patient should be treated in the same manner as described in Chapter 3 (see "Heart Attack").

Unfortunately, the bypass graft may close up in 15 to 20 percent of patients (20 to 30 percent in some reports). When this occurs, the patient may begin to experience angina again, and the chest discomfort may be even worse than before CABS. Some patients with advanced CAD may develop CHF, various cardiac arrhythmias, and cardiogenic shock. These complications must be treated in the usual manner (see Chapter 3). A small number of patients may develop complications involving the lungs, kidneys, brain, and liver (e.g., pneumonia, pulmonary embolism, renal failure, stroke). Excessive hemorrhage and infection may occur in some cases. Significant hypertension may occur with any type of cardiac surgery. It has been shown that *new* hypertension can occur in 30 to 50 percent of patients immediately following CABS. Increased sympathetic activity is considered the mechanism that causes new high BP in this circumstance, but the exact underlying cause is not clearly understood. When hypertension is produced after CABS, it should be treated in the usual manner (see Chapter 5).

Follow-Up Care after CABS

As soon as CABS is completed, the patient is transferred to the recovery room and then is moved again to the surgical cardiac care unit, as the patient's condition permits, for very close observation with continuous monitoring (e.g., ECG, BP). During this immediate postoperative period, the surgical and medical teams usually take care of the patient together, very closely. Any type of complication should be recognized and treated immediately. For example, some patients may require various antiarrhythmic agents (see Table 6.2), whereas others may require an artificial pacemaker or DC shock (see Chapters 16 and 18). CHF and cardiogenic shock should be treated in the usual manner (see Chapters 6 and 7). Any surgical complications (e.g., hemorrhage, wound infection) must be treated by the surgical team immediately. When the immediate postoperative period is over and no significant complication is observed, the patient's physical activity will be gradually and progressively increased in a similar manner as described after heart attack (see Chapter 3). The medical team gradually takes over the major role in postoperative care when the patient is going to be discharged from the hospital soon. As soon as the patient's condition becomes stable, he or she may be transferred to the ordinary hospital ward; the average hospital stay is about ten days.

Before discharge, it is highly recommended to have the Holter monitor ECG in order to make certain there are no significant cardiac arrhythmias. Of course, any significant arrhythmia should be treated (see Table 6.2 and Chapter 9). In addition, it is preferable to perform the exercise ECG test before discharge so that the functional capacity can be determined. This information will be extremely valuable after discharge from the hospital before participating in various physical activities (see Chapters 20 and 21). Of course, the patient cannot be discharged until all and any complications are under control and until the patient's physical condition is suitable for ordinary or minimal daily activities.

After discharge, the patient will be seen by the surgeon once or twice, and then a cardiologist or family physician will take over responsibility for long-term care. A precaution similar to the one described for heart attack victims has to be followed by all cardiac patients after CABS. When angina pain recurs, the patient has to be evaluated immediately, and the coronary arteriogram may have to be repeated in certain patients. Remember that underlying CAD and the process of atherosclerosis are by no means cured by CABS. Some patients may require one or more cardiac drugs even after successful bypass surgery.

Costs Involved with CABS

Before scheduling CABS, the usual costs involved in the surgery should be discussed with the patient and family members. By doing so, unnecessary misunderstanding and frustration can be avoided. The average cost of CABS is about $12,500 for each patient, and the total annual cost of this surgical treatment is estimated to be more than a billion dollars in the United States. Fortunately, the cost of CABS is paid by most medical insurance companies, at least in part (depending upon coverage), but the financial aspect cannot be ignored when the individual has no medical (health) insurance at all. Unnecessary worry about the financial burden is, of course, harmful for CAD. Thus, every individual should have some form of health insurance all the time.

CORONARY ANGIOPLASTY

As an alternative treatment to coronary artery bypass surgery, percutaneous transluminal coronary angioplasty (often called "coronary angioplasy") can be performed in selected cases of symptomatic coronary artery disease. The technique of coronary angioplasty was developed originally by Dr. Andreas Grüntzig and his colleagues in Switzerland, and approximately 1,000 coronary angioplasties have been performed worldwide (more than 500 cases in the United States) at this writing.

The best candidates for coronary angioplasty are those whose disease is limited to one important coronary artery and who have been symptomatic for less than two years. When coronary artery disease has existed for many years, there is a greater probability of rigid coronary artery stenosis, leading to less or no effectiveness of coronary angioplasty. Patients with multivessel coronary artery disease are *not* considered candidates for coronary angioplasty, because relieving only one of multiple lesions is unlikely to relieve the symptoms. Coronary angioplasty is likely to succeed only when the stenotic (narrowed) area is discrete and not totally occluded (blocked). When there is considerable calcification in the coronary arterial wall, coronary angioplasty is contraindicated because the stenosis will be too rigid to be affected by the procedure. Likewise, coronary angioplasty is *not* recommended for left main coronary artery stenosis, because long-term (one-year) results suggest that coronary artery bypass surgery is found to be superior to coronary angioplasty. Coronary angioplasty is difficult to perform when dealing with a very distal coronary artery lesion or stenosis involving a small and tortuous branch of the coronary artery.

As far as the technique for coronary angioplasty is concerned, a guiding catheter is introduced through a systemic artery and is advanced to the orifice of the narrowed coronary artery, in a manner similar to cardiac catheterization and coronary arteriogram. Then an inner balloon catheter is advanced to the stenotic area. When inflated, the balloon compresses atherosclerotic plaque, leading to relief of the stenosis in the involved coronary artery.

By and large, all patients who are under consideration for coronary artery bypass surgery can be screened for possible coronary angioplasty. Then the best candidates suitable for coronary angioplasty (as discussed previously) will be selected. Thus, all possible candidates for the procedure are significantly symptomatic, and all of them have already had coronary arteriography.

Since angioplasty's chance of success is estimated at approximately 60 percent, in addition to the possible development of complications (e.g., perforation or dissection of a coronary artery), cardiac surgeons must be available immediately (within one to two hours) for an emergency coronary artery bypass surgery.

Coronary angioplasty is performed by a cardiologist, specially trained in this field, in the cardiac catheterization laboratory. As far as the patient's sensation is concerned, there is no significant difference between coronary angioplasty and coronary arteriography except for a brief moment of angina during balloon inflation. In general, coronary angioplasty involves about a three-day hospitalization, and the patient may return to full activity if the procedure is successful.

The incidence of complications (as already mentioned) associated with coronary angioplasty has been in the range of 5 percent, and the mortality for well-selected patients is not more than 1 percent.

Coronary angioplasty is considered an investigational (experimental) procedure at present, and the short-term therapeutic result is reported to be favorable. Further investigations will be necessary for evaluation of the long-term efficacy of coronary angioplasty. There is a strong possibility that coronary angioplasty may become a routine therapeutic approach for a selected group of symptomatic coronary artery disease patients within one or two years as an alternative to coronary artery bypass surgery.

SURGERY FOR COMPLICATIONS ASSOCIATED WITH HEART ATTACK

Various surgical procedures are indicated for some heart attack victims when there are significant complications that are difficult or impossible to manage medically. Some surgeons have performed infarctectomies (resection of the infarcted or damaged heart muscle) when the patient develops cardiogenic shock or CHF following a heart attack, but the mortality rate is reported to be extremely high. Therefore, these operative procedures should still be considered experimental, and they may be performed only as a last resort. Ventricular aneurysmectomy (resection of the ventricular aneurysm) is recommended only when the patient suffers from considerable and persistent CHF and when there is well-demarcated paradoxical motion (abnormal movement of a portion of the pumping chambers of the heart confirmed by ventriculography—an X-ray movie showing the movement of the heart chambers during each heart cycle). Resection is *not* recommended, however, for a minor asymptomatic ventricular aneurysm or for diffuse, flabby, and irregular hypokinesis (markedly reduced movement of the pumping chambers as a result of poor contractile force in the heart muscle shown by ventriculography).

Surgical repair is indicated for ventricular septal defect or mitral insufficiency as a result of papillary muscle dysfunction or rupture of the chordae tendineae (see Chapter 3) after the lesion is stabilized (preferably for four to ten weeks) if significant CHF persists. For significant mitral regurgitation, replacement of the mitral valve is indicated. Some patients may require two or more different types of cardiac operations, such as CABS plus mitral valve replacement or ventricular septal defect repair, consecutively on the same day.

26

HEART
TRANSPLANTATION

Heart transplantation means that the entire heart of the cardiac patient is replaced by the heart of someone else, because far-advanced heart disease is so severe that it is no longer treatable using all available medical and surgical therapy. In other words, a recipient receives a donor's (often an accident victim) heart to replace the diseased heart so that the surgically implanted donor's heart will function for the recipient. Although heart transplantation is still considered experimental by many physicians, it should be considered therapeutic in view of its markedly improved survival rate in recent years. An improved survival rate is greatly enhanced by the proper selection of a recipient, refinements in surgical technique, and early recognition, prevention, and treatment of rejection phenomena. The current survival rate at one year is reported to be near 70 percent, with a 30 to 40 percent survival rate at five years. The longest survival is reported to be more than ten years. The survival rate after heart transplantation is comparably favorable to that of kidney transplantation. The rehabilitation to normal or near-normal heart function following transplantation has been observed in 90 percent of one-year survivors.

At this writing, more than 400 human heart transplants (some patients required more than one transplant) have been performed since the first heart transplantation in late 1967. Without question, the Stanford University (Stanford, California) cardiac transplantation program, directed by Dr. Norman Shumway, has led the world. At least two-thirds of all heart transplants (213 heart transplants for 195 patients) have been accomplished by the Stanford team. There are three other medical centers that have carried out major heart transplantation programs. They include the Groote Schuur Hospital in Capetown, South Africa, directed by Dr. Christiaan Barnard; Hôpital de la Pitié in Paris, France; and the Medical College of Virginia in Richmond, Virginia. Each of these medical centers has performed more than twenty-five heart transplants. In addition, there are new heart transplantation centers, which include the University of Arizona, Tucson; University of Wisconsin, Madison; Columbia University, New York, New York; and Downstate Medical Center, Brooklyn, New York.

It is difficult to estimate the number of potential heart transplant recipients, but about 75,000 patients will be evaluated for possible heart transplantation per year in the United States alone. The Stanford transplantation team predicts that approximately twenty-five transplants will be performed annually in the future at their institution. Heart transplantation is considered only for critically ill patients with far-advanced heart disease and intractable CHF (class IV functional class according to the New York Heart Association criteria) when all available medical and surgical treatment cannot improve cardiac condition. There are many factors that prevent heart transplantation, but one of the important considerations is the patient's age. By and large, heart transplantation is recommended for patients below fifty years of age.

HISTORICAL CONSIDERATIONS

The first heart transplantation was accomplished in an experimental animal study by Carrel and Guthrie in 1905 in America. They sutured a canine donor to the neck vessels of another dog; this heterotopic (outside the normal or usual heart position in the chest cavity) graft functioned for about two hours before blood clotting. Following this, heterotopic heart transplants were performed by a number of surgeons using various locations, including the neck, abdomen, and thorax. An invaluable contribution, indispensable for further development in total heart transplantation, was accomplished by Lower and Shumway of Stanford University in 1960. Their surgical technique was orthotopic (placement of the heart in the normal position) transplantation of the canine heart. In their series of eight consecutive canine heart transplants, five recipient dogs were able to live for six to twenty-one days. Without doubt, their surgical technique in experimental animal studies for the next several years created the sound foundation for the achievement of human heart transplantation in the late 1960s.

The rejection phenomenon after heart transplantation of canine hearts was recognized by these pioneers of the Stanford surgical team while they were attempting to prolong life in recipient dogs. They noted a progressive reduction of the amplitude of the QRS complex on the ECG, usually starting several days before death from rejection. Prolongation of survival to as long as one year was accomplished when these animals received immunosuppressive therapy (treatment for a foreign-body rejection phenomenon) with methylprednisolone (a form of cortisone) and azathioprine (Imuran). Unfortunately, some animals died from drug toxicity (primarily infection) during immunosuppressive therapy.

Human heart transplantation was attempted for the first time in January 1964. The heart of a 96-lb chimpanzee was orthotopically transplanted into a sixty-eight-year-old man with far-advanced CAD. Unfortunately, he died within one hour after the transplantation. Almost four years later, the first successful human heart transplantation was accomplished in December 1967 by Dr. Christiaan Barnard (South Africa) using a donor's heart in a fifty-four-year-old man. He died eighteen days later from pneumonia. At almost the same time, in December 1967, Dr. Adrian Kantrowitz (U.S.A.) transplanted a heart into an infant with tricuspid atresia (a form of congenital heart disease), but this baby died twelve hours later. The second heart transplantation by Barnard, performed on January 3, 1968, led to long-term survival.

The first heart transplantation at the Stanford University Medical Center was performed on January 6, 1968, on a fifty-four-year-old man with cardiomyopathy. He died fifteen days later as a result of gastrointestinal hemorrhage and gram-negative sepsis (a form of generalized bacterial infection). The second case performed at the Stanford University center took place on May 1, 1968, on a forty-year old man, who also died three days later from hypoxemia. Up to this point, significant discouragement among cardiac surgeons was inevitable in view of the high mortality rate and short survival after heart transplantation. Nevertheless, progressive improvements in many areas, including surgical technique, better selection of recipients and donors, and early recognition, prevention, and treatment of rejection phenomena, have been accomplished in order to attain longer survival after heart transplantation.

PROPER INSTRUCTIONS TO POTENTIAL RECIPIENTS AND FAMILY MEMBERS

When a patient is considered suitable for heart transplantation from a medical viewpoint, the potential recipient and family members should be properly informed regarding all aspects of the surgery. The risk-benefit ratio should be clearly indicated. The potential recipient must be willing to accept a 30 to 40 percent three-month mortality rate and must fully understand the complexity, consequences, and various complications. He or she should be informed that only one patient in the world's literature has survived for more than ten years and that the five-year survival rate is 30 to 40 percent. The patient should know that lifelong immunosuppressive therapy and the use of Persantine and Coumadin (a kind of blood thinner) are indicated after heart transplantation.

Serious potential complications (discussed shortly) after heart transplantation should be explained to the patient. Some patients develop recurrent infections and hemorrhage as a result of the lifelong immunosuppressive therapy. Others may also develop Cushing's syndrome (defined previously—see Chapter 5) and diabetes mellitus as a result of continuous corticosteroid therapy. After heart transplantation, impotence (the inability to achieve erection and/or ejaculation) has continued to be a common complication for over 50 percent of male patients. It is mandatory to have close and lifelong medical follow-ups by a competent physician who is fully familiar with all aspects of heart transplantation.

INDICATIONS FOR HEART TRANSPLANTATION (SELECTION OF RECIPIENTS)

The proper selection of recipients for heart transplantation is extremely important for longer survival. By and large, the ideal recipient is a young patient (below age fifty) who is dying of end-stage heart disease in spite of all available medical and surgical treatment, but who is otherwise healthy both physically and mentally (meaning no disease of any organ other than the heart). These potential recipients should have a poor prognosis for surviving the next six to twelve months, and they suffer from intractable CHF. In the Stanford series, eleven patients between the ages of twelve and twenty-one years have had heart transplantations, and their overall survival from one month to four years was 64 percent. Most of the young recipients have had cardiomyopathies. Most commonly (in 55 percent of the recipients), heart transplantation has been performed in patients with advanced CAD. The remainder have had cardiomyopathies of various origins and uncorrectable congenital heart lesions.

Contraindications for heart transplantation have to be carefully evaluated; otherwise, a good survival rate cannot be expected. In general, common contraindications include severe irreversible pulmonary hypertension with increased pulmonary vascular resistance greater than three to four times normal, lung diseases including pulmonary infarction (dead lung tissue as a result of blood clot in the lungs), active infection, diabetes mellitus requiring insulin injection, cachexia or any other debilitating systematic disease, mental disorders, and malignancy. It is important to remember that right ventricular failure rapidly develops after heart transplantation when there is significantly increased pulmonary vascular resistance. In addition, some other contraindications are a positive cross-match test between the recipient's serum and the donor's lymphocytes, ABO blood type incompatibility, and inappropriate size between the recipient's and the donor's heart. It is contraindicated to transplant a small donor's heart into a large recipient's heart. On the contrary, a large donor's heart into a small recipient's heart creates no problem. In fact, there may be some beneficial effects of transplanting a large donor's heart into a small recipient. Unfortunately, significant numbers of potential recipients die at various transplantation centers while they are waiting for donors or while they are being evaluated.

DONOR SELECTION AND MANAGEMENT

The proper selection of cardiac donors is critical for successful heart transplantation and long survival. The ideal cardiac donors should be young, healthy individuals who died suddenly from some form of accident or brain hemorrhage. Male cardiac donors are preferably younger than thirty-five, whereas female donors should be younger than forty years of age. In the Stanford program, the average age of the donors has been twenty-seven years. When potential cardiac donors are older than the age limits mentioned, coronary arteriography should be performed to rule out CAD even if there is no history of heart disease. Most potential cardiac donors are accident victims and have injuries to various organs, particularly the brain. Therefore, any possible trauma to the chest, especially the heart, should be carefully evaluated; various medications given and procedures provided during CPR should be reviewed in depth. It is important to ascertain the exact duration of cardiopulmonary arrest and hypotension that may have damaged the heart considerably. If possible, a careful history regarding the presence or absence of any heart disease should be obtained from relatives of the potential cardiac donor. When there is any evidence of significant heart damage or known heart disease, the victim's heart cannot be used in a transplant. When the potential cardiac donor is found to have a normal heart and when there is no contraindication, he or she is accepted.

From the medicolegal viewpoint, it is extremely important, before removing the potential donor's heart, to follow acceptable criteria and to confirm the definition of brain death, which varies slightly from state to state. The Harvard criteria are frequently utilized to define brain death. In general, the criteria include (1) no spontaneous movements or breathing, (2) no reflexes, (3) unreceptivity and unresponsivity; and (4) a flat electroencephalogram (EEG—a recording of brain waves).

As far as proper management of the potential donor's heart is concerned, generally there are two approaches. Most commonly, the potential donor's heart is removed in an adjacent operating room in conjunction with the recipient procedure so that there will be the shortest possible cardiac ischemia time of thirty to forty-five minutes. The second method, which has been used more often since 1977, involves donor cardiectomy (removal of the donor's heart) at a distant hospital; the heart is then transported very rapidly by airplane to the transplantation center. Of course, the donor's heart has to be well treated (i.e., myocardial preservation using a topical or coronary flush-cooling technique) before and during transportation. In the latter method, the donor's heart can be more readily available so that unnecessary waiting by potential recipients after acceptance into a heart transplantation program can be minimized.

In the Medical College of Virginia program, the transplantation team will fly to the donor hospital to obtain the heart when an acceptable donor is located. When a potential recipient for heart transplantation is approved by the team, the patient's blood type is communicated to fifty-two different transplant centers in the eastern United States for blood matching. Following this procedure, when an acceptable donor is located, the legal definitions of death should be satisfied and all medicolegal permissions obtained before actual management of the donor's heart. The donor's heart is stored in the iced saline and is transported rapidly to the transplantation center. This team has successfully transplanted hearts into twenty-two patients using this method of donor heart procurement without major complications, with a mean ischemic time of 3.5 hours and a mean waiting time of ten to fourteen days.

At present, the safe period for storage of the donor's heart is not clearly established. Needless to say, the shortest storage time will enhance the results of heart transplantation and prolong survival.

SURGICAL TECHNIQUE AND IMMEDIATE POSTOPERATIVE CARE

When a suitable donor's heart is selected and all necessary preparations are made, the surgical technique itself is not extremely complicated. The technique of orthotopic (placement of the heart in the normal position) transplantation has been modified slightly since its original description by Lower and Shumway. After placing the recipient on cardiopulmonary bypass, the recipient's heart is removed from the body, leaving the posterior walls of the right and left atria with their venous connections in place. The atria of the donor's heart are opened posteriorly and sutured to the corresponding structures of the residual atria of the recipient; finally, the great vessels are anastomosed (end-to-end anastomosis of the aorta, end-to-end anastomosis of the pulmonary artery, and so forth). The usual immediate postoperative care is similar to that after other major cardiac surgery.

After approximately thirty minutes of resuscitation of the beating transplanted heart, cardiopulmonary bypass is discontinued. Intravenous infusion of isoproterenol or dopamine (both agents increase pumping action) is started in order to improve cardiac output. As a rule, broad-spectrum antibiotics are administered before the initial incision in order to prevent infection. Immunosuppressive therapy is initiated with azathioprine (Imuran) by mouth preoperatively in a daily dosage of about 2 mg/kg (150 mg/day). As soon as cardiopulmonary bypass is discontinued, immunosuppressive therapy is continued with 500 mg of methylprednisolone (a cortisonelike agent) intravenously every eight hours until the patient is able to take medications by mouth. When the patient begins to take medications orally (usually the first day after transplantation), prednisone (also a cortisonelike drug) is started by mouth in a dosage of 100 mg/day. The prednisone is tapered by 5 mg/day until the daily dosage becomes 1 mg/kg. Then a maintenance dose of this drug is continued for the first four to eight weeks. At the same time, when the patient is able to take drugs orally, Imuran is also started with the same dosage as already described; the drug should be continued indefinitely as long as toxic effects on bone marrow and/or liver are not observed. The dosage of Imuran has to be reduced when liver toxicity occurs or when the white blood cell count is reduced significantly. Various rehabilitation efforts, including physical therapy, occupational therapy, and psychosocial counseling with the patient and family, are begun during the first postoperative week.

EARLY POSTOPERATIVE COURSE AND MANAGEMENT

Most patients are hospitalized for approximately two months following heart transplantation, and during this period an aggressive immunosuppressive therapy is the most important part of preventing and treating the rejection phenomenon. High doses of methylprednisolone, prednisone, and Imuran are given as outlined previously, and the dosages have to be adjusted according to the patient's response. In addition, the early rejection phenomenon is reduced considerably when antithymocyte globulin is administered for the first two to three months after transplantation.

Common manifestations of the rejection phenomenon include a reduction in the amplitude of the QRS voltage, atrial tachyarrhythmias, and gallop rhythm. Among these findings, the reduction of the QRS voltage is the most frequent and a sensitive sign of the rejection phenomenon. Therefore, ECGs have to be taken frequently, and any change in the QRS voltage has to be carefully evaluated. The rejection phenomenon is usually confirmed by muscle biopsy (microscopic examination of tissue) of the right ventricular subendocardium (inner layer of the right pumping chamber).

When acute and significant rejection phenomena are diagnosed, the dosages of immunosuppressive agents have to be increased. Fortunately, the rejection phenomenon can be reversed in 90 to 95 percent of the cases with high doses of methylprednisolone and antithymocyte globulin. As expected, aggressive immunosuppressive therapy leads to serious infectious complications. Most patients suffer about two or three episodes of infectious complications during the first year after transplantation. Infection is the most common cause of death following heart transplantation. Infection accounts for 62 percent of all deaths in the first three months after transplantation, and for 46 percent of deaths after the first three months in the Stanford series. Infections most commonly occur in the lungs, accounting for 47 percent of all types of infections, but any organ may be involved. Infections in the bloodstream and urinary tract are the next most common complication. Tuberculosis may be reactivated, and kidney infection may recur. Therefore, sputum and urine culture tests must be obtained before surgery. Skin tests for tuberculosis and various fungus infections are also valuable, especially when these diseases are suspected.

Various preventive measures for infections include prophylactic antibiotics, reverse isolation, adjustment in room ventilation (e.g., the use of increased-pressure air-conditioning with a good air-filter system or an electric air-cleaner), and special nursing care. Cephalosporin and gentamycin are given one hour prior to heart transplantation and for forty-eight hours after surgery as prophylactic antibiotic therapy. Mouthwashes with tetracycline and amphotericin-B are used for the first several weeks after surgery. When the patient has to be in the hospital outside his or her room even for a few minutes, a mask has to be worn to avoid any infection in the respiratory tract. Chest X-ray films are taken daily for approximately two weeks following heart transplantation and then two to three times per week until discharge. When any sign of infection is noted in the chest X-ray film, sputum culture tests are obtained immediately to identify the causative bacteria, and an appropriate antibiotic is administered accordingly. In general, high doses of antibiotics are required, and multiple drugs are often indicated for prolonged periods in all posttransplantation patients when any form of infectious complication occurs.

LATE POSTOPERATIVE COURSE AND LONG-TERM TREATMENT

All patients should have lifelong medical care under a competent physician after heart transplantation. After discharge from the hospital, patients require medical checkups once or twice weekly for the next three to six months. During this early postdischarge period, patients are closely observed for signs of rejection of infection as the dosage of prednisone is tapered to an average of 0.4 mg/kg at one year. When a late rejection phenomenon occurs after discharge, the oral prednisone dosage is doubled, with tapering dosages during a two-week period. In the Stanford series, after one year, there is an average of one rejection phenomenon per 365 patient days and one episode of serious infection per 445 patient days. Therefore, it is essential to have continuous medical surveillance at two- to four-week intervals.

Adequate functional capacity is maintained in the transplanted heart at rest and even during physical exercise. Although the transplanted heart is denervated (lacks nerve control), near-normal cardiac output is maintained so long as there is no rejection phenomenon or any other major complication. During physical exercise, stroke volume (the amount of blood ejected by the pumping chambers) rises first; then increased levels of circulating catecholamines speed up the heart rate. Consequently, the transplanted heart has the capability of maintaining near-normal heart function in 90 percent of long-term survivors in the Stanford series. Thus, many posttransplantation patients have returned to productive, active lives.

Another major complication is the development of accelerated coronary atherosclerosis in the transplanted heart in a small number of patients. This complication usually occurs within eighteen to forty-eight months following transplantation, and the accelerated atherosclerotic process is considered to be due to rejection-induced injury to the coronary artery. It is not uncommon to observe markedly elevated blood cholesterol levels (350 to 450 mg percent), even when these patients follow strict low-fat and low-calorie diets. The patient is unable to experience chest pain because the transplanted heart is denervated even when there is far-advanced coronary artery narrowing causing angina pectoris or even heart attack. As a consequence, sudden death may occur from serious ventricular arrhythmias or acute CHF secondary to a massive, painless heart attack as a result of accelerated atherosclerosis. Therefore, close medical supervision with frequent ECGs and blood tests (to determine cholesterol levels) is essential.

SURVIVAL AND PROGNOSIS

Since all patients who have received heart transplants have suffered from far-advanced heart disease with intractable CHF, a high mortality rate is certainly expected. Nevertheless, the one-year survival rate approaches 70 percent, with a 30 to 40 percent five-year survival rate. When patients survive the critical first three months after heart transplantation, the one-year survival rate approaches 80 percent. After one year, the annual survival rate is progressively reduced by 4 to 6 percent a year. At this writing, there is only one patient in the world who has survived more than ten years after transplantation.

FINANCIAL ASPECTS

The average cost for initial hospitalization for heart transplantation ranges from $60,000 to $70,000 in the Stanford program. At the Medical College of Virginia, the cost is slightly less. In the University of Arizona program, the average cost of initial hospitalization for three transplant patients was reported to be only $21,600 per patient. The average cost for medications, various tests, and medical surveillance after the first year is estimated at about $2,000 to $3,000.

27

A PRACTICAL
MEDICAL GUIDE

• The same disease process involves both angina pectoris and heart attack but to different degrees. Irreversible heart muscle damage occurs in heart attack, but angina pectoris does not cause permanent damage. Heart attack is often preceded by angina pectoris.

• Heart attack is the number one killer in the modern world, and at least 600,000 people die of heart attacks annually in the United States alone. About half those 600,000 deaths occur before the patient reaches the hospital.

• Immediate and proper medical attention is extremely important because a few minutes may mean the difference between life and death. Many heart attack victims die needlessly when the heart is only minimally damaged, primarily because of delayed medical attention. Sudden death often occurs even if heart damage is minimal because of "electric failure" of the heart. Medical attention is often delayed because patients and family members misinterpret the symptoms. Unnecessary delays can be avoided when the general public is adequately educated and motivated.

• When cardiopulmonary arrest is not immediately treated (within four minutes), brain damage is often permanent even if heart function returns to normal. In this case, the patient becomes a semiinvalid.

360

• When proper medical attention is provided immediately, many heart attack victims recover completely and may return to previous activities, including productive jobs.

• Heart attack can be prevented in many ways, by controlling and even eliminating various risk factors.

• Cigarette smoking and birth control pills have a cumulative effect in speeding up the process of atherosclerosis and the development of CAD and other thromboembolic phenomena.

• All cardiac patients with known CAD should try even harder to control or eliminate various risk factors. A heart attack victim who smokes cigarettes after recovery is being not only foolish but also rather suicidal.

• There are many excellent medications for heart attack and its complications (CHF, cardiac arrhythmias, cardiogenic shock), but the most important therapeutic approach is physical and mental rest, especially during the first few weeks.

• CABS is the most common major surgery performed in America today; more than 70,000 CABS operations are performed annually. CABS not only improves the quality of the patient's life but can prolong the life span of many patients as well.

• CABS is primarily indicated for severe angina (with or without previous heart attack), in spite of full medical treatment, that interferes in the daily life of the patient.

• The angina symptom is entirely eliminated after CABS in at least 60 percent of cases. CABS improves the symptom of angina considerably in at least 90 percent of the cases. Surgical mortality is not more than 1 to 3 percent, and the incidence of perioperative MI is 5 to 15 percent.

• The graft of CABS remains open in 70 to 80 percent of cases after five years.

• It is essential to perform coronary arteriography before CABS.

• The saphenous vein graft is the most common approach to CABS.

• It is essential to follow the doctor's advice very closely after discharge, and physical activity has to be increased very gradually as is tolerated under medical guidance. A sudden or excessive physical work load is hazardous to the heart.

• In general, the individual's physical capacity can be easily determined judging from the work load he or she is able to perform in the exercise ECG test. The exercise work load or energy expenditure is expressed with the MET concept, and the exercise ECG test result can easily be applied to various daily activities (see Tables 3.11 and 3.13).

• Although the speed of recovery after a heart attack may vary considerably, depending upon various factors, young people with mild heart attack can recover completely within four to eight weeks.

• When any new symptom occurs during the recovery period, immediate medical attention should be sought. The patient or a family member should call the medical emergency number 911 or an ambulance to go to a nearby hospital ER when the clinical situation seems urgent; his or her physician should be notified promptly.

• It is highly desirable for the general public, especially all family members of heart attack victims, to learn how to perform CPR.

• Any physical activity that requires work loads with a heart (pulse) rate beyond 130 beats/min. should be avoided during the recovery period after a heart attack.

• Sexual activity may be resumed about seven to eight weeks after a heart attack in most cases. However, any sexual relationship with a person other than one's usual partner should be avoided because extraordinary work loads are often required. Sexual activity should be avoided within two to three hours after a meal and/or alcohol consumption.

• Extraordinary physical activity of any kind should be avoided within two to three hours after a meal and/or alcohol consumption.

• The following activities should be avoided after recovery from a heart attack:

1. Sudden and vigorous physical exercise of any form.
2. Competitive sports such as an intense tennis game (singles).
3. Isometric activities such as lifting heavy objects, pushing or pulling a disabled car or similar object, opening a stuck window, and so forth.
4. Walking, running, or other physical activities in a very cold or very hot and humid environment (snow shoveling on a cold day is the worst physical activity).
5. Walking or other forms of physical activities should be avoided when the patient is tired, emotionally disturbed, or suffers from any cardiac symptom. Exercise does not cure any cardiac symptom or fatigue.
6. Straining during a bowel movement.
7. Intense arguments or fistfights.

• Driving an automobile is allowed ten to twelve weeks after a heart attack in most cases. However, driving in heavy traffic, especially during rush hours, should be avoided.

• After a heart attack, most people may be able to return to their previous jobs within two to three months.

• CABS by no means cures or prevents atherosclerosis or underlying CAD. Therefore, constant precautions with close medical supervision are necessary even after CABS.

• Angina pectoris is chest pain as a result of insufficient blood supply to the heart muscle secondary to narrowing of one or more coronary arteries. Typical angina is usually provoked by an extraordinary physical activity, and the chest pain usually subsides upon resting or taking NG.

• Angina usually lasts from a few minutes to ten or twenty minutes. When angina lasts longer than twenty minutes or the pain persists even after resting or after taking two or more NG, a heart attack should be suspected, and immediate medical attention should be sought.

• Angina pectoris is most commonly due to coronary artery stenosis as a result of atherosclerosis, but it may be due to spasm involving one or more coronary arteries. Not uncommonly, coronary artery stenosis (fixed lesion) and spasm co-exist. Coronary artery spasm alone may cause a heart attack.

• For long-term medical treatment of angina pectoris, propranolol (Inderal) and many long-acting nitrates are frequently used in conjunction with intermittent sublingual NG.

• NG should always be fresh (not more than six months old), and they should be kept in a relatively cool place away from direct sunlight.

• When BP is abnormally elevated (above 140/90 mmHg in adults), it is called *hypertension.* Conversely, the term *hypotension* is used when BP is lower than normal. Hypotension is a common manifestation of shock.

• Elevated diastolic blood pressure is more serious clinically than elevated systolic pressure, but most hypertensive patients have elevation of systolic as well as diastolic pressure.

• It is important to recognize and treat hypertension because it often leads to an increased risk of heart attack, angina pectoris, CHF, kidney failure, and stroke.

• One of every six American adults has high BP (at least 20 million people, and possibly as many as 35 million), but half of them are not aware of it. Thus, a medical checkup is necessary from early childhood, especially when high BP or heart disease runs in the family.

• Although the exact cause of hypertension is unknown (called "essential" hypertension) in 90 percent of the cases, high BP can be relatively well controlled with a low-salt diet, weight reduction, and various antihypertensive medications.

• High BP may be completely curable when an identifiable cause or known underlying disease is found (called "secondary" hypertension) and corrected.

• There is a bidirectional relationship between kidney disease and hypertension. Namely, various kidney disorders frequently cause high BP, and high BP often produces damage to the kidneys that may lead to kidney failure.

• Hypertension is often produced by oral contraceptives in sensitive women. Dicontinuation of oral contraceptives is sufficient to treat high BP in this circumstance in most cases.

• Common manifestations of high BP include epistaxis (nose bleeds), headache, and dizziness, but many hypertensive individuals may be asymptomatic, especially in mild cases.

• When one or more antihypertensive medications are prescribed, these drugs must be taken regularly and indefinitely, and periodic medical checkups are necessary.

• Thiazide diuretics (water pills) are the most commonly used drugs for hypertension, and propranolol (Inderal) is also frequently prescribed.

• CHF means that the heart is unable to pump enough blood to meet the demands of the body. Thus, CHF is a final expression of deteriorating function of the heart; it is by no means a complete diagnosis of heart disease.

• CHF is primarily due to two major mechanisms: (1) impairment of myocardial contractile force (e.g., heart attack, cardiomyopathy) and (2) mechanical abnormality (e.g., valvular heart diseases and various congenital heart diseases).

• The most common cause of CHF is hypertension.

• CHF is classified into four categories, from functional class I to IV according to the New York Heart Association criteria. Functional class I is the mildest form, whereas class IV is the worst case.

• The earliest symptom of CHF is dyspnea on exertion, and it is soon followed by fatigue, nocturnal dyspnea, orthopnea, and ankle edema. In severe cases, acute pulmonary edema may develop, and it may be fatal unless treated promptly.

• The objectives of treatment for CHF are to eliminate or correct the underlying cause, increase the force and efficiency of the heart's pumping action, and reduce abnormal retention of sodium and water.

• A specific search should be made for surgically correctable cardiac lesions, especially when CHF fails to respond to conventional medical therapy.

• Many mild cases of CHF can be managed successfully with restriction of salt intake and physical activity, digitalis, and diuretics.

• It is important to take prescribed medications regularly even when the patient feels well. The most common reason for worsening of CHF is a failure to follow medical advice and to take medications regularly.

• Heart transplantation may be considered only for individuals below fifty years of age, with far-advanced CHF as a result of irreversible heart disease in spite of all available conventional medical and surgical treatment.

• The definition of cardiogenic shock is an arterial BP of less than 90 mmHg or a systolic fall greater than 80 mmHg in a patient with previously known hypertension. Cardiogenic shock is the most serious complication of a heart attack, and its high mortality rate still exceeds 75 to 80 percent.

• The patient with cardiogenic shock is restless with altered sensorium as a result of reduced blood flow to the central nervous system; the skin is pale, cyanotic (blue or purplish color), cool, and moist. Urine output is reduced as a result of impaired blood flow to the kidneys, and it is generally less than 20 ml/hour.

• As soon as the diagnosis of cardiogenic shock is made, every effort should be exercised to raise BP, at least above the 90 mmHg systolic level, using various vasopressor drugs in order to restore vital organ perfusion.

• A third heart sound is commonly heard in young people (called the "physiologic third heart sound"), but the presence of the third heart sound among older individuals usually indicates CHF (less commonly, mitral regurgitation). This sound in older people is called "a ventricular gallop sound" or "S_3 gallop."

• A heart murmur is an abnormal noise generated by the heart, and it is commonly produced by diseased heart valves or congenital heart lesions.

• Many healthy people may have a slight heart murmur, especially young individuals—called a "functional murmur." Thus, the presence of heart murmur does not necessarily indicate heart disease. Conversely, many cardiac patients do not have heart murmurs.

• Any individual with a loud heart murmur must be evaluated by a competent physician to determine the cause.

• Heart murmurs are expressed according to intensity (loudness), frequency (pitch), configuration (contour), quality, duration, direction of radiation (transmission), and timing of the cardiac cycle.

• Pericardial friction rubs are hallmarks of pericarditis. These friction rubs are very high-pitched sounds, scratchy in quality, and they seem close to the ears. They are usually best heard with the patient leaning forward after exhaling completely.

• Artificial heart valves produce characteristic loud heart sounds upon opening and closing.

• In the normal heart, cardiac impulses arise from the primary pacemaker (sinus node); cardiac impulses activate the artria followed by ventricular activation. In normal adults, this electric event occurs regularly at about 60 to 75 beats/min. The heart rate increases during physical exercise or emotional excitement.

• The term *cardiac arrhythmia* is used to designate any form of abnormal heart-beats or rhythms. Thus, cardiac arrhythmia may be due to abnormal conduction of cardiac impulses and/or to abnormal cardiac impulse formation in the heart.

• The presence of cardiac arrhythmia per se is not necessarily indicative of heart disease; many healthy people may have a variety of abnormal heart rhythms from time to time. Conversely, cardiac patients may not have cardiac arrhythmia.

• Extremely slow (less than 40 beats/min.) or rapid (more than 160 beats/min.) heart rhythm is clinically significant. The underlying cause should be determined, and proper management should be provided.

• The artificial cardiac pacemaker is often indicated for very slow heart rhythm (complete heart block and SSS), especially when the patient is symptomatic (e.g., syncope or near-syncope).

• For very rapid heart rhythm, various medications are usually indicated. Many cardiac patients with chronic tachyarrhythmias require one or more antiarrhythmic medications for many months or years, and even indefinitely.

• When the clinical situation is extremely urgent because of lift-threatening arrhythmias (e.g., VF), immediate application of DC shock is the treatment of choice.

• No treatment is indicated for benign or mild cardiac arrhythmias (e.g., extra heartbeats) that occur only occasionally.

• Excessive coffee or alcohol consumption or cigarette smoking may provoke various cardiac arrhythmias, even in healthy people. The term *holiday heart syndrome* is used to describe the sudden occurrence of various cardiac arrhythmias during weekends or holidays as a result of heavy alcohol consumption.

• The most common causes of almost every type of cardiac arrhythmia are recent heart attack and digitalis toxicity.

• Congenital heart disease is a form of cardiovascular disease that is present at birth, resulting from a developmental abnormality; its incidence is reported to be 8 to 10 per 1,000 live births.

• Ventricular septal defect is the most common congenital cardiac lesion if mitral valve prolapse syndrome is not included.

• Mitral valve prolapse syndrome is considered a form of congenital heart disease; its incidence is estimated to be 10 to 15 percent of the general population. The syndrome often causes atypical chest pain that may mimic angina pectoris or even heart attack.

• Clinical manifestations vary considerably depending upon the nature and severity of various congenital lesions. Some complex cardiac malformations are incompatible with life, whereas some benign lesions are entirely asymptomatic. Some congenital heart lesions (e.g., small ventricular septal defect) may be cured spontaneously.

• Prophylactic antibiotics are recommended before dental or surgical procedures for most patients with congenital heart lesions and RHD in order to prevent bacterial endocarditis.

• Many children may recover completely from rheumatic fever without any permanent damage to the heart valves, whereas others may eventually develop RHD months or even years later.

• Rheumatic fever is the most common cause of valvular heart disease, and mitral stenosis is the most common valvular lesion.

• Rheumatic fever is an inflammatory disease that develops as a delayed response to pharyngeal infection with group A streptococcus. The disease process involves primarily the heart, joints, central nervous system, skin, and subcutaneous tissues.

• In typical cases, acute rheumatic fever is characterized by migratory polyarthritis; fever and carditis, often associated with Sydenham's chorea; subcutaneous nodules; and erythema marginatum (pinkish rash).

• Rheumatic fever most commonly affects children between the ages of five and fifteen years; the overall incidence of RHD is third, behind coronary and hypertensive heart disease.

• The diagnosis of rheumatic fever is established with a reasonable certainty when two or more of Jones's major criteria (carditis, polyarthritis, chorea, erythema marginatum, and subcutaneous nodules) are present. Likewise, rheumatic fever can also be diagnosed with a high probability when there is one major criterion and two minor criteria. Elevation of the ASO titer is the most reliable laboratory test to support the diagnosis.

• Once the diagnosis of rheumatic fever is made, bed rest is the most important aspect of general care. Drug therapy consists of penicillin, salicylate, and corticosteroids. The most effective method of administration is a single intramuscular injection of 1.2 million units of benzathine penicillin (Bicillin).

• RHD may involve any heart valve, and it is frequently associated with various cardiac arrhythmias, especially AF.

• No treatment is required for asymptomatic patients with mild valvular lesions. However, the surgical approach (e.g., valve replacement) has to be considered for symptomatic patients with advanced RHD. When any surgical approach is considered, it is essential to perform cardiac catheterization before surgery.

- After replacement of the diseased valve with an artificial heart valve, anti-coagulant therapy should be continued indefinitely. Of course, periodic blood tests (e.g., prothrombin time) are mandatory during anticoagulant therapy.

- Cardiomyopathy is a disease process involving the heart muscle predominantly or entirely; it is commonly due to unknown causes (called "idiopathic" cardiomyopathy). Various known disease processes or toxic substances may produce cardiomyopathies (e.g., alcoholic cardiomyopathy).

- Clinical manifestations and outcome are very similar regardless of the causative factor in cardiomyopathies. In advanced cases of cardiomyopathy, severe CHF occurs and is eventually fatal in many cases unless treated properly. Only symptomatic and supportive treatment is available, but underlying disorders or causative factors should be treated or eliminated simultaneously. For selected patients, heart transplantation may be considered.

- Inflammation or infection in the heart includes myocarditis, pericarditis, and endocarditis. Although inflammation or infection is the most common cause, these disease processes may be due to various chemical or physical agents, drugs, radiation, trauma, and neoplasms.

- Viral infection is the most common cause of myocarditis or pericarditis. In many cases, the exact cause is not found, especially in pericarditis (termed "idiopathic pericarditis").

- Common clinical findings of acute myocarditis and/or pericarditis include fever, weakness, anorexia, general malaise, palpitations, chest pain, dyspnea, and edema. In advanced cases, CHF and various arrhythmias often occur. Management of viral myocarditis or pericarditis is supportive and symptomatic.

- When acute pericarditis is severe and long-standing, it frequently leads to pericardial effusion and is often followed by constrictive pericarditis.

- The term *postcardiotomy syndrome* is used when acute pericarditis occurs as a result of surgical trauma following a major cardiac operation. Most cases recover completely, but markedly symptomatic patients may require corticosteroids or Indocin.

- Hemopericardium (bloody pericardial effusion) is most commonly due to tuberculosis or malignancy.

- Cardiac tamponade is the most serious life-threatening complication of pericardial effusion and acute pericarditis, regardless of the causative agents or underlying disorders. Cardiac tamponade is produced by the accumulation of fluid in the pericardium in amounts sufficient to cause significant obstruction to the inflow of blood to the ventricles. Cardiac tamponade causes marked reduction of cardiac output and systemic venous congestion; a fatal outcome is often unavoidable unless treated immediately.

• For a massive pericardial effusion, a pericardial tap is indicated. For cardiac tamponade, rapid aspiration of pericardial fluid by pericardial tap is the only life-saving measure. For constrictive pericarditis, pericardiectomy (resection of the pericardium) is the treatment of choice.

• Endocarditis is defined as infection involving the endocardium (the inner lining of the heart chambers).

• Endocarditis primarily affects damaged heart valves; less commonly, the infection involves congenital defects or artificial heart valves. When the causative bacteria are highly virulent, a normal heart may be affected. Bacterial endocarditis is often fatal unless properly and immediately treated with appropriate antibiotics.

• The infection caused by microorganisms with high pathogenicity (e.g., *Staphylococcus aureus*) is usually acute, whereas the infection caused by low-virulence bacteria (e.g., *Streptococcus viridans*) is generally subacute. *Streptococcus viridans* is the most common bacteria to produce endocarditis involving congenital or rheumatic heart valve lesions.

• Common clinical manifestations of endocarditis include fever, heart murmurs, anemia, hematuria, splenomegaly, petechiae (pinpoint- to pinhead-size hemorrhage spots on the skin), and embolic phenomena.

• The most important diagnostic test for bacterial endocarditis is the blood culture that confirms the presence of a causative bacteria in the bloodstream. Blood cultures are positive in over 95 percent of patients with acute endocarditis and in 85 to 95 percent of patients with SBE. In general, three to five blood cultures are necessary for each patient.

• As soon as the diagnosis of endocarditis is established or strongly suspected, an appropriate antibiotic should be initiated promptly. Bactericidal antibiotics (agents capable of killing and destroying bacteria) should be used rather than bacteriostatic antibiotics (agents inhibiting the growth or multiplication of bacteria). In general, antibiotics should be continued for four to six weeks for SBE, and six to eight weeks for acute endocarditis.

• Although tumors of the heart are relatively uncommon, they should be recognized early because cardiac tumors can be cured completely by surgery in most cases.

• Over three-fourths of all primary tumors of the heart are benign, and half of these occur inside the heart chambers. Myxomas are the most common primary cardiac tumors (nearly always in the atria), and surgical cure is expected in most cases.

• The diagnosis of cardiac tumors is confirmed accurately by echocardiography or angiocardiography, which demonstrates a space-occupying lesion.

• Traumas of various kinds may damage the heart in many ways. Cardiac damage may involve various heart valves and related structures, heart muscles, pericardium, and coronary arteries. In addition, cardiac arrhythmias are commonly produced by a variety of traumas. Of course, cardiac rupture due to severe trauma is invariably fatal.

• The most serious manifestation of syphilis is the involvement of the cardiovascular system and central nervous system, which usually takes place about ten to thirty years after the appearance of the primary lesion, chancre.

• The fundamental lesion of cardiovascular syphilis is aortitis, and aortic regurgitation occurs in approximately 10 percent of cases with untreated syphilitic aortitis. A full course of antisyphilitic treatment with penicillin should be given to all patients.

• CPR can be performed by one person, but it is preferable to have a team, especially in the hospital. Mouth-to-mouth resuscitation to restore breathing and closed cardiac massage to initiate heartbeats are the most important aspects. Artificial respiration should be performed at a rate of 12/min., and every fifth chest compression should be followed by a lung ventilation.

• Approximately 250,000 people have artificial pacemakers in the United States alone, and 25,000 to 40,000 new patients will require pacemaker implantation annually. The energy source is a lithium battery that lasts ten to twelve years.

• Some patients may need artificial pacemakers for only a few days or weeks, but many people require pacemaker implantation permanently.

• All patients with artificial pacemakers should have periodic medical checkups indefinitely, because certain complications and malfunctions may occur. Artificial pacemaker follow-up care facilities are available in most modern countries.

• Any special diet program without medical supervision is hazardous because a nutritional imbalance with a deficiency of vitamins and/or minerals may be produced; even death may result from severely restricted diet programs (e.g., liquid protein diets).

• A low-cholesterol and low-saturated-fat diet with low caloric intake is highly recommended for all patients with CAD and for those with risk factors. Any fat that hardens by refrigeration after cooking is an animal fat that should be removed. Cardiac patients should eat more fish and poultry (without skin) in place of the meat of four-legged animals. Salty foods should be avoided by all cardiac patients, especially those with high BP and/or CHF.

• Exercise programs, especially those involving vigorous physical activities, should be designed under medical supervision even for healthy people. It is highly recommended that everyone have a complete medical checkup, including exercise ECG test, before starting an exercise program, especially after age forty, when there is a family history of heart disease or sudden death, or when the individual has a history of dizziness, palpitations, near-syncope, syncope, or chest pain.

• Complete evaluation is mandatory for all cardiac patients before an exercise program, and a medically supervised program is recommended. Remember that sudden or vigorous physical activity may be fatal for cardiac patients, especially those recovering from a heart attack.

• Cigarette smoking is bad for health in many ways. In heart attack victims below forty years of age, the sole major risk factor is heavy cigarette smoking.

• The most harmful effects of cigarette smoking for heart disease are primarily due to nicotine and carbon monoxide.

• When there is long-standing chronic lung disease from heavy smoking, the right ventricle progressively enlarges; eventually, right ventricular failure will occur.

• Alcohol is said to protect against heart attack in certain cases, but this view is not uniformly accepted by most physicians.

• Excessive alcohol intake may cause various cardiac arrhythmias, elevation of BP, depression of pumping action of the heart, elevation of blood triglyceride level, and cardiomyopathy. In most cardiac patients, not more than two cocktails or two bottles of beer are recommended per day. Alcohol is by no means a substitute for nitroglycerin to relieve chest pain. In cardiac patients, extraordinary physical activity or sexual intercourse should be avoided within two to three hours after drinking alcoholic beverages.

• In recent studies, Anturane has been found to be protective against sudden death in patients with previous heart attack. Likewise, Persantine and aspirin are reported to be beneficial in preventing sudden death and a new coronary event in patients with previous heart attack. Further investigations will be nececcary for a final conclusion.

GLOSSARY

Ambulatory (Holter monitor) ECG test. A non-invasive diagnostic test that records the electrical activity of the heart for twenty-four hours using a portable tape recorder to detect any abnormality of heart rhythm.

Anastomosis. Surgical bypass graft.

Aneurysm. A bulging and thinning of a blood vessel wall or a heart chamber wall.

Aneurysmectomy. Surgical resection of an aneurysm.

Angina pectoris. Chest pain or chest discomfort caused by insufficient blood supply to the heart muscles as a result of narrowing of the coronary artery(ies).

Anorexia nervosa. Severe malnutrition with extreme emaciation as a result of self-induced starvation in order to lose weight; it may lead to death.

Antagonistic effect. Opposing effect.

Anti-anginal drugs. Medications used for the prevention and treatment of angina pectoris (e.g., propranolol or nitroglycerin).

Anti-arrhythmic agents. Medications such as quinidine or procainamide (Pronestyl), used for the prevention and treatment of various cardiac arrhythmias.

Anticoagulants (blood-thinning drugs). Medications that interfere with or prevent coagulation of blood (blood clot formation). Common anticoagulants include Coumadin and heparin.

Anti-hypertensive agents. Medications, such as hydrochlorothiazide, used for the treatment of hypertension.

Arrhythmia. Abnormal heartbeats or rhythm.

Artery. A blood vessel that supplies nutrients and oxygen-rich blood from the heart to various organs and tissues.

Artificial cardiac pacemaker. Electronic device that activates the heart using batteries—may be used temporarily or may be implanted permanently. It is most commonly used in the treatment of various slow heart rhythms, particularly complete A-V (heart) block or sick sinus syndrome.

Atherosclerosis. Hardening of the arteries—the usual cause of angina pectoris and heart attack.

Atria. Plural of *atrium.*

Atrial fibrillation. Chaotic, irregular, and rapid cardiac rhythm arising from the atria.

Atrial premature contractions. Extra heartbeats arising from the atria.

Atrial septal defect. A hole in the muscle wall between the atria—a common form of congenital heart disease.

Atrial tachycardia. Rapid and regular heart rhythm arising from the atria.

Atrium. Receiving chamber of the heart.

A-V junctional tachycardia. Rapid and regular heart rhythm arising from the A-V junction.

Bactericidal antibiotics. Antibiotics (e.g., penicillin) capable of killing and of destroying bacteria.

Bacteriostatic antibiotics. Antibiotics (e.g., erythromycin) inhibiting the growth or multiplication of bacteria.

Beriberi heart disease. Cardiomyopathy (heart muscle disease) as a result of vitamin-B_1 (thiamine) deficiency.

Beta-blocking agents. Medications such as propranolol (Inderal) that are commonly used in the treatment of various cardiac arrhythmias, angina pectoris, and hypertension.

Bifascicular block. A combination of right bundle branch block and a block in one of the divisions of the left bundle branch system.

Bilateral bundle branch block (BBBB). A serious heart block—a block of both right bundle branch and left bundle branch systems including bifascicular block and trifascicular block. Complete BBBB causes complete A-V (heart) block.

Blood pressure. Pressure within the artery. The systolic pressure is the pressure during the pumping phase of the ventricles, whereas the diastolic pressure is the pressure during the expansion period of the ventricles.

Bradyarrhythmia (also *Bradycardia*). Abnormally slow heart rhythm.

Brady-tachyarrhythmia. A combination of a slow heart rhythm and rapid heart rhythm—often a late manifestation of the sick sinus syndrome.

Cardiac arrest. Little or no heart function as a result of ventricular fibrillation or no heartbeating at all.

Cardiac catheterization. Invasive diagnostic cardiac test performed by a specially trained cardiologist. Catheters are introduced into the heart chambers and large blood vessels via arm or groin blood vessels. Diagnosis of various heart diseases can be made by measuring pressures in various locations within the heart chambers and blood vessels.

Cardiac tamponade. Life-threatening heart condition secondary to sudden accumulation of large amounts of fluid or blood in the pericardial sac, leading to marked impairment of the pumping action of the heart.

Cardiogenic shock. Life-threatening complication of a heart attack—common manifestations include hypotension, clammy skin, unclear mental state, markedly reduced urine output, and very poor pumping action of the heart.

Cardiomegaly. Enlarged heart.

Cardiomyopathy. Heart muscle disease.

Cardiopulmonary. Heart and lungs.

Cardiopulmonary arrest (collapse). Cessation of heart and lung functions.

Cardioverter. Electric shock machine; defibrillator (DC shock machine).

Catheter. Small plastic tube.

Chordae tendineae. Structures supporting the mitral valve.

Coital death. Death during sexual intercourse.

Coitus. Sexual intercourse.

Collateral circulation. Reserve blood vessels.

Complete A-V (heart) block. A disturbance of normal conduction from the atria to the ventricles preventing electrical impulses from traveling through the heart muscle and conduction system, causing a very slow heart rhythm.

Coronary angiogram or arteriogram. An X-ray study in which dye (a chemical) is injected through catheters into the heart chambers and coronary arteries. The X-ray films taken during dye injection demonstrate the degree and the location of coronary artery narrowing or blockage.

Coronary artery. A blood vessel in the heart that supplies nutrients and oxygen-rich blood to the heart muscles.

Coronary artery bypass surgery. Anastomosis of one or more coronary arteries that are narrowed or blocked, using a saphenous vein (leg vein).

Coronary artery disease. Heart disease due to narrowing or blockage of coronary artery(ies) from atherosclerosis; commonly used to designate angina pectoris and myocardial infarction.

Cor-pulmonale. Heart disease secondary to lung disease.

Corticosteroids. Cortisone-like medications commonly used in the treatment of various inflammatory processes, such as pericarditis following a heart attack or coronary artery bypass surgery.

Cyanosis. Purplish-bluish discoloration of mucous membrane or skin as a result of insufficient supply of blood and oxygen.

Degenerative-sclerotic change in the conduction system. Normal conduction tissue is replaced by a fibrotic tissue. Often an aging process and a part of atherosclerotic process—leading to various forms of heart block.

Diastole. Expansion period of the ventricles.

Diastolic murmur. A heart murmur that occurs during the expansion period of the ventricles (pumping chambers).

Digitalis. An inotropic agent that strengthens the pumping action of the heart (better known as "heart pill"), and it is the most important drug in the treatment of heart failure. In addition, digitalis is commonly used in the treatment of various rapid heart rhythms, particularly atrial fibrillation.

Digitalis intoxication. Digitalis poisoning.

Dilatation. Expansion.

Direct current shock. Electric shock for rapid heart rhythm.

Diuretic. Water pill—increases the flow of urine.

Dyspnea. Shortness of breath.

Echocardiogram. Non-invasive test using the principle comparable to sonar detection in submarines for the diagnosis and evaluation of various abnormalities in the structures and functions of the heart.

Ectopic beats or rhythms. Heartbeats or heart rhythms arising from any location other than the sinus node—may originate from the atria, A-V junction, or the ventricles.

Ectopic focus. Any location of the heart other than the sinus node.

Edema. Fluid accumulation resulting in swelling—commonly due to heart failure.

Electrocardiogram. A recording of the electrical activity of the heart.

Electrolyte imbalance. Abnormal value of one or more electrolytes (e.g., sodium, potassium, chloride, calcium, etc.) in the blood.

Embolism. Blood clot formation in the blood vessel leading to disturbance of blood circulation to various organs, such as the lungs.

Endocarditis. Bacterial (most commonly staphylococcal and streptococcal) infection of the inner lining of the heart chambers. Endocarditis often affects damaged heart valves and congenital defects.

Exercise ECG test. A non-invasive diagnostic test for coronary artery disease using a motor-driven treadmill or bicycle.

Extrasystoles. Premature heartbeats arising from the atria, A-V junction, or ventricles.

Functional capacity. Ability of performing physical activity.

Gallop rhythm. Abnormal extra heart sounds causing triple or sometimes quadruple sounds that are somewhat comparable to the canter of a horse.

Heart block. Slower than usual conduction or no conduction of the cardiac impulse.

Heart failure. A condition in which the heart is unable to pump blood adequately so that various symptoms (e.g., shortness of breath, leg edema, etc.) occur. Hypertension is the most common cause of heart failure.

Heart murmur. Abnormal noise generated by a blood flow through a damaged heart valve or a congenital defect of the heart.

Hemodynamic monitoring. The measurement of pressures in various heart chambers and large blood vessels and the determination of oxygen content in blood samples obtained from these chambers and blood vessels.

Hemopericardium. Accumulation of blood in the pericardial sac.

Hemothorax. Accumulation of blood in the chest cavity.

Hydrochlorothiazide (Esidrix or Hydrodiuril). The most commonly used diuretic, very effective in the treatment of heart failure. In addition, the drug is also frequency used in the treatment of hypertension.

Hyperlipidemia. Elevated levels of cholesterol and/or triglycerides in the blood.

Hypertension. Elevated blood pressure—the most common cause of heart failure and the major risk factor for a heart attack.

Hyperthyroidism (thyrotoxicosis). Increased function of the thyroid gland—a common cause of rapid heart rhythms, particularly atrial fibrillation.

Hypotension. Lower then normal blood pressure—a common sign of cardiogenic shock.

Hypothyrodism (myxedema). Decreased function of the thyroid gland—frequently causes pericarditis and pericardial effusion.

Inotropic agents. Medications such as digitalis and isoproterenol (Isuprel), used in order to improve the pumping action of the heart.

Ischemia. Insufficient blood supply to the tissues.

Lipids. Cholesterol and triglycerides.

METs. Metabolic units or metabolic equivalents—multiple of the basal metabolic unit.

Myocardial imaging. Nuclear scanning or radioisotope study of the heart—a very useful diagnostic test to detect heart muscle damage or areas of myocardial ischemia.

Myocardial infarction. Heart attack—a portion of the heart muscle is dead as a result of blockage of one or more coronary arteries; this leads to no blood supply to the heart muscle.

Myocardial ischemia. Insufficient blood supply to the heart muscle as a result of coronary artery narrowing leading to angina pectoris.

Myocarditis. Infection or inflammation of the heart muscle.

Myocardium. Heart muscle.

Occlusion. Blockage.

Pansystolic (or holosystolic) murmur. Heart murmur that occupies the entire period of the pumping action of the heart.

Papillary muscle. Tissue supporting the mitral valve.

Penicillin shock. Death or near-death following administration of penicillin. A manifestation of severe allergic reaction to the drug.

Pericardial effusion. Fluid accumulation in the pericardial sac.

Pericardial friction rub. A sensation similar to that of touching a purring cat—an important sign of pericarditis.

Pericardiocentesis (pericardial tap). Aspiration of pericardial fluid via a needle inserted into the pericardium—the best therapeutic approach for massive pericardial effusion or cardiac tamponade.

Pericarditis. Infection or inflammation involving pericardium—commonly due to virus infection, but it may occur following a heart attack or coronary artery bypass surgery.

Pericardium. Sac surrounding the heart.

Peri-operative myocardial infarction. Myocardial infarction (heart attack) occurring during or immediately following a heart surgery (usually coronary artery bypass surgery).

Peripheral pulse. Pulse in the arms or legs (e.g., pulse in the wrist).

Pneumothorax. Collapse of a partial or entire lung(s) as a result of accumulation of air in the chest cavity.

Propranolol (Inderal). A beta-blocking drug effective in treating abnormal heart rhythm, hypertension, and angina pectoris.

Prothrombin time determination. A blood test to determine the degree of coagulability (stickiness).

Pulmonary edema. Fluid accumulation in the lungs—usually due to severe heart failure.

Pulmonary embolism. Blood clots in the lungs.

Quinidine. A drug that controls and treats abnormal heartbeats and rhythm.

Rheumatic fever. An inflammatory disease that develops as a delayed response to pharyngeal infection with group A streptococcus (a kind of bacteria). Rheumatic fever involves primarily the heart, joints, central nervous system, skin, and subcutaneous tissues.

Rheumatic heart disease. A variety of valvular lesions months or many years following single or repeated attacks of acute rheumatic fever. Mitral stenosis (narrowing of the mitral valve) is the most common valvular lesion.

Sick sinus syndrome. Dysfunctioning of sinus node, resulting in abnormally slow heart rhythm leading to dizziness, near-syncope, or syncope.

Sinus node. Natural pacemaker of the heart.

Stenosis. Narrowing.

Syncope. A loss of consciousness as a result of temporary cessation of respiration or circulation, or very slow or rapid heart rhythm.

Synergistic effect. Intensifying effect.

Systole. Contraction (pumping) period of the ventricles.

Systolic murmur. A heart murmur that occurs during a pumping period of the ventricles (pumping chambers).

Tachyarrhythmia (or Tachycardia). Rapid heart rhythm.

Thromboembolic phenomenon. Blood clot formation.

Thrombophlebitis. Painful and swollen tissues over inflamed veins; often leads to blood clot formation.

Thrombosis: Blood clot formation within a blood vessel.

Trifascicular block: A combination of right bundle branch block and left anterior as well as posterior division of the left bundle branch system. Complete trifascicular block causes complete A-V (heart) block.

Vasodilator agents: Medications such as sodium nitroprusside (Nipride) or hydralazine (Apresoline), used in the treatment of severe heart failure and cardiogenic shock.

Vasopressor agents: Medications such as metaraminol (Aramine) or norepinephrine (Levophed), used in the treatment of cardiogenic shock.

Vein: A blood vessel that carries back oxygen-poor blood and waste products from various organs and tissues to the heart. Venous blood is darker than arterial blood.

Ventricle: Pumping chamber of the heart.

Ventricular fibrillation: Life-threatening, chaotic, irregular, and ineffective heart rhythm arising from the ventricles—the most common cause of cardiac arrest and frequently a precursor of sudden death.

Ventricular premature contractions: Extra heartbeats arising prematurely from the ventricles.

Ventricular septal defect: A hole in the muscle wall between the ventricles—a common form of congenital heart disease. Ventricular septal defect may be caused by a heart attack—a life-threatening complication.

Ventricular tachycardia: Regular and rapid cardiac rhythm arising from the ventricles—serious arrhythmia.

Wolff-Parkinson-White (WPW) syndrome: A heart condition that predisposes to a very rapid heart rhythm—a form of congenital heart disease.

BIBLIOGRAPHY

Chung, E. K.: *Cardiac Emergency Care, Second Edition*, Philadelphia, Lea & Febiger Pub., 1980.

Chung, E. K.: *Artificial Cardiac Pacing: Practical Approach*, Baltimore, Williams & Wilkins Co., 1979.

Chung, E. K.: *Exercise Electrocardiography: Practical Approach*, Baltimore, Williams & Wilkins Co., 1979.

Chung, E. K.: *Electrocardiography: Practical Applications with Vectorial Principles*, Second Edition, Hagerstown, Md., Harper & Row Pub., 1980.

Chung, E. K.: *Quick Reference to Cardiovascular Diseases*, Second Edition, Philadelphia, J.B. Lippincott Pub., 1982.

Chung, E. K.: *Non-Invasive Cardiac Diagnosis*, Philadelphia, Lea & Febiger Pub., 1976.

Chung, E. K.: *Ambulatory Electrocardiography: Holter Monitor Electrocardiography*, New York, Springer-Verlag Pub., 1979.

Chung, E. K.: *Controversy in Cardiology*, New York, Springer-Verlag Pub., 1976.

Chung, E. K.: *Principles of Cardiac Arrhythmias, Second Edition*, Baltimore, Williams & Wilkins Co., 1977.

Chung, E. K.: *Digitalis Intoxication*, Netherlands, Excerpta Medica, 1969.